Classic Cases
in Medical Ethics

Classic Cases in Medical Ethics

Accounts of the Cases and Issues that Define Medical Ethics

FIFTH EDITION

Gregory E. Pence
Professor of Philosophy
School of Medicine and Department of Philosophy
University of Alabama at Birmingham

Boston Burr Ridge, IL Dubuque, IA Madison, WI New York
San Francisco St. Louis Bangkok Bogotá Caracas Kuala Lumpur
Lisbon London Madrid Mexico City Milan Montreal New Delhi
Santiago Seoul Singapore Sydney Taipei Toronto

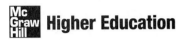

Higher Education

CLASSIC CASES IN MEDICAL ETHICS: ACCOUNTS OF THE CASES THAT SHAPED
AND DEFINE MEDICAL ETHICS

Published by McGraw-Hill, a business unit of The McGraw-Hill Companies, Inc., 1221 Avenue of the
Americas, New York, NY, 10020. Copyright © 2008, 2004, 2000, 1995, 1990, by The McGraw-Hill
Companies, Inc. All rights reserved. No part of this publication may be reproduced or distributed in
any form or by any means, or stored in a database or retrieval system, without the prior written
consent of The McGraw-Hill Companies, Inc., including, but not limited to, in any network or other
electronic storage or transmission, or broadcast for distance learning. Some ancillaries, including
electronic and print components, may not be available to customers outside the United States.

This book is printed on acid-free paper.

2 3 4 5 6 7 8 9 0   DOC / DOC   0 9 8

ISBN: 978-0-07-353573-9
MHID: 0-07-353573-7

Editor-in-chief: *Emily Barrosse*
Publisher: *Lisa Moore*
Senior sponsoring editor: *Mark Georgiev*
Development editor: *Marley Magaziner*
Executive marketing manager: *Pamela S. Cooper*
Production editors: *Melissa Williams and Jill Eccher*
Manuscript editor: *Dale Boroviak*
Senior production Supervisor: *Rich DeVitto*
Senior designer: *Violeta Diaz*
Cover design: *Jenny El-Shamy*
Typeface: *10/12 Palatino*
Compositor: *International Typesetting and Composition*
Printer: *R. R. Donnelley & Sons*

Library of Congress Cataloging-in-Publication Data

Pence, Gregory E.
   Classic cases in medical ethics : accounts of the cases that have shaped and define medical
   ethics/Gregory Pence.—5th ed.
      p. ; cm.
   Includes bibliographical references and index.
   ISBN-13: 978-0-07-353573-9 (alk. paper)
   ISBN-10: 0-07-353573-7 (alk. paper)
   1. Medical ethics—Case studies.   I. Title
[DNLM: 1. Bioethical Issues—United States. 2. Ethics, Medical—history—United States.
3. Ethics, Clinical—history—United States. 4. History, 20th Century—United States.
5. Patient Rights—legislation & jurisprudence—United States. 6. Social Justice—
ethics—United States.
W 50 P397c 2008]
R724.P36 2008
174'.2—dc22   2007012849

www.mhhe.com

Preface

I first started writing this book for my students 20 years ago when I had already been teaching the emerging field of bioethics for 10 years. I wrote this book for them because existing texts failed to convey the excitement of real cases in bioethics. In this fifth edition, I tried to keep the good parts of past editions ("If it's not broke, don't fix it") and to add to, or improve, them.

Every reviewer used some chapters and not others, so it was difficult to cut any chapter. I decided to edit every chapter, sometimes reducing the number of words by a third, while retaining the essence of each. In addition, I added relevant cases and new issues to each chapter.

Like previous editions, this edition was tested on my undergraduates and medical students during 2006. As in the past, my students freely told me of mistakes and biases, improving the book.

If we date the start of modern bioethics to the 1962 God Committee, we're almost at half a century of bioethics. Professors today must both teach about new issues (face transplants) while showing how they build on previous cases (heart and hand transplants). And sometimes one issue ties them together: a desire to be first in surgery.

Personally, I believe that knowing about real cases and how they were resolved is real education in ethics for people who will one day make medical decisions. Like the spreading ripples of a stone in a pond, more and more cases build up spheres of knowledge that are as close as we can teach to what Aristotle called *phronesis* or practical wisdom.

As always, I would like to hear your comments and can be reached at my email address: pence@uab.edu.

Gregory E. Pence
pence@uab.edu

v

Acknowledgments

In doing this fifth edition, my steadfast research assistant of three different summers, Emily Taylor, has been invaluable as a seasoned critic, editor, and proofreader. One day in a few years, she will be a good physician. Assisting Emily in the summer of 2006 were Shalini Vaid and Derek Patterson, who were great in finding facts, new articles, proofing, and showing up every day.

I also would like to thank Stuart Rachels of the University of Alabama for many suggestions over the last decade, and my student Sara Singhal for proofing the page proofs and saving me from many errors.

Medical students Jessica Steinkampf and John Allen also helped to proof the text. Mrs. Minnie Randle and Pamela Williams in my office always provided cheerful, efficient support.

I would also like to thank the following reviewers for their careful comments on the book and my proposals:

Deborah R. Barnbaum, Kent State University
Charles E. Cardwell, Pellissippi State Technical Community College
Joyce Kloc Babyak, Oberlin College
Ryan E. Walther, Norwich University
Donna J. Werner, St. Louis Community College (Meramec)

About the Author

GREGORY E. PENCE is a Professor of Philosophy in the School of Medicine and Department of Philosophy at the University of Alabama at Birmingham (UAB), where he has taught for 30 years. With McGraw-Hill, he wrote *The Elements of Bioethics (2006) and edited Classic Works in Medical Ethics (1995).*

Rowman & Littlefield published his *Who's Afraid of Human Cloning?* in 1998, *Re-creating Medicine: Ethical Issues at the Frontiers of Medicine* in 2000, *Designer Food: Mutant Harvest or Breadbasket of the World?* in 2002, and *Cloning After Dolly: Who's Still Afraid?* in 2005, as well as his anthologies: *Flesh of My Flesh: Ethical Issues in Human Cloning—A Reader* (1998) and *The Ethics of Food: A Reader for the 21st Century* (2000). With G. Lynn Stephens, he wrote *Seven Dilemmas in World Religions* (Paragon, 1995). A frequent writer of op-eds in national newspapers, *Brave New Bioethics* (2004) collects these.

At UAB, he served for 22 years on its Institutional Review Board, and for much lesser terms, on its Hospital Ethics Committee and Animal Use and Care Committee. In 1994, he won UAB's highest award for undergraduate teaching. He directs UAB's BS/MD program.

He delivered the Soundings Lecture at Castleton State College, the Thornton Lecture at Alma College the Seidman Trust Lecture at Rhodes College, the Rutland Lecture at Clemson University, and the Howard/Keegan Lecture at Texas A&M University. He has talked in China, Israel, Switzerland, London, Portugal, Brazil, and at a hundred hospitals and universities in America. He has discussed bioethics on CNN, National Public Radio, and national television, and has testified before committees of the U. S. Congress and California Senate.

In 2006, he was awarded a Pellegrino Medal for his lifetime work in medical ethics and in 2007, Medical Ethics was chosen by first-year medical students at UAB as one of their 3 best courses.

Brief Contents

Contents

Part Two
CLASSIC CASES ABOUT THE BEGINNINGS OF HUMAN LIFE

Part Three
INTERLUDE FOR ETHICAL THEORY

Part Four
CLASSIC CASES ABOUT RESEARCH

Part Five
CLASSIC CASES ABOUT INDIVIDUAL RIGHTS VERSUS
THE PUBLIC GOOD

CHAPTER 1

Requests to Die

Elizabeth Bouvia and Larry McAfee

T his chapter discusses Elizabeth Bouvia and Larry McAfee, two people with nonterminal physical disabilities who tried to die, who won important cases in court, and whose outcomes surprised onlookers. It also discusses the rationality of suicide, structural discrimination against people with disabilities, relief of depression and symptoms, autonomy, disability culture, and philosophers in history on rational suicide.

THE CASE OF ELIZABETH BOUVIA

In 1983, Elizabeth Bouvia's father drove her from Oregon to Riverside General Hospital in California, where psychiatrists diagnosed her as suicidal and admitted her as a voluntary patient. Wanting "just to be left alone and not bothered by friends or family or anyone else and to ultimately starve to death," she had already attempted suicide once.[1] "Death is letting go of all burdens," she claimed. "It is being able to be free of my physical disability and mental struggle to live."

Almost totally paralyzed from cerebral palsy, Elizabeth was 25 years old. She had never had the use of her legs, although she could use her right hand to operate a battery-powered wheelchair and to smoke cigarettes. She could control her facial muscles to chew, swallow, and speak.

Her life had never been easy. Her parents divorced when she was five years old. Her mother raised her for the next five years, after which she abandoned her to a children's home. The following account comes from two physicians:

> For their 18th birthday, some children receive cars and gifts. When [Elizabeth] turned 18, her father, a postal inspector, told her that he would no longer be able to care for her because of her disabilities. The chief of psychiatry at Riverside says that what she did next showed great drive and promise. She gathered her requisite amount of state aid and lived on her own in an apartment with a live-in nurse. Although she earlier had dropped out of high school, she completed her general equivalency degree and went on to graduate from San Diego State University with a bachelor's degree in 1981. She even entered a master's program at the university's School of Social Work, but left in 1982 over a disagreement about her field work placement. . . .

1

For eight months, she worked as a volunteer in the San Diego placement program, but she has never been employed for salary or wages. . . .

During the last year, Ms. Bouvia faced a series of devastating events. In August, 1982, she married an ex-convict, Richard Bouvia, with whom she had been corresponding by mail. Together they conceived a child, but a few months later she suffered a miscarriage. . . .

Her husband's part-time job did not provide enough income for the two to live decently, so they called her father to ask for help. He declined to aid them, Richard Bouvia said. They next went to Richard Bouvia's sister in Iowa to ask for help. That did not work out for long, and soon they ended up back in Oregon, where Richard Bouvia still could not find work. At that point, he abandoned her, stating—according to pleadings in the case—that he "could not accept her disabilities, a miscarriage, and rejection by her parents.". . .

A few days later, Elizabeth Bouvia got a ride to Riverside General and wheeled herself into the emergency room, complaining that she wanted to commit suicide.[2]

In addition to her problems with her husband and father, she had severe degenerative arthritis, a painful condition. As she was an indigent resident of California (she had lived in Riverside as well as in Oregon), Medi-Cal, a state-federal program, paid for her medical care.

Donald Fisher, chief of psychiatry at Riverside Hospital, cared for Bouvia during her first four months there. Since he refused to let her starve herself to death, she contacted the American Civil Liberties Union (ACLU) and telephoned a reporter. Richard Scott of Beverly Hills, both a physician and a lawyer, represented her for free.

The Legal Battle: Refusing Sustenance

In a hearing before California probate judge John Hews, Dr. Fisher testified that because Bouvia might change her mind, he would not let her starve and would force-feed her: "The court cannot order me to be a murderer nor to conspire with my staff and employees to murder Elizabeth."[3] Bouvia asked Judge Hews to enjoin Dr. Fisher from forcibly feeding her.

Habeeb Bacchus, associate chief of medicine at Riverside Hospital and Bouvia's second physician, argued that "being allowed to die when there's no need for her to die—this is a dangerous precedent. Patients might wonder: 'Am I next slated to be allowed to die?'"[4]

Advocates for the disabled feared that if Bouvia died, other disabled people would do the same. A lawyer at the Law Institute for the Disabled asserted that Bouvia symbolized a "social problem" of disabled people who are told they cannot be productive and said, "She needs to learn to live with dignity."[5]

At this point, the case escalated into a public debate:

Disabled individuals held vigils at the hospital to convince her to change her mind. Bouvia's estranged husband hitchhiked to Riverside from Iowa, retained lawyers, and asked to be named her legal guardian. He charged the ACLU with using his wife as a "guinea pig." She filed for divorce. Columnist Jack Anderson's offer to raise funds for Bouvia's treatment was rebuffed. Richard Nixon sent a letter to Bouvia to "keep fighting." A meeting with President Reagan was discussed.

Two neurosurgeons offered free surgery to help her gain the use of her arms. A convicted felon volunteered to shoot her.[6]

Judge Hews allowed the forced-feeding. Admitting Bouvia's rationality, sincerity, and competence, he decided based on the "profound effect on the medical staff, nurses, and administration of the hospital," as well as the "devastating effect on other . . . physically handicapped persons."[7] Bouvia's lawyer said Hews accepted "the Chicken Little defense that the sky would fall if Ms. Bouvia wasn't force-fed."[8] Judge Hews held that since the patient was not terminally ill and could live for decades, "there is no other reasonable option."

The columnist Arthur Hoppe argued otherwise:

> I had the feeling that the judge, the doctor, and the hospital had found Elizabeth Bouvia guilty—guilty of not playing the game. It was as though the Easter Seal Child had looked into the camera and said being crippled was a lousy deal and certainly nothing to smile about.[9]

Boston University law professor George Annas blasted Hews:

> The judge's decision begs the question: Is there a reasonable option? In the adversary proceeding played out in California, no one seemed to search for reasonable options. The county, in fact, consistently took the most extreme position. It continually threatened to eject Ms. Bouvia from the hospital by force, and leave her out on the front sidewalk, hoping someone would pick her up and take her away. Almost from the beginning, the county and hospital made it clear that they did not care whether she lived or died but, because of their own fear of potential legal liability, would not let her die at Riverside Hospital.[10]

Elizabeth appealed, and throughout it, she continued to be force-fed. When aides inserted plastic tubing in her mouth, she bit through the tubing, so thereafter three attendants held her down while another inserted tubing through her nose into her stomach and pumped in a liquid diet. Annas commented on this gruesome scene:

> I do not believe competent adults should ever be force-fed; but efforts at persuading the individual to change his or her mind, and offering oral nutrition should continue. If a court determines, however, that invasive forced-feeding is required, . . . then to [prevent] hospitals from becoming the most hideous torture chambers, some reasonable limit must be placed on this "treatment."[11]

Elizabeth Bouvia lost her first appeal and left Riverside Hospital in 1984. Various commentators interpreted differently what happened next. Two physicians wrote in a medical journal:

> The standoff continued until April 7, when Ms. Bouvia unexpectedly checked herself out of the hospital. The hospital bill for the 217 days, excluding physicians' fees, was more than $56,000, paid by Riverside County and by the State of California. Ms. Bouvia went to the Hospital del Mar at Playas de Tijuana, Mexico, known for amygdalin (Laetrile) treatments for cancer. She believed the staff would help her die. Her new physicians, however, became convinced that she wanted to live. Two weeks later, Ms. Bouvia left the hospital, hired nurses, and moved to a motel. Three days later, with friends, a reporter, and an intern from Hospital del Mar at her side, she gave up her plan to starve herself to death and took solid food. Ms. Bouvia said that she wanted treatment, including surgery to

reduce muscle spasms. As of August 1985, Ms. Bouvia's location and plans were
not known. Her case was complicated further by the revelation that the newspaper reporter who covered the case most closely had a contract with Ms. Bouvia for
a book, television, and movie rights to her story.[12]

This account emphasizes Elizabeth Bouvia's unexpected departure from the hospital, her expensive hospital bills at public expense, the agreement of Mexican with
American physicians in refusing to allow her to die, her seemingly arbitrary decision
to give up starving herself, and the contract for book and film rights to her story.

In contrast, lawyer George Annas writes:

> Two years ago this column dealt with Elizabeth Bouvia's unequal and doomed strug-
> gle. . . . After losing both in the hospital and in the courtroom, Ms. Bouvia fled to
> Mexico on April 7, 1984, to seek her death. She was soon persuaded that Mexican
> physicians and nurses would be no more sympathetic to her plan than those at River-
> side, and so returned to California. Because of the brutal force feeding she had
> endured at Riverside, she was afraid to return there. Since no other facility would
> admit her unless she agreed to eat, she resigned herself to eating and entered a "pri-
> vate care" location. There she remained, without incident, for more than a year.[13]

An advocate for dignified dying, the Hemlock Society's Derek Humphry,
wrote even more sympathetically:

> Her troubles multiplied. The graduate school where she had been studying
> refused to readmit her, and her brother was drowned in a boating accident. Not
> long after, Elizabeth had a miscarriage, and she learned her mother was dying of
> cancer. . . . Determined once again to be in charge of her fate, she asked her father
> to take her to the county hospital in Riverside, near Los Angeles (an area where
> she had friends), for an examination. She checked herself into the psychiatric ward
> and told physicians she wanted to die by starvation. Elizabeth specifically asked
> that, until she died, she was to be looked after normally and given painkillers
> when her arthritis was troublesome.[14]

Disability advocate Paul Longmore offered a very different perspective on
Bouvia's case, arguing that it reflected rank prejudice against the disabled. He
wrote:

> The very agencies supposedly designed to enable severely physically handi-
> capped adults like her to achieve independence . . . become yet another massive
> hurdle they must surmount, an enemy they must repeatedly battle but can never
> finally defeat. . . .
> [When she tried to go on internship,] the SDSU [San Diego State University]
> School of Social Work refused to back her up. They wanted to place her at a center
> where she would only work with disabled people. She refused. Reportedly, one of
> her employers told her she was unemployable, and that, if they had known just how
> disabled she was, they would never have admitted her to the program. . . .
> The attorneys brought in three psychiatric professionals to provide an
> independent evaluation. None of them had experience or expertise in dealing
> with persons with disabilities. In fact, Elizabeth Bouvia had never been exam-
> ined by psychiatric or medical professional qualified to understand her life
> experience. . . .

Her examiners prejudicially concluded that because of her physical condition she would never be able to achieve her life goals, that her [physical] disability was the reason she wanted to die, and that her decision for death was reasonable. . . . [Judge Hews] too declared that Ms. Bouvia's physical disability was the sole reason she wished to die.[15]

Each account appeared in scholarly journals, implying objectivity, yet the physicians portray her as irresponsible; Annas and Humphry portray her as a heroine fighting a cold bureaucracy; Longmore portrays her as a victim of a prejudiced system and of misguided, do-gooder lawyers. Physicians refer to her as "Bouvia," Humphry calls her "Elizabeth," and Longmore uses "Elizabeth Bouvia" or "Ms. Bouvia." The physicians say that "she got a ride" to Riverside, as if she had hitchhiked to some arbitrary location; Humphry says that her father took her to a place "where she had friends." Longmore emphasizes her desire to be independent; Humphry emphasizes her physical pain and social trauma. Longmore suggests that society is prejudiced against disabled people and thus that Elizabeth Bouvia's disability is not so much her problem as society's problem. Humphry writes from a point of view inside Elizabeth Bouvia; the physicians write from the viewpoint of hospital staff members who deal with problematic patients. Longmore critiques an inadequate system that forces terrible, desperate decisions.

In 1985, Bouvia entered Los Angeles County-USC Medical Center, where physicians installed a morphine pump to control pain caused by her worsening arthritis. Because she declared she would eat, she was not force-fed.

After two months, physicians transferred her to nearby High Desert Hospital, another public hospital. Although she ate there, her physicians decided that she wasn't eating *enough* and again force-fed her. They reasoned that "since she is occupying our space, she must accede to the same care which we afford every other patient admitted here, care designed to improve and not detract from chances of recovery and rehabilitation."[16] Critics objected: must all patients who occupy High Desert Hospital's space do as they are told?

Bouvia petitioned courts to stop her forced-feeding. At this time, she weighed only 70 pounds. A consultant on nutrition noted that a weight of 75 or 85 pounds "might be desirable." Her physicians wanted her to weigh about 110 pounds.

At a hearing, Judge Warren Deering interpreted her low weight as "not motivated by a bona fide right to privacy but by a desire to terminate her life."[17] He said the right to privacy did not cover suicide by starvation and ordered forced-feeding because "[s]aving her life [was] paramount."

Bouvia appealed and the California Court of Appeal ruled in her favor: "A desire to terminate one's life is probably the ultimate exercise of one's right to privacy."[18] This Court found "no substantive evidence to support the [lower] court's decision."

Judge Deering had been concerned that Bouvia could live for decades more, but his concern was dismissed: "This trial court mistakenly attached undue importance to the amount of time possibly available to her, and failed to give equal weight and consideration for the quality of that life; an equal, if not more significant, consideration."

The appeals court concluded:

This matter constitutes a perfect paradigm of the axiom: "Justice delayed is justice denied." Her mental and emotional feelings are equally entitled to respect. She has been subjected to the forced intrusion of an artificial mechanism into her body against her will. She has a right to refuse the increased dehumanizing aspect of her condition. . . . The right to refuse medical treatment is basic and fundamental. It is recognized as part of the right of privacy protected by both the state and federal constitutions. Its exercise requires no one's approval. It is not merely one vote subject to being overridden by medical opinion. . . .

[A precedent has been established that when] a doctor performs treatment in the absence of informed consent, there is an actionable battery. The obvious corollary to this principle is that a competent adult patient has the legal right to refuse medical treatment. [Moreover,] if the right of the patient to self-determination as to his own medical treatment is to have any meaning at all, it must be paramount to the interests of the patient's hospital and doctors. . . . The right of a competent adult patient to refuse medical treatment is a constitutionally guaranteed right which must not be abridged. . . .

In Elizabeth Bouvia's view, the quality of her life has been diminished to the point of hopelessness, uselessness, unenjoyability, and frustration. She, as the patient, lying helplessly in bed, unable to care for herself, may consider her existence meaningless. She is not to be faulted for so concluding. . . . As in all matters, lines must be drawn at some point, somewhere, but that decision must ultimately belong to the one whose life is in issue.

For the first time, a federal appellate court said that a competent adult patient had a constitutionally guaranteed right to refuse medical treatment and that it must not be abridged. This court also had strong words about forced-feeding:

We do not believe it is the policy of this State that all and every life must be preserved against the will of the sufferer. It is incongruous, if not monstrous, for medical practitioners to assert their right to preserve a life that someone else must live, or more accurately, endure, for "15 or 20 years." We cannot conceive it to be the policy of this State to inflict such an ordeal upon anyone.

The court concluded "no criminal or civil liability attaches to honoring a competent, informed patient's refusal for medical service."

If nothing else, Elizabeth Bouvia, frail, small, alone, and barely able to move, won a remarkable victory for other patients. Preceding the U.S. Supreme Court's *Cruzan* decision by five years, she wrested from the courts the first clear statement that competent, adult patients have a constitutional right to refuse medical treatment to die.

After her victory, Bouvia did not kill herself. When some caring people offered to help her die, she changed her mind. Most importantly, by giving her control over her life, they gave her a reason to live.

A decade after her victory in court, she described her body as "gnarled and useless."[19] She lived in California on Medi-Cal, in a private hospital room with 24-hour-day care at a cost in 1994 of $300 a day. A morphine pump controlled her pain, and she weighed 100 pounds. She said her life was "a lot of needles and bags," and she spent her time watching television. "I wouldn't say I'm happy, but I'm physically comfortable, more comfortable than before. There is nothing really to do. I just kind of lay here."

Robert Scott, the physician and lawyer who represented Bouvia, battled depression most of his life and committed suicide in 1992. When he did, Bouvia said, "Jesus, I wish he could have come in and taken me with him."

In 1996, Bouvia appeared on "60 Minutes" on the tenth anniversary of a previous "60 Minutes" story on her. For a decade, she had lived in Riverside County Hospital, but in 1997, her new pro bono attorney Griffith Thomas, M.D., got her disability payments put into a trust fund that allowed her to live in her own apartment with 24-hour-a-day in-home assistants. Even though it was cheaper for the public to do this than housing her in a hospital, it took a decade for someone to make this arrangement for her.

Elizabeth in 1996 still had pain each day and needed a morphine drip. She wished to be left alone and did not intend to be alive for another story by "60 Minutes" in 2006. Not thankful for being forced to live, she felt ambivalent about being alive.

THE CASE OF LARRY MCAFEE

At 29 years old, Larry McAfee in 1985 became almost completely paralyzed (a C-2 quadriplegic) in a motorcycle accident. He had studied mechanical engineering at Georgia State University in Atlanta. On a dirt road, he flew over his motorcycle, snapping his neck and crushing his two top vertebrae. Left with use only of his eyes, mouth, and head, he could not clear his throat and sometimes choked. He could not breathe on his own and needed a ventilator. He lacked control over his bladder and bowels and could feel no pleasure from sexual activity. He was unmarried.

McAfee had a $1 million health insurance policy, and remained for over a year at the expensive Shepherd Spinal Center in Atlanta, where the average stay for C-1 to C-4 patients is 19 weeks. After that year, he moved to an apartment in Atlanta, where he insisted on certified nurses who were three times more expensive than home health aides. After living like this for 16 months, he exhausted his insurance. His family offered to take care of him, but he refused to be a burden on them.

With no resources, he became eligible for Medicaid, the fund in each state that pays for medical care for the indigent. McAfee wanted Georgia Medicaid to pay for his care in his apartment and refused to enter a state nursing home, but Georgia officials instead transferred him to a nursing home in Ohio. This facility could care for respirator-dependent C-1 patients, and it accepted McAfee on a temporary basis until Georgia could find a bed for him.

Only a small number of nursing homes in America admit ventilator-dependent patients. Even fewer take such patients on Medicaid because Medicaid's reimbursement is not enough to cover the number of staff needed to care for such patients.

In Ohio, McAfee wouldn't make appointments for vocational rehabilitation. The administrator there said, "Larry was very demanding, wanted things precisely the way he wanted them. . . . I had nurses toward the end who just couldn't work with him anymore because they were just extremely, extremely frustrated."[20] He noted that McAfee's family and friends were all in Georgia.

McAfee claimed that he had been housed in Ohio with demented, senile, and brain-damaged patients who were being cheaply warehoused with only one or two staff for as many as 40 patients. The easiest way to warehouse such patients is to keep them heavily sedated. McAfee said that he experienced intense loneliness and received inadequate personal care. "You're just a sack of potatoes," he said.[21]

After two years, when it became clear that McAfee had been dumped on them, Ohio officials angrily hustled him onto a plane and left him in the emergency room at Grady Memorial Hospital in Atlanta.

After he returned to Atlanta, and because no other facility in Georgia would take him, McAfee spent several miserable months in the intensive care unit of Grady Memorial Hospital. In 1989, Briarcliff Nursing Home in a suburb of Birmingham, Alabama, finally accepted him as a patient, and he transferred there.

Russ Fine, a disability advocate and director of the Injury Control Research Center at the University of Alabama at Birmingham, listened when McAfee called his weekly radio talk show, hosted by Russ and his wife, Dee. According to Russ, McAfee's treatment on Medicaid represented "everything that's wrong about the system that serves disabled people."[22]

On first meeting McAfee, Fine found him lying in bed staring at the ceiling, with no voice-activated telephone and no television. All he could do was stare "at whatever happened to be in front of his face. From a quality of life standpoint, it was a devastating commentary on a society with a very advanced health-care system."[23]

A reporter once arrived to find McAfee's urinary catheter not connected to a container and spilling urine on the floor. Fine says, "These facilities were not equipped to take care of a patient such as Larry, with labor-intensive health-care requirements."[24]

In 1989, four years after the federal court ruled for Elizabeth Bouvia, McAfee filed suit in federal court in Atlanta to exercise his right to die. Because his ventilator had once been dislodged accidentally and he had experienced terrifying suffocation, McAfee did not want it disconnected. Instead, he had designed a puff-sip switch for his IV line that enabled him to take lethal drugs by blowing and sucking in a specific pattern.

In 1989, after a heart-wrenching 45-minute hearing in Fulton County Superior Court, Judge Edward Johnson found in McAfee's favor. Johnson ruled that physicians could prescribe lethal drugs that McAfee would take, using his switch to die.

Everyone assumed that with his legal victory, McAfee would kill himself within days. Like Elizabeth Bouvia, he did not. Russ Fine had convinced McAfee to stay alive. But when he did, his financial problems began.

Social Security, besides financing medical care for Americans over 65 with Medicare, provides financial assistance to disabled people as Supplemental Security Income (SSI). In 1992, SSI payments averaged $362 a month and were paid to 5.4 million elderly, disabled, or blind Americans.[25] McAfee qualified for SSI assistance.

In 1989, Fine persuaded Birmingham's United Cerebral Palsy to let McAfee live temporarily in its nine-person group home for the severely disabled that had a supported-employment program. McAfee stayed there on and off until late 1990, but because he required expensive nurses, he soon had to look elsewhere to live.

Federal regulations surrounding Medicaid block the use of its payment for people like McAfee in group homes. Disability advocates claimed that this structural discrimination forces people like McAfee and Bouvia to live in public hospitals or to be warehoused in huge public nursing homes. When President George Bush refused a waiver of these Medicaid regulations to help McAfee, the Georgia legislature created an independent-living facility for him and the five other patients as an exception to Georgia's disability law and Medicaid plan. McAfee then lived in Augusta, near its medical school.

In 1993, his accident and fight were portrayed in *The Switch*, a CBS movie. To keep his disability payments, McAfee could not accept any money from the movie.

A few months later, Georgia "forgot" to fund McAfee's group home in its state budget. Once again, Fine held Georgia's feet to the fire for McAfee, pointing out that the cost per person in the group home was only $52 a day. Georgia found funds to continue the home for another year.

In 1993, a kink in his urinary catheter caused urine to back up. Being paralyzed, he could not feel what was happening; the backup caused toxicity and high blood pressure. This caused two devastating strokes.[26] He survived, but the strokes injured his brain, and he was left with just a little short-term memory.

He had planned to leave the group home for his own apartment but instead was transferred to a long-term nursing home. When he won the right in court to use his switch and before he lost his ability to use it, this was just the kind of place he had wanted to avoid.

Larry McAfee died in 1995, ten years after his accident, not by his own hand but after being comatose for many months.

THE CASE OF DAX COWART

Twenty-nine-year-old bachelor Dax (Donald) Cowart suffered burns over two-thirds of his body in 1973 in Texas. Treated against his will for 14 months in a burn unit in Parkland Hospital in Dallas, Dax's physicians ignored his refusal to be treated. Instead, they honored the wishes of his mother, who overruled him. He was left blind, disfigured, and with only partial use of his fingers.[27]

After winning $1 million from an out-of-court settlement with a gas company (that was responsible for his burns), he hired a plane, flew to Mexico, and spent several hours on a landing strip with a gun in his hand, debating whether to kill himself. Like Elizabeth Bouvia and Larry McAfee, once he obtained the power to do so and control of his life, he decided not to kill himself.

Instead, he graduated from law school in 1986 and later married a nurse he had known previously when both of them were in high school. He became interested in ham radio and raising golden retrievers. Since then, he has been active as a trial lawyer and has won cases for plaintiffs in lawsuits.

In retrospect, he rejects the decision of his physicians to keep him alive. He frequently tells his story in public, emphasizing the cruelty of his physicians, who made him endure 14 months of terrible pain. He argues that even though he is glad to be alive today, his physicians were wrong to treat him against his wishes.

As he once said to this author, "If I should be so unlucky as to be burned that way again, and if I knew what was waiting at the end, I wouldn't go through that pain to get there."[28]

BACKGROUND: PERSPECTIVES ON SUICIDE

Greece and Rome

Ancient Greek aristocrats strove not simply to live, but to lead lives of nobility, honor, excellence, and beauty. Believing that "the unexamined life is not worth living," they thought the "important thing is not to live but to live well." They thought that study of philosophy would provide wisdom to approach death (*philosophy* means "love of wisdom" in Greek). Plato records Socrates as saying, "True philosophers make dying their profession, and . . . to them of all men, death is least alarming. . . . So if you see one distressed at the prospect of dying, it will be proof that he is a lover not of wisdom but of the body."[29]

Socrates died famously. Sentenced to die for his political beliefs, he could have fled Athens, but chose instead to drink hemlock, a poison. At his death scene, he discussed death with a friend.

The friend said that if one is convinced of life after death, it is easy not to fear death, but if the soul is "dispersed and destroyed on the very day that the man himself dies [and] may be dissipated like breath or smoke, and vanish away, so that nothing is left of it anywhere. . . . [no] one but a fool is entitled to face death with confidence, unless he can prove that the soul is absolutely immortal and indestructible."

Socrates replied that the soul may be immortal, but if it is not, then death is like a sleep from which one never awakes. If so, we should not fear it, because no one will exist to feel pain or to miss life.

Hemlock acts as a poison by decreasing circulation at the extremities, creating distal numbness, and eventually stopping the heart. During Socrates' abstract discussion about death, the hemlock was working, moving up from his toes to his ankles. As the discussion ends, the state poisoner finds that Socrates' thighs are numb and says that, in minutes when the poison reaches the heart, Socrates will die.

As his friends begin to cry, Socrates says, "Calm yourselves and try to be brave!" He dies moments later. His admiring follower, Plato, and the author of this account, writes, "Such . . . was the end of our comrade, who was, we may fairly say, of all those whom we knew in our time, the bravest and also the wisest and most upright man."

Centuries later in Rome, emperor Marcus Aurelius (portrayed in the 2000 movie *Gladiator*) wrote that suicide surpassed undignified dying. This Roman Stoic defended the argument for the open door: "If the room is smoky, if only moderately, I will stay; if there is too much smoke, I will go. Remember this, keep a firm hand on it, the door is always open."[30]

Another Stoic, Seneca, wrote about old age: "If it begins to shake my mind, if it destroys my faculties one by one, if it leaves me not life but breath, I will depart the putrid or the tottering edifice."[31]

In the 20th century, existentialist philosopher Jean-Paul Sartre revived the argument for the open door.[32] He emphasized that choice—even the choice of staying alive each day—is inescapable. He famously wrote, "Not to choose is always still a choice."

Christianity and Voluntary Death

The Bible does not explicitly prohibit suicide, and seems to condone the suicides of Saul and Judas. During the fourth century, Augustine condemned suicide, basing his condemnation on the sixth commandment, "Thou shalt not kill" (Exodus 20:13).

Augustine distinguished between private killing and killing endorsed by God or divine authority. Killing undertaken on one's own authority is never right, but when God commands killing, humans must obey. So Abraham had to obey when God commanded him to kill his son, Isaac. Individuals who so kill are instruments in God's hand.

This reasoning underlies the permissibility of killing in capital punishment and in just wars. The worldly Ambrose had already said that Christians could kill in war, and Augustine went further by condoning war against heretics. Frederick Russell in *The Just War in the Middle Ages* says that through Augustine's interpretation of killing for Christians, "the New Testament doctrines of love and purity were accommodated to the savagery of the Old Testament and pacifism was defeated."[33]

Augustine does not explain how he knows when God orders humans to kill and when God orders humans to abstain. In particular, how do we know that God forbids suicide for people with terminal illness?

The 13th-century philosopher and theologian Thomas Aquinas held that suicide is sinful. It is so because it left no time for repentance; because life is a gift from God and only God can take it back; because it deprives the community of talented people; because it deprives children of their parents; and because it is unnatural, going against the instinct of self-preservation.

Three thinkers who allowed suicide were the French essayist Michel de Montaigne in the 16th century, the Dutch philosopher Baruch Spinoza and the English poet John Donne in the seventeenth. Montaigne concluded his essay "To Philosophize Is to Learn How to Die" by saying, "If we have learned how to live properly and calmly, we will know how to die in the same manner."[34] Spinoza wrote, "A free man, that is to say, a man who lives according to the dictates of reason alone, is not led by the fear of death."[35] Donne wrote, "When the [terminal] disease would not reduce us, [God] sent a second and worse affliction, ignorant and torturing physicians."[36]

Hume   In the 18th century, Scottish philosopher David Hume argued that suicide "is no transgression of our duty to God." Hume hated vanity and observed, "The life of a man is of no greater importance to the universe than that of an oyster."[37]

In his "Essay on Suicide," Hume disagreed with Augustine and Aquinas. For dying patients, Hume argued, voluntary death is not a sin: "A house which falls by its own weight, is not brought to ruin by [God's] providence."[38] Hume argued that if God made the world through the laws of causality—the laws of biology, medicine, and physics—then disease belonged to the natural working of such laws.

Hume attacked the idea that suicide is blasphemous. Immanuel Kant argued that we have a station in life assigned to us by God and which we must not give up, but Hume replied, "It is a kind of blasphemy to imagine that any created being can [by taking his own life] disturb the order of the world. Any suicide is insignificant to the workings of the universe and it is blasphemy to think otherwise." To Hume, only narcissists believe that the world's smooth functioning requires their continued existence.

In his "Essay," Hume disputed Aquinas's argument that suicide harms the community:

> A man who retires from life does no harm to society; he only ceases to do good; which, if it is an injury, is of the lowest kind. All our obligations to do good to society seem to imply something reciprocal. I receive benefits of society, and therefore ought to promote its interests; but when I withdraw myself altogether from society, can I be bound any longer? But [even] allowing that our obligations to do good were perpetual, they have certainly some bounds; I am not obliged to do a small good to society at the expense of a great harm to myself: when then should I prolong a miserable existence, because of some frivolous advantage which the public may perhaps receive from me?

Kant   Hume's contemporary, the German philosopher Immanuel Kant, opposed suicide for several reasons. First, for Kant an act is right if it represents or is based on a rule that can be universalized, that is, a rule we would want everyone to act on. Kant argued that suicide cannot be universalized because its motive is self-interest (for instance, escaping pain), and for Kant, self-interest can never justify moral decisions.

Second, suicide is immoral because people should always be treated as ends in themselves, never as mere means. Kant reasoned that treating oneself as an end-in-itself entails recognizing one's free will as an absolute (rather than as a relative) value, but destroying oneself entails destroying that freedom of will. "Man's freedom cannot subsist except on a condition which is immutable. This condition is that man not use his freedom against himself to his own destruction."[39]

Third, a person "who does not respect his life even in principle cannot be restrained from the most dreadful vices." If I do not respect my own life, I will not respect anything else. To respect the sacred value of the lives of others, I must respect the sacred value of my own.

Finally, Kant wrote, "Human beings are sentinels on earth and may not leave their posts until relieved by another beneficent hand. God is our owner; we are His property."[40]

John Stuart Mill   In one of the most famous passages in political philosophy, John Stuart Mill expressed "one very simple principle" in his 1859 essay, *On Liberty*. It grounds the political and ethical autonomy that enables competent patients to end their own lives. Mill writes that

> One very simple principle [is] entitled to govern absolutely the dealings of society with the individual in the way of compulsion and control, whether the means

used is physical force in the form of legal penalties, or the moral coercion of public opinion. That principle is, that the sole end for which mankind are warranted, individually or collectively, in interfering with the liberty of action of any of their number, is self-protection. That the only purpose for which power can be rightfully exercised over any member of a civilized community, against his will, is to prevent harm to others. His own good, either physical or moral, is not a sufficient warrant. . . . The only part of the conduct of any one, for which he is amenable to society, is that which concerns others. In the part which merely concerns himself, his independence is, of right, absolute. Over himself, over his own body and mind, the individual is sovereign.[41]

According to this principle, so long as others are not harmed, we can do whatever we want with our own lives and bodies.

Mill distinguished between *self-regarding* and *other-regarding* acts, and argued that we may censure others only for their other-regarding acts. Paradoxically, Mill's analysis can be used both for and against suicide. On one hand, taking one's own life is clearly self-regarding; suicide is often described as the ultimate personal issue. On the other hand, suicide is other-regarding because it deeply affects others, especially when they believe they should have acted differently to prevent it. If a suicidal person desired to make others feel guilty, sorry, or incompetent, then Mill's principle condemns him.

The Modern Era   When American feminist Charlotte Perkins Gillman killed herself in 1935, she left a note saying that she preferred "chloroform to cancer." In an essay published posthumously, she wrote: "The record of a previously noble life is precisely what makes it sheer insult to allow death in pitiful degradation. We may not wish to 'die with our boots on,' but we may well prefer to 'die with our brains on.'"[42]

A century ago, only the poor and people without families went to a hospital to die. Before the Harrison Act of 1914, Americans could purchase heroin and opiates to lessen the pain of terminal cancer and to die at home on their own terms. Today, physicians control such drugs, death has been medicalized, and most people die in hospitals or nursing homes.

The nature of deadly diseases has also changed. Before World War II, most people died of sudden-onset, acute diseases such as pneumonia and cholera. Today, people live longer and die slowly from chronic diseases such as emphysema, diabetes, dementia, cancer, and coronary artery disease. Because such diseases slowly erode the quality of life, death at a time of one's own choosing remains a moral issue.

The Concept of Assisted Suicide

One question raised by the cases of Elizabeth Bouvia and Larry McAfee is what to call their intended action: suicide, rational suicide, assisted suicide, euthanasia, voluntary death, or self-deliverance? Let us clarify some terms here.

First, *euthanasia* usually means the killing of one person by another for merciful reasons. The preceding cases do not involve euthanasia, then, since in each case the death would be initiated by the person herself or himself.

Second, it is inaccurate to say that a terminally ill patient who forgoes medical treatment "commits suicide." It is true that the definition of suicide is now often broadened to include indirect ways of bringing about one's own death.[43] Nevertheless, we should distinguish between: (1) cases where an underlying disease is incrementally leading to death, and thereby in choosing not to do everything possible, the patient accepts death at an earlier date; and (2) cases where a competent adult without a terminal illness causes his or her own death. The second kind of case is appropriately called suicide.

One reason to maintain the distinction between forgoing treatment in terminal illness and committing suicide is that if a death is classified as a suicide, life insurance companies refuse to pay benefits. Another reason is that in all states it is illegal to assist in a suicide.

The issue for physicians and nurses in the Bouvia and McAfee cases is therefore best called *assisted suicide*. Neither Bouvia nor McAfee had a terminal disease, hence the term *suicide*. They could not easily kill themselves, and so they needed help from others, especially medical staff members: hence the term *assisted*.

ETHICAL ISSUES: FOR AND AGAINST
ASSISTED SUICIDE

Easy to Kill Oneself?

Why don't patients such as Elizabeth Bouvia and Larry McAfee simply go off somewhere and kill themselves? Answer: it's difficult to commit suicide when you want to die painlessly and aesthetically, and when you need to be sure that you accomplish what you intend. When you are disabled, it's almost impossible to kill yourself without someone's help.

During the Iran-Contra hearings in 1987 during the administration of Ronald Reagan, national security advisor Robert McFarlane took between 30 and 45 10-milligram tablets of Valium. When he didn't die, people inferred that he didn't want to die. An equally plausible explanation is that he didn't know how to kill himself; most people don't. In 1985, physician Robert Rosier didn't know how much morphine to give his terminally ill wife to help her die. If physicians don't know, what about the rest of us?[44]

Whenever a suicide is botched, people infer ambivalence, but this may be mistaken. Emergency medicine is full of stories of bizarre survivals.[45] The hand holding the gun wobbles a fraction of an inch and leaves the would-be suicide a drooling zombie. Because the drugs they take for courage also relax muscles and soften impact, some jumpers survive the fall from the Golden Gate Bridge.[46] One jumper hit a parked car and not only did not die, but did not even lose consciousness.

Although suicide attempts by teenagers increased 300 percent between 1967 and 1982, only one in 50 attempts succeeded.[47] The elderly know more and succeed one in three times; Miami Beach leads America in successful suicides. Women attempt suicide more than men, but are less successful. Men use violent means (such as guns) whereas women use drugs.

Methods available for committing suicide present a grim picture. Valium and other benzodiazepines usually are taken in insufficient quantities to cause death and merely make people permanently comatose or brain-injured.

People using other methods are just as likely to end up in the ER as dead. Carbon monoxide (CO) poisoning may not work because the car can stall or run out of gas, or the CO concentration may not be enough to produce death, so that the person ends up in a coma.

Slitting one's wrists in a warm tub is not easy: the cuts are painful and must be made deep and in the right place. Nor is this method certain: in the time between unconsciousness and death, the arm may move out of the water and the blood may coagulate. One ER physician observes, "Most slashers just get a trophy: a claw hand."

Some people who don't kill themselves properly with medication wake up in the ER with a nasogastric tube down their throat, into which syrup of ipecac is pumped to induce vomiting. This is followed by injections of saline solution and gastric lavage—alternate flooding and suctioning out of the stomach—and then granulated charcoal is pumped in to absorb the remaining toxins. These procedures are painful, messy, and unpleasant, especially for those who return to consciousness while they are in progress.

People may be reluctant to use certain methods if they want to spare the feelings of others, or if they want to be found in a reasonably dignified state after death. A drug overdose not only decreases respiration but also relaxes bowels and bladders. Jumping off a building or shooting oneself in the head leaves a big mess. Hanging is not so great either: difficult to do correctly—because the neck may not break and the victim, kicking in agony as he partially asphyxiates, may not die—and undignified, because it relaxes bowel and bladder control. Men who die by hanging are also found with an erect penis.

Rationality and Competence

The play and movie, *Whose Life Is It, Anyway?* dramatized one issue of these cases. Its quadriplegic hero, Ken Harrison, wants to die and offers rational arguments for suicide to his psychiatrist. However, because Harrison is intelligent and sane enough to formulate a convincing case for suicide, his psychiatrists decides he's too intelligent and sane to die. Harrison can convince the psychiatrist of his rationality only by deciding to live.

In Elizabeth Bouvia's case, psychiatrist Nancy Mullen testified that since Bouvia was suicidal, she was incompetent to make decisions about her life. Mullen said that she could conceive of no situation where a person could make a competent decision to take her own life.[48] Carol Gill, a clinical assistant professor of occupational therapy who used a wheelchair, criticized the ACLU for accepting the decision of "a handful of medical experts" that Bouvia was competent when she decided to starve herself.[49]

These experts may have begged the question of rational suicide. A question is begged when the answer is assumed to be true rather than proved. In these cases, the question or point is whether a decision to die rather than lead an unsatisfactory life is irrational: whether it indicates misinformation or faulty reasoning.

Just assuming that a decision to die is always irrational—or incompetent—begs that question.

This is not to say that a decision to die is always rational. Elizabeth Bouvia may have been depressed, and psychological tests might have shown this. But Mullen and Gill did not base their arguments on such tests. They were not her therapists and were not treating her. They reacted to the content of Bouvia's decision rather than to psychological tests. Indeed, three psychiatric professionals who tested Elizabeth found her competent.[50]

In America, a patient is legally competent until proven otherwise in a hearing. No patient can be held in a hospital against her will without having been proven legally incompetent. In practice, hospitals sometimes break such laws. Although Dax Cowart was never declared incompetent, he was treated against his will for 14 months in a burn unit.

Autonomy

At the start of bioethics, autonomy fueled the patient's rights movement. Applied to the right to die, a person who has not been proven incompetent has an autonomous right to end his life.

Opponents of assisted suicide argued that Bouvia and McAfee did not want to die because they did not kill themselves quietly but made dramatic demands on public institutions. They were "acting out" and pleading for attention. In such cases, physicians must not accede to wishes of unstable patients, because doing so may not represent the patient's best interests. It would be foolish and cruel to assist in the suicide of every distraught patient who came to an ER wishing to die.

The Roman Catholic Church opposes autonomous suicide. In 1990, Father Kevin O'Rourke argued that humans are not in control of their lives.[51] O'Rourke argued that God has a plan for each person, and it never includes suicide.

One problem with uncritical acceptance of autonomy is the famous SUPPORT study (Study to Understand Prognoses and Preferences for Outcomes and Risks of Treatments). It studied predictions about advance directives and end-of-life care and discovered that competent people do not accurately predict what they will later find acceptable or unacceptable as quality of life.[52] People who predicted that they would rather die than go on a ventilator most often did *not* choose to die but instead went on a ventilator. It's one thing to say abstractly that one would "rather be dead than live like that," but when actually faced with death, most people decide to live, even with bad quality of life.

Moreover, in rehabilitation medicine there is the equally famous *adaptation effect,* in which after some time, patients like Larry McAfee or Dax Cowart, who were disabled in accidents, adapt their views about acceptable quality of life. What they once considered unacceptable then becomes acceptable. For most patients, it can take six months or more for this effect to occur.

Given the fallibility of the predictions of competent people about their actual wishes at the end of their lives, if we have a person with severe disabilities whose life seems to have some pleasure and not too much pain, then letting her die cannot be justified solely by appealing to her present wishes. Chances are too high that she is incorrectly forecasting her future preferences.

On the other side, supporters of assisted suicide argue that providing such assistance finishes a continuum of good medical care. Normally, leaving a patient untreated is abandonment and is considered unethical (and for physicians, a crime). But when quality of life diminishes, the fact that a patient does not have a terminal disease is irrelevant. The real issue is whether a quality of life is acceptable to the person who must endure it, and that is an evaluative judgment that can be made only by the patient herself. If physicians refuse to assist in suicide and make this evaluation for patients, that is vile paternalism.

Although autonomy creates bad results in some cases, honoring it leads to the greatest good for the greatest number. The death rate for humans is 100 percent. Each of us will die and each of us wants control over how we do so. We value autonomy in our life and in our dying.

If physicians ignore autonomy, patients can be "flogged to death" with unnecessary tubes, surgery, and radiation. Such barbaric end-of-life treatment differs little from involuntary commitment of competent people in psychiatric wards, a practice condemned even in the former Soviet Union.

Autonomy is both an ethical and a political value in bioethics. As we have seen, both Kant and Mill argued for autonomy as the source of values and individual choices.

Unlike Kant, Mill argued that the state should have no power to force an individual to act in his own best interest. In essence, Mill saw individual rights as conditions limiting what government may do to citizens.

The key question was not whether Elizabeth Bouvia was demonstrably competent or incompetent, but where the onus of proof should lie. For rugged individualists and Libertarians, who abhor the growing powers of government and physicians, this onus should be on those who would take away autonomy.

In 1990, the U.S. Supreme Court decided in its *Cruzan* decision that no state may pass a law limiting the right of competent patients to decline medical treatment, even if declining treatment would hasten death. *Cruzan* built on the *Bouvia* and *McAfee* decisions, and was a victory for the right of competent adults to control how they died.

Treating Depression, Pain, and Symptoms Well

Although not every decision to die is irrational, many suicidal people suffer from treatable depression. Humane physicians will not let patients die because of chemical imbalances in their brains.

This is especially true of the three patients of this chapter, who were young, nonterminal, competent adults. Although it is understandable to want to die after being horribly burned or after losing physical abilities, people in the throes of depression do not understand how much better they can come to feel. Antidepressants can lift moods and change outlooks on life, and therefore should be given to all nonterminal patients who wish to die.

A different clinical issue concerns relief of symptoms. In this regard, psychiatrist and palliative care physician John Shuster says it is always important to ask patients who want to die, "What is the chief symptom that makes you want to die?"[53] He observes that often that chief symptom is not what outsiders would predict. One of his patients suffered obviously from air hunger but that was not his chief complaint. Instead, he missed going to a public park with his trailer, so visits to the park were quickly arranged by hospital volunteers. Moreover, with well-financed coverage, almost any symptom can be controlled, including pain, air hunger, itchiness, fatigue, and even boredom.

Social Prejudice and Physical Disabilities

Disability advocate Paul Longmore, who was quoted earlier and who is himself a ventilator-dependent quadriplegic, opposes voluntary death for people with disabilities. He believes that the Bouvia case shows how a prejudiced system destroys the independence of disabled people, rather than nurturing it.

By creating intolerable conditions for disabled people, society paints them into a corner. Such patients are left with only one autonomous decision that is consistent with their former autonomous selves: they can decide to die. Every other decision is made for them by others who keep them passive and dependent. In Longmore's words:

> Given the lumping together of people with disabilities with those who are terminally ill, the blurring of voluntary assisted suicide and forced "mercy" killing, and the oppressive conditions of social devaluation and isolation, blocked opportunities, economic deprivation, and enforced social powerlessness, talk of their "rational" or "voluntary" suicide is simply Orwellian newspeak. The advocates of assisted suicide assume a nonexistent autonomy. They offer an illusory self-determination.[54]

To see Elizabeth Bouvia as simply a case of a right to die is to miss the heart of a much bigger issue. What made Elizabeth Bouvia want to die was the cumulative effect of centuries of prejudice against people who are physically disabled—prejudice that is virulently expressed in modern American society which idealizes youth, beauty, sex, athleticism, fitness, and wealth. Other values also make life worthwhile, such as caring for others, erudition, creativity, and community, but our culture does not idealize such values.

Longmore attacks films that encourage disabled people to view killing themselves as a rational response to their low quality of life. He cites *Annie Hall*, *Elephant Man*, and especially *Whose Life Is It, Anyway?* He claims that watching the latter depressed Elizabeth Bouvia. He hated *Million Dollar Baby*.

Some critics of autonomy see Bouvia's case as a failure on the part of society: a lack of caring, a case where she slipped through the cracks of an impersonal system. They see her as a tragic figure not because of her physical situation but rather because of her *social* situation. Even as a hospitalized patient, she remained alone, and it was her aloneness that underlay her fierce assertion of her right to tear herself away from life.

Structural Discrimination Against the Disabled

In 1990, the Americans with Disabilities Act (ADA) went into effect. This legislation represents one of the most sweeping changes in American law. Although not always enforced, its long-term effects will integrate Americans with disabilities into normal life.

Raising the issue of inadequate resources puts physicians in an awkward place. On the one hand, they do not want to be instruments of torture to disabled people who want to die. On the other hand, they do not want to acquiesce to unnecessary deaths of the disabled because a prejudiced, cheap society has the wrong attitude toward people with disabilities. In this regard, it is important to recognize that most institutions are still not anywhere near in compliance with the ADA.

The catch is that to provide great care, the patient must be rich or have good insurance, or society must be generous. If the true measure of a society's humanity is how it treats its least well-off members, then our society is not humane, at least toward the disabled.[55]

As a result of childhood polio, Paul Longmore's arms are paralyzed, his spine is curved, and he uses a ventilator as much as 18 hours a day. He is an associate professor of history at San Francisco State University. His success would not have been possible without being able to live independently on his own, which required lots of home health care aides. Fortunately, California's generous Medicaid program paid for his domestic aides (costing $15,000 a year) and he managed to avoid being disqualified from Medicare disability, which paid for his ventilator (costing $12,000 a year). Had he lived in Georgia or Michigan, Longmore too, might have wanted to die; he would not have been able to find a group home and "probably would have found [his] life unendurable."

A more subtle issue concerns depression stemming from inadequate resources for the disabled. Do we want to encourage society to be financially stingy by being ethically/morally generous in allowing disabled people to kill themselves? Do we want to give some families an easy way out of paying for expensive care? It seems that ethics requires some safeguards against making assisted suicide too easy, as shown by the three cases in this chapter where the patients decided to live when they obtained control of their case or better resources.

Longmore maintains that Elizabeth Bouvia's problems resulted in part because she did not receive the maximum payments she was entitled to; he says that her county is notorious for its stinginess in benefits to disabled people. The hospital where she was supposed to do her internship refused to comply with laws designed to ensure her disability rights.

Elizabeth was discouraged from seeking work or marrying, because when a disabled person takes a job or marries, her benefits are reduced. California's In-Home Supportive Services program allowed Elizabeth to manage her own life at home while she was single; when she married, however, she became ineligible for the program: her husband was now expected to care for her. Given these circumstances, Longmore thinks it is no wonder that Bouvia was later divorced or that she became discouraged about completing her training. Even in the unlikely event that she was able to overcome discrimination and find a job, she would then lose the benefits that allowed her to live on her own at home. Longmore concludes:

> This is a woman who aimed at something more significant than mere self-sufficiency. She struggled to attain self-determination, but she was repeatedly thwarted in her efforts by discriminatory actions on the part of the government, her teachers, her employers, her parents, and her society. Contrary to the highly prejudiced view of the appeals court, what makes life with a major physical disability ignominious, embarrassing, humiliating, and dehumanizing is not the

need for extensive physical assistance, but the dehumanizing social contempt toward those who require such aid.

The case of Larry McAfee also raises structural issues about rights of people with disabilities, although this case was clouded by his personality. Was he a demanding, spoiled patient, as some people described him, or was he a heroic figure who would rather die than live in the institutional squalor of publicly funded nursing homes?

Russ Fine believes that McAfee's desire to die resulted from his inadequate care. Public officials were controlling costs by requiring patients like McAfee to live in the most cost-effective facilities, but McAfee said that if he couldn't get his own apartment he would rather die. According to Fine, McAfee "was very vocal about inferior nursing care, which was the rule, not the exception, in these marginal health-care facilities that had accepted these contracts."[56]

Once, Fine had brought him a Thanksgiving dinner and the two were watching a televised football game while waiting for McAfee's family to arrive. Fine was drowsing in an armchair when he suddenly realized that McAfee had stopped breathing. By the time the family arrived, nurses and aides were swarming over McAfee, trying to get him breathing. When he finally revived, Fine saw tears streaming out of his eyes. "He didn't really want to die," Fine concluded. "He was just terrified."[57]

It should be noted that McAfee, like Bouvia, wanted to work, but getting paid for working would have made him ineligible for most publicly funded assistance in housing or Medicaid.

Cases such as Bouvia's and McAfee's suggest that society often does give severely disabled people only three limited, grim choices: to become a burden on their families or friends, to live miserably in a large public institution, or to kill themselves.

In small-group homes, a few home health aides can help disabled residents lead productive lives. Both Bouvia and McAfee wanted such arrangements, and giving them this would have been cheaper than the care they received in hospitals. (Elizabeth Bouvia's care cost at least $300 a day between 1986 and 1996.)

Not many group homes exist. A major reason is a reaction called NIMBY—"not in my back yard"—neighborhood resistance to such homes. In the case of group homes for the disabled, such resistance seems to be based on prejudice. Neighborhoods argue that group homes create dangerous situations and lower property values, but this does not seem convincing for homes for people with disabilities. Prejudice should not be allowed to prevent communities from giving their disabled citizens better choices than imprisonment in hospitals or death.

The Rule of Rescue

The campaign to obtain a presidential waiver for Larry McAfee provoked criticism. Two citizens complained when McAfee said that he would not return to a nursing home to "vegetate" and wanted Georgia to pay for his private apartment.[58] They wrote:

> But why should McAfee be the only one singled out and given special attention, not to be in a nursing home, or that Medicaid should "open up" for? . . . McAfee "understands" that life is preferable, but it must be life with some dignity; in this case, his way or no way. McAfee says that if someone else won't pay for him to live where and how he chooses, he'd rather be dead. What about all the other people in the same situation?[59]

Critics like these hold that American society rescues only someone like McAfee who gets into the national spotlight; it ignores all the others whose needs are just as great. In McAfee's case, there were some 75,000 to 85,000 others.

McAfee and Bouvia illustrate the *rule of rescue*. When one person's plight is made prominent by the news media, society tends to feel compelled to rescue that person, even if the rescue entails spending enormous amounts of scarce medical resources. In contrast, obscure people quietly go "unrescued" and live in abysmal conditions until they die. The rule of rescue in effect turns some crucial decisions over to the media: the editors of local newspapers and television news departments become gatekeepers, determining who will and will not be rescued. This is hardly the most rational way to distribute scarce medical resources. (Chapter 13, about the God Committee, further discusses the rule of rescue.)

Disability Culture

During the last decades, people with disabilities increasingly protested against society's discrimination. They asserted their right to 24-hour-a-day attendants, public transportation, and good housing.[60] People with disabilities think they have a condition, not an illness. For them, "disability culture" is not a bad thing, but a source of pride and identity.

They argue that the disabled community is the only minority that anyone may join at any time. Just as James Meredith had to sue in 1962 to become the first black person admitted to the University of Mississippi, so quadriplegic Edward V. Roberts had to sue to be admitted to the University of California. Has society more successfully integrated the races than the disabled?

People with disabilities abound who see their life as a call-to-action to help their less assertive disabled friends. They despise Mattel's "Share-a-Smile Becky" in a wheelchair (sold in some hospitals' gift shops) and demonstrate outside classes of Princeton bioethicist Peter Singer, whose views on quality of life, they fear, would allow society to easily kill the disabled or deny them adequate resources.

Disability groups also heckled the Hemlock Society (now called Compassion in Dying) accusing it of being too sympathetic to the assisted death of nonterminal patients. They cite psychologist Faye Girsh, the Society's executive director who testified on behalf of Bouvia, on behalf of Jack Kevorkian when he killed some nonterminal women beset by economic hardship; on behalf of George DeLury who in 1996 in Manhattan killed his wife in the late stages of multiple sclerosis; and on behalf of Canadian Robert Latimer, who in 1993 killed his 12-year old daughter who had cerebral palsy. Disability groups accused Girsh and her Society of being on the side of rich, well-insured, autonomous elites, not interested in securing better conditions for the disabled.

Conclusion

As our cases showed, requests to die from young, nonterminal patients involve more than simply viewing physicians as cruel if they refuse to honor these requests on demand. There are more issues beneath the surface, including issues about justice in the design of medical and social services in our society for people with disabilities and issues about adequate treatment of depression and symptoms.

FURTHER READING AND RESOURCES

"A Man of Endurance" *20/20* television show on March 22, 1999 on Donald Cowart's case. Call 1-800-CALL-ABC to order tape (around $30).

"Elizabeth Bouvia: 10 Years Later," *60 Minutes* Special, www.cbs.com

Pat Milmoe McCarrick, "Active Euthanasia and Assisted Suicide," Scope Note 18, *Kennedy Institute of Ethics Journal* no. 1 (March 1992).

James Rachels, *The End of Life*, Oxford University Press, Oxford, 1986.

CHAPTER 2

Comas

Karen Quinlan, Nancy Cruzan, and Terri Schiavo

The famous case of Terri Schiavo exploded across the world in 2005, but it had a pedigree, building on the previous cases of Nancy Cruzan and Karen Quinlan. The Quinlan case started in 1975 in New Jersey courts. Fifteen years later in 1990, the U.S. Supreme Court finally defined basic rights of dying patients. Fifteen years after that, the Schiavo case showed that problems still remained about treatment of incompetent patients at the end of life.

The Quinlan case sparked the public's interest in medical ethics and its many questions: Does a person die when only machines keep her body alive? Can families alone decide when medicine ceases to be treatment and becomes torture? Can physicians? Does killing patients differ from intentionally letting them die? In making decisions, what role should courts take? What should be the standard of brain death? The definition of personhood? How should we safeguard incompetent patients from overzealous families? When, if ever, should we force families to accept medical realities?

THE QUINLAN CASE

In April 1975, after just turning 21, a perky, independent young woman named Karen Quinlan became comatose from drinking alcohol after taking either barbiturates or benzodiazepines, or both.[1] Karen had also been dieting, and at admission, weighed only 115 pounds.

Benzodiazepines, antianxiety drugs such as Valium, Librium, Ativan, and Xanax, act on specific nerve receptors in the brain and are considered safer than barbiturates. The latter have been around since 1912, when physicians first used phenobarbital.

Both benzodiazepines and barbiturates intensify with alcohol, an effect called *synergism*. Alcohol *potentiates* these drugs, and an empty stomach increases the effects. Actor River Phoenix unintentionally killed himself in 1993 by mixing barbiturates, alcohol, and benzodiazepines.

Karen lost her brain from a synergistic reaction of barbiturates, benzodiazepines and alcohol, taken on an empty stomach. These drugs suppressed her breathing, caused loss of oxygen to her brain, and after 30 minutes, destroyed her higher brain.

At St. Clare's Hospital, a Catholic institution in Denville, New Jersey, a small ventilator, also called a ventilator, kept Karen breathing. It also prevented aspiration of vomit, which could cause pneumonia.

Respirators began to be used in medicine during the 1960s and by 1975 had become common in cases of emergency and trauma. The respirator's use in this case showed that the *criteria of death* needed clarification. Because the brain must have a fresh supply of oxygenated blood to live, lack of such oxygenated blood (anoxia) quickly damages the brain and over enough time, destroys it. The traditional definition of death—where the body stops breathing and the person is declared dead—indirectly *assumed* brain death to be inevitable, but now a respirator prevented this.

Karen's appearance shocked her sister, who said:

> Whenever I thought of a person in a coma, I thought they would just lie there very quietly, almost as though they were sleeping. Karen's head was moving around, as if she was trying to pull away from that tube in her throat, and she made little noises, like moans. I don't know if she was in pain, but it seemed as though she was. And I thought—if Karen could ever see herself like this, it would be the worst thing in the world for her.[2]

Sometimes Karen would choke, sit bolt upright with her arms flung out and her eyes wide open, appearing to be in intense pain. Eventually her breathing stabilized, but even then she didn't breath deeply enough to sigh. Without breathing to a sigh, the lower sacs of her lungs risked infection. Hence she was put on a larger respirator for a "sigh volume." This larger respirator required a tracheotomy (a hole cut surgically in the throat or trachea) to which her mother, Julia Quinlan, reluctantly agreed.

This more powerful respirator altered her appearance. At a later hearing, her lawyer testified about Karen in September 1975 that:

> Her eyes are open and move in a circular manner as she breathes; her eyes blink approximately three or four times per minute; her forehead evidences every noticeable perspiration; her mouth is open while the respirator expands to ingest oxygen, and while her mouth is open, her tongue appears to be moving in a rather random manner; her mouth closes as the oxygen is ingested into her body through the tracheotomy and she appears to be slightly convulsing or gasping as the oxygen enters the windpipe; her hands are visible in an emaciated form, facing in a praying position away from her body. Her present weight would seem to be in vicinity of 70–80 pounds.[3]

Karen Quinlan, of course, was in a coma, but what does that mean? The word "coma" is vague. Despite popular belief at the time, under New Jersey law in 1975 Karen was not brain-dead, which required *all* of her brain to be not functioning.

Karen Quinlan was in a serious form of coma called *persistent vegetative state* (PVS). PVS is a generic term covering a type of deep unconsciousness that, if it persists for a few months, is almost always irreversible. In this case, her eyes were *disconjugate,* i.e., they moved in different, random directions at the same time. Despite eye movements, she was thought to be *decorticate:* Karen's brain could not receive input from her eyes. She had slow-wave—not isoelectric or "flat"—electroencephalograms (EEGs).

At one time, a patient in such a condition would simply starve to death; but in the late 1960s, crude intravenous and nasogastric feeding tubes began to be used. Initially, an intravenous tube fed Karen, but as her condition persisted, the rigidity of her muscles made it difficult to insert and reinsert such a tube into her veins. Five months after her admission, in September 1975, she required a nasogastric feeding tube.

The Quinlans never allowed a picture to be taken of Karen in PVS. So the public never saw a realistic picture of a PVS patient with a shaved head on her respirator and feeding tube.

In the fall of 1975, the Quinlan parents decided that Karen would never regain consciousness, so they decided to remove the respirator and let Karen's body die. They had no idea that their struggle to reach this decision would be the easy part.

The Quinlans averred that Karen had twice said that if anything terrible happened to her, she did not want to be kept alive as a vegetable on machines. But was she really a "vegetable?" We now know that a rare patient may recover from PVS.

Recall that the use of respirators in the Quinlan case revealed new ethical problems about brain death. In combination with a feeding tube, the question arose of how active could ethical physicians be in *withdrawing* such devices? To physicians and family members, such withdrawals may *feel* like killing a vulnerable patient. The Catholic Church asserted such. Were such feelings justified? Isn't it a physician's job to look out for vulnerable patients? What if the patient's family feels differently than the physician? How should such a conflict be resolved?

Robert Morse and Arshad Javed, a resident in internal medicine and a fellow in pulmonary medicine, were the physicians of record in this case and, when the Quinlans asked them to disconnect Karen's respirator, they wanted to block charges of criminal misconduct. Why was that?

First, in 1975 the American Medical Association (AMA) equated withdrawing a respirator for death to occur with euthanasia, and then equated that with murder. Note that in 1975, no federal or state court had decided anything about death and dying or clarified the rights of dying patients or their families.

Second, the physicians feared that if the Quinlans later changed their minds, they could sue for malpractice. One common definition of malpractice is "departure from normal standards of medical practice in a community" and in 1975—when almost all physicians felt it their duty to continue treatment until the very last moment of life—actively assisting in the death of a comatose patient would have been such a departure.

Paul Armstrong, a Legal Aid lawyer for indigent clients, represented Karen Quinlan and her parents. Armstrong was a young, inexperienced lawyer interested in big issues of constitutional law.

Dr. Morse testified that no medical precedent allowed him to disconnect Karen's respirator. The neurologist Julius Korein testified that he had seen about 50 patients in PVS and that all of them were better off than Karen; he described Karen as having no mental age at all and as being like "an anencephalic monster."[4] Famous neurologist Fred Plum confirmed Korein's diagnosis; Plum described Karen as "lying in bed, emaciated, curled up in what is known as flexion contracture.

Every joint was bent in a flexion position and making one tight sort of fetal position. It's too grotesque, really, to describe in human terms like fetal."[5]

The lower-court judge decided that Karen's respirator should not be disconnected because her wishes had never been written down, so Karen's true wishes were unknown. He further ruled that her parents' testimony about her wishes (substituted judgment) could not be taken as final if it entailed her death. He also ruled that the right to die could not be found in the U. S. Constitution.

Several weeks later, the New Jersey State Supreme Court heard the case on direct review. These justices expressed surprise when physicians distinguished between disconnecting a respirator and not starting it. Additionally, lawyers for the physicians argued that once a physician accepted a patient, an absolute duty to pursue the patient's welfare became "attached" to the physician, such that the physician could never pursue death.

In contrast, neurologist Julius Korein testified that physicians privately used "judicious neglect" in letting terminal patients die and that this was an unwritten standard of the time in medicine. The justices pressed the hospital's lawyers about the physician-patient relationship. Why couldn't Morse and Javed allow Karen to be transferred to another hospital, where other physicians could disconnect her? The lawyers for the hospital hemmed and hawed, but finally just said that St. Clare's thought it would be immoral to do so. The justices found all these lines of reasoning "rather flimsy."

The U.S. Supreme Court in 1965 had first recognized a right to privacy in *Griswold* v. *Connecticut,* when it found state laws unconstitutional that banned physicians from giving contraceptives to married couples. The *Griswold* court said for a state government to say women and couples couldn't use contraception to avoid having children violated the *fundamental liberty to lead one's personal life as one saw fit* that the Constitution assumed such liberty, and that such liberty made the lives of Americans the envy of people around the world.

This decision marked the start of a split in American life about the role of the federal government enforcing quasi-religious values in family and personal life that still continues today in divisions between "red" and "blue" states and in divisions in bioethics. Under the misleading phrase "family values," social conservatives attempted to block expansion of choice at the start of life about birth control pills, intrauterine devices (which block implantation of embryos), abortion, and in vitro fertilization. At the end of life, in both the Quinlan (1975) and Schiavo (2005) cases, they tried to block choices of spouses and parents about discontinuing treatment of incompetent patients.

In January 1976, after two months of deliberation, the New Jersey Supreme Court ruled unanimously in favor of the Quinlans. The Constitution's implied right to privacy (liberty) allowed the family of a dying incompetent patient to decide to let that patient die by disconnecting life-support. Because the Supreme Court of the United States had not yet made a comparable decision, New Jersey was thus the first to apply the right to privacy in a case of letting die. The New Jersey court also allowed Joseph Quinlan to become Karen's guardian, gave legal immunity to Morse and Javed for disconnecting Karen's life-support, and suggested (though it did not require) an advisory role for ethics committees in hospitals composed mostly of laypeople to help in future cases.

This last suggestion is interesting because the ensuing decades have seen a proliferation of hospital ethics committees (HECs). But the court may have been guilty of a fantasy here in thinking that such committees could help the legal system. For consider: how many laypeople in 1975 would have understood, before all the publicity, the real issues of the Quinlan case? Moreover, some of the real issues emerged only after the legal battle.

Pulling the Plug or Weaning from a Respirator?   In April 1976, four months after the higher-court decision, a respirator helped Karen Quinlan's body breathe. By then, decubitus ulcers had eaten through her flesh, exposing her hip bones. Why Karen was still alive at this point is one of the least understood and most interesting aspects of this case.

According to the Quinlans, Morse resisted implementing the decision of the New Jersey Supreme Court, because "this is something I will have to live with for the rest of my life."[6] The head nun was more blunt: "You have to understand our position, Mrs. Quinlan. In this hospital we don't kill people."[7] To this, Julia Quinlan replied, "Why didn't you tell me 10 months ago? I would have taken Karen out of this hospital immediately."

The administrators at St. Clare's were not alone in their position. Catholic hospitals saw the Quinlan decision as another step down a slippery slope that had started three years earlier with the American legalization of abortion in 1973. During the trial, the Vatican theologian Gino Concetti criticized the Quinlans: "A right to death does not exist. Love for life, even a life reduced to ruin, drives one to protect life with every possible care."[8] A pulmonary specialist at Catholic University in Rome said that removal of the respirator "would be an extremely dangerous move by her doctors, and represents an indirect form of euthanasia."[9]

Instead of simply disconnecting Karen's respirator, Morse and Javed weaned her from it. "Weaned" means they gradually trained the body off the machine by building up different muscles. The tired, confused Quinlans and their inexperienced lawyer did not understand what this meant, and the real implications would become painfully clear over the next 10 years. Eventually, Javed had Karen off the respirator for four hours; then, after intensive work over many weeks, for 12 hours. By late May of 1976, Karen was off the respirator altogether.

A more experienced lawyer would have obtained a *writ of habeus corpus* ("you should have the body"), which protects Americans from false imprisonment. This writ can be issued by a local judge and works quickly. If the Quinlans had gotten one, they could have transferred Karen to a hospital where she would have been quickly allowed to die.

This weaning confused the public: Some people took it to mean that Karen had gotten better; others, that Karen's physicians had "pulled the plug," but a miracle had prevented her death. Both impressions were false.

St. Clare's hospital now wanted Karen transferred and New Jersey's Medicaid office forced a nursing home to accept Karen in June 1976. At this point, Karen had been in PVS for 14 months.

After more than 10 years in this nursing home, Karen Quinlan's body expired in June 1986. For several months before that, Karen had had pneumonia, and the Quinlans had declined antibiotics to reverse it.

Substituted Judgment and Kinds of Cases.   The *Quinlan* decision ran two different kinds of cases together.[10] As noted, the Court based its decision partly on the right to privacy, a right that in medical contexts would presumably apply only to competent patients. But the standard of *substituted judgment* also grounded *Quinlan*, according to which relatives or friends could substitute their judgment for that of an incompetent patient.

Consequently, this decision had at least two major problems. First, how did a family's right to exercise substituted judgment derive from *Griswold*? Critics felt that the New Jersey court had jumped too quickly from married people's right to control their own reproduction (the situation in *Griswold*) to parents' right to let an adult, comatose incompetent child die—especially because no intervening decisions had been made about whether competent adults had a right to hasten their own death by refusing medical treatment. Given that quick, big jump, critics wondered what was next. Giving parents the right to make life-or-death decisions for never-competent patients? For retarded babies?

Second, substituted judgment is a notoriously subjective criterion.[11] It presumes that decisions made by a patient's family will reflect what the patient herself would have wanted done. In the Quinlan case, like the later Cruzan and Schiavo cases, it was unclear whether these women had really expressed a wish not to have their lives prolonged or whether the families just wished it so.

Finally, the right to privacy most obviously applies to competent patients and their rights to determine their own medical destinies. Ideally, our courts would have first laid out that right and then tackled incompetent patients. But life is messy and things didn't happen that way, so the *Quinlan* decision tackled incompetent patients first. It took 15 more years before things were straightened out, when the U. S. Supreme Court finally decided the Cruzan case.

THE CRUZAN CASE

The Cruzan case led to a landmark decision by the United States Supreme Court in June 1990.[12] Before this decision, 20 states had recognized the right of competent patients to refuse medical life-support, and all these states (with the exception of New York and Missouri) had recognized the right of surrogates to make decisions for incompetent patients.[13] The *Cruzan* decision first explicitly recognized the rights of competent dying patients.

On January 11, 1983, 24-year-old Nancy Cruzan lost control of her car at night on a lonely, icy country road in Missouri.[14] Thrown 35 feet from the car, she landed face down in a water-filled ditch. Paramedics arriving on the scene found that her heart had stopped. Injecting a stimulant into her heart, they restarted it, but because her brain had been anoxic for 15 minutes, Nancy did not regain consciousness.[15]

For seven years, Nancy remained in this state. Over time, her body became rigid, her hands curled tightly, and her fingernails became claw-like. Like Karen Quinlan, Nancy could take nothing by mouth and somebody turned her every two hours to prevent ulcers. She drooled much of the time, causing her hair, pillow and sheets to be wet. Her care cost the state of Missouri $130,000 a year.

Where the Quinlan case focused on withdrawal of a respirator, the Cruzan case, like the Schiavo case 15 years later, focused on withdrawal of a feeding tube. Because she could not swallow, Nancy could not be fed by mouth. Loss of ability to swallow signals a key decision in the care of incapacitated patients, especially those with dementia or neurological diseases. Before feeding tubes began to be used in the 1960s, the natural course for such patients was death by starvation. With a feeding tube, this natural deterioration of the body can be put on hold for years, even decades.

Legally or morally, is a PVS patient owed food and water forever? Karen Quinlan's parents thought so; they never withdrew the nutrition that kept her body alive. Nancy's parents, Joe and Joyce Cruzan, thought otherwise: they sought permission in court to disconnect her feeding tube.

In discussing the Cruzan case, it is necessary to understand standards of legal evidence. The minimum standard is *preponderance of evidence*; a more rigorous standard is *clear and convincing evidence;* the most rigorous standard—the standard used for serious felonies—is *beyond a reasonable doubt.*

Preponderance of evidence simply means that there is more evidence one way than the other; in some cases, this simply means there is some evidence rather than none. *Clear and convincing* denotes more rigorous evidence and with dying, it requires an advanced directive (living will) or durable power of attorney. Finally, *beyond a reasonable doubt* requires the most evidence and, of course, is used in trials of homicide to establish guilt and where the accused is presumed innocent.

The Cruzans won their case in probate court; but upon direct review, the Missouri Supreme Court reversed the decision, and this reversal had to do with the standard of clear and convincing evidence. Because Nancy had no advanced directive and because only her parents and a sister testified about her alleged wishes, the Cruzans did not produce enough evidence to be "clear and convincing" about Nancy's true wishes. In particular, Joe Cruzan emphasized that Nancy was a fighter and strong-willed, and therefore wanted to die, but it was hard for the Justices to see why Nancy's strong will wouldn't make her want to fight to return to life.

The Missouri Supreme Court concluded that the state had an interest in preserving life, regardless of quality of life, and no matter how strongly the family felt otherwise, that before medical support could be withdrawn from an incompetent patient, its standard of clear and convincing evidence had to be met. Missouri felt it had a duty to protect an incompetent adult child against parents who might be merely seeking financial and emotional closure.

In reviewing this Missouri decision, the United States Supreme Court did much more than adjudicate this particular case. Indeed, it made three very important declarations.

First, and most important, it recognized a right of *competent* patients to decline medical treatment, even if such refusal led directly to their death. The Supreme Court decided in *Cruzan* for the first time that the Constitution gave competent Americans freedom to refuse unwanted medical support.

Second, the Supreme Court found that withdrawing a feeding tube did not differ from withdrawing any other kind of life-sustaining medical support. Some state laws, which permitted forgoing or withdrawing respirators but not artificial nutrition, were hence unconstitutional.

Third, with regard to *incompetent* patients, the Supreme Court held in Cruzan that a state *could, but need not,* pass a statute requiring the clear and convincing standard of evidence about what a formerly competent patient would have wanted done. Because Missouri had such a standard, its law was constitutional. Because the Cruzan family had not met that standard, Nancy's feeding tube could not be removed.

Cruzan said nothing about never-competent patients, such as people with profound mental retardation. Because of past abuses, it is reasonable to expect that in these cases only state laws with the most rigorous standards of proof would pass the Supreme Court's review. For such cases, the Supreme Court will probably require the standard of beyond a reasonable doubt.

Reactions to the Supreme Court *Cruzan* decision ran along two lines: legal commentators welcomed it; medical commentators hated it.

Most legal scholars supported the new conservative position of the Rehnquist Court on its role with regard to the Constitution. The proper function of the Supreme Court, according to the law professor Charles Baron, was not as a super legislature over the states or even to promulgate uniform rules of state law. Instead, the U.S. Supreme Court should only strike down state laws that conflict with either federal law or the U.S. Constitution.[16] So not every bad or undesirable state law is unconstitutional.

Texas law professor John Robertson went so far as to say that Nancy Cruzan could not be harmed and hence had no interests in the case. He argued that the real claim in *Cruzan* had nothing to do with Nancy Cruzan's right to die or her right to privacy (her liberty interests); instead, the case was about the Cruzan family's right to be free of the emotional burden of maintaining her body in a state institution.[17]

Both Baron and Robertson agreed that the previous legal standard of *substituted judgment* was a mockery "[leading] us to pretend that we are merely complying (however reluctantly) with the wishes of the patient. The result in most states is mere lip service to substituted judgment. Almost any evidence is deemed sufficient to establish a preference for death over PVS and/or families are empowered to express patient preferences for death—with few questions asked."

In contrast, another standard used in such cases was that of *best interests of* the patient. So in the Cruzan case, would the best interests of Nancy be to live on in such a state and subject her family to such a burden? Most people would say no, although this judgment is not open-and-shut since the State of Missouri argued that Nancy's best interests entailed continued feeding.

A different kind of reaction came from physicians who worked with families of vegetative patients. Neurologist and bioethicist Ronald Cranford of Minnesota, who would later testify in the Schiavo case, predicted that "many families will experience the utter helplessness of the Cruzans." Allowing the standard of clear-and-convincing evidence would "place an enormous burden on society, which will spend hundreds of millions of dollars each year for a condition that no one in their right mind would ever want to be in."[18]

Hospice physician Joanne Lynn emphasized that in Missouri and New York, "the suffering of the patient and family, the costs, the kind of life that can be gained, are all to count for nothing. If life can be prolonged, then it will have to be."[19]

Nancy had been divorced just before her accident, and many of her friends knew her only by her married name, Nancy Davis. When her case first became widely known, her friends had not realized who she was. After the major decision, the case was reheard in a lower court and Nancy's old friends testified. In that hearing, the lower court decided that Nancy Cruzan's parents had met the clear-and-convincing standard.[20] So five months after the Supreme Court decided *Cruzan*, on December 14, 1990, physicians legally removed Nancy Cruzan's feeding tube, and her body died.

THE HUGH FINN CASE

Controversy erupted in 1998 when the Republican governor of Virginia disputed a wife's right to remove the feeding tube of her husband, Hugh Finn, who had been in PVS for three years.[21] Hugh Finn, a former television anchorman in Louisville, Kentucky, had prepared a document stating that he would not want to live in a persistent vegetative state sustained by a feeding tube. Unfortunately, before he could sign it, a terrible automobile accident severed his aorta and left his brain anoxic for many minutes. His resulting coma left him unable to eat, care for himself, or communicate.

Or so it seemed, until a nurse claimed that, when she smoothed his hair, he had said "Hi" to her. So Hugh's brother, John, challenged a request by Hugh's wife, Michelle, to remove Hugh's feeding tube. Hugh's parents joined John in the suit. They lost in court, but Governor James Gilmore asked the Virginia Supreme Court to continue Finn's feeding tube. Gilmore stated that its removal would be "mercy killing or euthanasia." The high court disagreed, deciding that removal would merely "permit the natural process of dying" and would not be euthanasia.

Hugh Finn's body died shortly thereafter, but Governor Gilmore had set a precedent for escalating a private family dispute about a dying patient into a sensationalized, national debate. Seven years later, Governor Jeb Bush in Florida escalated another such dispute to a much bigger national debate.

THE TERRI SCHIAVO CASE

During the months of 1990 when the U. S. Supreme Court was deciding its *Cruzan* decision, an even bigger coma case was beginning. On February 25, 1990, Terri Schiavo, a 27-year-old, anorexic Caucasian woman went into a coma because of anoxia, a lack of oxygen to her brain, perhaps from a heart arrhythmia caused by extreme hypoalkemia (an imbalance of potassium in her body), causing severe hypoxic ischemic encephalopathy (brain damage).[22]

There is evidence that Terri Schiavo suffered from anorexia before her heart attack. People with such eating disorders may suffer from an imbalance of potassium. According to documents filed in her malpractice suit, a three-stage imbalance of potassium led to Terri's heart attack, which led to anoxia and subsequent brain damage.

Many diets today contain too little potassium; the average American woman consumes less than half of the 4700 milligrams a day considered to be adequate.[23]

Among other medical conditions, chronic lack of potassium can cause heart attacks and strokes. Moreover, blood tests for potassium can be normal even when real symptoms occur from chronic potassium insufficiency. As a result, physicians often fail to diagnose a chronic lack of potassium.

To keep her alive, physicians inserted a PEG (percutaneous endoscopic gastronomy) feeding tube. When a patient lacks the reflex to swallow, a PEG tube is placed through the abdominal wall into the stomach, allowing a nutritious, slushy mixture to feed the patient. PEG tubes are sometimes inserted to buy time after an emergency, with the implicit understanding that they may be temporary and may be removed later.

Once attached, feeding tubes can be emotionally difficult for people to remove. Years later, removal of the feeding tube became the central issue of this case.

Two months later in April, her husband Michael transferred Terri from the hospital to a rehabilitation center. In May, and with no objection from her parents, Robert and Mary Schindler, he became her legal guardian. Later, her parents took her to their home to care for her, but were overwhelmed by the task and returned her to the center. Later, Michael flew Terri to California for a two-month experiment with a "thalamic stimulator implant" in her brain. Later, at the Mediplex Rehabilitation Center in Brandon, Florida, and for months 13–18 into her coma, three shifts of workers worked 24 hours a day trying to rehabilitate Terri.

In July 1991, Terri went to Sable Palms, a skilled care facility, where neurologists continued to test her and where speech, occupational, and physical therapists worked on her for another three years, from 1991 to 1994.

Michael Schiavo and Terri's parents stopped living together in May 1992. That August, Michael received a settlement from the malpractice case against Terri's obstetrician for failing to diagnose her potassium imbalance. He got $750,000 from the hospital for a trust fund specifically for Terri's care and $300,000 for loss of her companionship.

The three adults fought over this money. Michael owed the Schindlers $10,000 and the Schindlers believed they were entitled to part of the $300,000 for loss of spousal companionship. After the dispute, their relationship soured.

Based on what several physicians told Michael, at this point Terri had no chance of meaningful recovery. Michael agreed to a "Do Not Resuscitate" order for Terri, but her parents violently disagreed and he later rescinded the order.

The Schindlers then tried to remove Michael as Terri's guardian, but a court-appointed special guardian investigated and determined that Michael had acted appropriately toward Terri, which the court accepted.

Four years passed, during which Terri's condition did not improve. During this time, and in order to help care for Terri, Michael became certified as a licensed respiratory therapist.[24]

In May 1998, eight years after Terri's heart attack, Michael asked a court to allow removal of the PEG tube so that Terri could die. Michael testified that, while watching television many years before, Terri had once remarked that she wouldn't want to live in a vegetative state. The Schindlers responded that their daughter wanted to live and that they didn't want the money for themselves but to be set aside for Terri's care.

Nearly two years after Michael Schiavo's request to have Terri's feeding tube removed, Judge George Greer in 2000 approved the request. He ruled that clear and convincing evidence existed that Terri would not have chosen to live under such circumstances. Legally, this ruling lacked support, because Terri's parents disputed this claim and because she had no living will.

The Schindlers appealed, which took a year, but they lost. They appealed again, this time to the Florida Supreme Court, which in April 2001 denied their appeal.

Over the next few years, the Schindlers began to allege that Michael caused Terri's condition, perhaps because of domestic abuse. An autopsy after her death proved that no such abuse occurred. Moreover, if Terri had arrived at an emergency room with this kind of trauma, surely Michael would have been reported (as required by law) to authorities for domestic violence, battery, or possible manslaughter. Nor, if such evidence existed, would the hospital and its physicians have settled a malpractice case or allowed Michael to become Terri's guardian.

The Schindlers also testified that, even if she had asked them to do so, they would not remove Terri's feeding tube under any circumstances. They said that even if she developed gangrene and all her limbs had to be amputated, they would still keep her alive.[25]

A year later in the fall of 2003, having exhausted all appeals in Florida, the Schindlers appealed in federal court to prevent removal of Terri's feeding tube. The Schindlers appealed to the public through the media, and several physicians publicly joined their side, including a pathologist and a physician who hoped to try exotic "coma stimulation" therapies.

Lawyers for Florida Governor Jeb Bush, a Catholic, filed a brief on the side of the Schindlers; Governor Jeb Bush praised the parents in the media for defending their daughter's right to life. President George W. Bush praised his brother's stand. The Advocacy Center for Persons with Disabilities filed a lawsuit claiming that removal of Terri's PEG tube would abuse a person with disabilities. The anti-abortion group, Life Legal Defense Fund, helped the Schindlers hire lawyers, eventually paying bills of $300,000.

Three neurologists, including distinguished neurologist Ronald Cranford, testified that Terri was in PVS (Cranford substituted "permanent" for "persistent" to emphasize the irreversibility of her condition). The Schindlers cited Terri's ability to swallow saliva as evidence that she was not in PVS; Cranford rebutted and testified that such swallowing was controlled by primitive functions of her brain stem.

Dr. William Mayfield, a pioneer in the field of medical radiology and a founder of the American College of Hyperbaric Medicine, testified that he believed that hyperbaric oxygenation therapy (HBOT) would benefit Terri. Neurologist Ronald Cranford retorted, "Increase the blood flood to dead tissue, and what do you get? Dead tissue."[26]

Physician William Hammesfahr, a champion of HBOT, testified for the Schindlers that Terri was not in PVS and would respond well to hyperbaric treatments, which were then his primary business. Hammesfahr, who seemed eager to appear on television, presented himself as an unappreciated genius, like Semmelweis, who was far ahead of the medical community and, hence, a pariah.[27]

The three neurologists found Hammesfahr unprofessional and noted that he required cash in advance for his hyperbaric treatments and had published no articles documenting the amazing successes he claimed from using his hyperbaric chambers.

Mayfield and Hammersfahr represented extreme, marginal positions in the medical community. The overwhelming medical consensus was that Terri had died long ago, that she had no chance of returning to any normal conscious state, and that dragging on the controversy was two steps backwards from the Cruzan case in moving towards an enlightened national policy about ending care for comatose patients.

At the last moment, a neurologist affiliated with the Mayo Clinic in Jacksonville, Florida, William Cheshire, visited Terri in her room and opined that Schiavo "may" have been in a minimally conscious state, although he did not extensively examine her.[28] Cheshire was director of Center for Bioethics and Human Dignity, a web-based bioethics center and passionate critic of assisted suicide.[29]

Another disagreement among these physicians concerned what Terri's movements meant. Ability to respond to a squeeze or pinch is consistent with PVS. In the Cruzan case, when neurologist Cranford examined Nancy, her lawyer William Colby described what happened:

> Cranford next grabbed hold of Nancy's stiff right leg and tried to bend it straight. Nancy grimaced. Then he reached for the soft skin on the inside of the upper part of her right arm, and held the pinch. Slowly, as if she were a robot, Nancy's head lifted off the bed and turned. Her face locked on her father's for about ten seconds, before she lowered just as slowly to the pillow.[30]

Despite being there and witnessing this phenomenon in this case, Dr. Cranford insisted that Nancy Cruzan's biography was over, that no one was conscious within the reflexes of her body, and that further treatment was futile.

In the fall of 2003, the Florida legislature passed a special bill, *Terri's Law*, that allowed the Governor to issue a one-time stay of a judge's order to remove a feeding tube in certain cases where a patient is in PVS. After its passage, Governor Bush immediately issued such a stay.

Michael and the American Civil Liberties Union appealed in state court and won, but Governor Bush appealed to a mid-level appellate court, lost, and appealed again to the Florida Supreme Court.

On September 23, 2004, Florida's Supreme Court ruled 7-0 that Terri's Law was unconstitutional. It based its decision upon two constitutional canons: the separation of powers and the unlawful delegation of authority. "It is without question an invasion of the authority of the judicial branch for the Legislature to pass a law that allows the executive branch to interfere with the final judicial determination in a case," wrote Chief Justice Barbara Pariente.[31]

About two months later, the top U. S. court let stand without comment the decision by the Florida Supreme Court against Terri's law.[32] Activists predicted Terri's imminent "brutal murder" and claimed (based on watching the widely seen videotape aired constantly on television) that she was a "purposefully interactive, alert, curious, lovely young woman who lives with a very serious disability."[33]

At the end of February 2005, 15 years after the case began, the Schindlers filed a variety of desperate motions in Judge Greer's court. Judge Greer ordered the feeding tube removed. The Schindlers appealed, but a Florida appellate court again rebuffed them.

Extraordinary events, of a kind never before seen in the history of modern bioethics, then ensued. As the Schlinders lost in court, they became desperate; they turned to the media for their cause, enlisting their other son and daughter to go on television. Catholic priests dressed in robes of monastic orders appeared with them. Anti-abortion activist Randall Terry showed up. People flooded Florida legislators with email and phone calls.

Activists and the Schlinders then turned to the U. S. Congress. First, House leaders tried to compel Terri to appear before a House committee as a witness, and fall under protection of the federal program that protects such witnesses. Judge Greer ignored this subpoena.

So activists next turned to Congressional leaders and President Bush. House Speaker Tom DeLay faced an ethics scandal and indictments in his home state of Texas for getting money in illegal ways, exactly the kind of scandal that had forced previous speaker Jim Wright out of Congress in 1989. (DeLay also failed to reveal that his family had agreed to remove a respirator from his father, who had been badly injured in an accident in 1988 at his Texas home.)[34]

In the Senate, Senator Bill Frist, the physician, may have planned to run for President in 2008 and may have wanted to align himself with the same culture-of-life constituency that had helped George W. Bush narrowly win. So the two of them worked to have Congress pass a federal version of Terri's Law, which they did, having President Bush fly back during a Congressional recess and sign a bill passed at midnight by a vote of 203 to 58.[35]

Some critics said that Senator Frist crossed a dangerous ethical line and committed virtual malpractice by declaring—merely by watching the edited video clip and never actually visiting or examining Terri—that Terri "did not seem to be" in a persistent vegetative state. As one critic fumed, "It's quackery. It'd be hilarious if it weren't so grotesque, how his presidential ambition and pandering to the right wing is clashing with his life's work."[36] Congressman Dave Weldon, a physician and also a pro-life Republican, agreed with Frist. So these high-ranking politician-physicians publicly contradicted the neurologists who had actually examined Terri.

Congressmen Frist and Weldon had one problem here: the federal government cannot order a physician to insert a feeding tube. The only thing it could do is order a federal judge to review the case again, which was done. The federal judge, James Whittemore, reviewed the whole case over two days and concluded, like two dozen appellate judges before him, that nothing was amiss, that Terri had no chance of recovery, that Michael was properly motivated, and that previous courts had made no errors. An appeal to the U. S. Court of Appeals for the 11th Circuit in Atlanta, a conservative group, produced the same conclusions.

During March 2005, media exposure escalated, producing what *Newsweek* later called "a public spectacle airing nonstop on cable and playing on front pages around the world."[37] Terri's supporters traveled to Pinellas Park, Florida, to hold prayer vigils, while others threatened to kill Michael and his lawyer, George Felos.

Various members and friends of both sides went on cable television shows and endlessly discussed the family's problems.

A juggernaut for Terri ensued: soon, four Schindlers, plus recovered coma patients, some physicians, activist monks, Patrick Mahoney, director of the Christian Defense Coalition, and anti-abortion activist Randal Terry all campaigned on television, radio, and the Internet against Michael Schiavo, who was media shy and only had his brother, Scott, and lawyer George Felos to help him.

The tactics in this case showed contempt for the truth and a willingness to say anything, do anything, to win. No matter what the facts, or the law, the attitude was: "Do what it takes to win." So Barbara Weller, an attorney working for the Schindlers said that she herself had seen Terri trying to talk, and thus went from a lawyer to a witness. Protestors called Judge Greer a "judicial murderer" and Republicans blasted the "imperial judiciary." The Reverend James Kennedy urged Governor Jeb Bush to ignore the federal judges the way Alabama's Governor George Wallace did in defying federal orders to integrate.[38] Soon after, the FBI arrested a man offering $250,000 to kill Michael Schiavo and $50,000 to do the same to Judge Greer. Another two people were arrested trying to break into the hospice.

For example, Terri was said to be "suffering terribly" by starving, even though physicians in palliative care repeatedly denied first, that when feeding tubes are removed, terminal patients suffer, and second, that in this case, any person still existed to suffer.[39]

The case again showed the limitations of the media, of television, of Internet and radio, because what made great visuals (people praying and screaming outside Terri's hospice), what made great drama (the Schlinders crying on television), and what made great tension (various people claiming that Michael was evil), distorted facts of the case. What had been a private family dispute suddenly became the War of Saints against Evil.

On March 18, the last appeal failed to the U.S. Supreme Court (which had already twice refused to review the case) and Terri's feeding tube was removed for the last time. Palliative care physicians predicted it would take about two weeks for Terri to die and emphasized that, in terminal patients such as Terri, it would not be painful. Opponents outside decried "murder by starvation." After 13 days, while protestors prayed and rallied outside, Terri's body expired, on March 31, 2005. An autopsy, ordered by Michael, showed she had not been abused.

What Schiavo's Autopsy Showed

Chief Medical Examiner for Pinellas County, Florida, Jon Thogmartin, MD, released Terri's autopsy on June 13, 2005. It answered some questions and left others as mysteries.

First, he cleared up the mysterious bone scan of 1991 introduced by the Schindlers in 1992 with the claim that Terri's coma had been caused by trauma, possibly by Michael. Here is what happened: when Mediplex admitted Terri in early 1991, her physicians there ordered a bone scan to rule out degenerative changes in her bones. The bone scan was done at nearby Manatee Memorial Hospital. There, the bone scan form *erroneously* listed Terri Schiavo as a case of "closed head injury" and said "the patient has a history of trauma." Thogmartin writes, "It appears that with little or no knowledge of the admitting diagnosis or clinical situation of Mrs. Schiavo, Manatee Memorial staff and radiologists completed the report.[40]

The coroner writes that it is true that the bone scan showed a compression fracture of the spine, but it was *due to osteoporosis,* a common condition in paralyzed patients. Moreover,

> In summary, any rib fractures, leg fractures, skull fractures or spine fractures that occurred concurrent with Mrs. Schiavo's original collapse would almost certainly have been diagnosed in February, 1990, especially with the number of physical exams, radiographs, and other evaluations she received in the early evolution of her care at Humana Hospital-Northside. During her initial hospitalization, she received twenty-three chest radiographs, three brain CT scans, two abdominal radiographs, two echocardiograms, one abdominal ultrasound, one cervical spine radiograph, and one radiograph of her right knee. No fractures or trauma were reported or recorded. . . . By far the most likely explanation for the bone scan findings in Mrs. Schiavo are prolonged immobility induced osteoporosis and complicating H.O. [hypertopic ossification[41]] in an environment of intense physical therapy.[42]

In sum, there was no evidence of trauma or abuse by anyone. Michael was wrongly accused of killing Terri. Everyone misunderstood what the 1991 bone scan revealed and how it had originally been mistakenly labeled.

The big surprise of the autopsy was that "Mrs. Schiavo's heart was anatomically normal without any areas of recent or remote myocardial infarction. Her heart (including the cardiac valves, conduction system and myocardium) was essentially unremarkable. . . ." That was a big surprise because, although the cause of her heart attack was debatable, few of Michael's supporters doubted that she had had one.

We cannot prove that either trauma or a heart attack caused Terri's coma. Probably, we will never know exactly what happened to her. Two crucial pieces of evidence are that she may have consumed as much as one gram of caffeine a day and that she had hypoalkemia. Perhaps this combination, after the extreme weight loss, stressed her heart too much that night.

According to reports filed by paramedics or police the night of her original collapse, no other drugs were found in her system.

Another surprise was that the autopsy showed no clinical evidence of bulimia, especially the kind of wear on the enamel of the back teeth that is often caused by this condition. Despite the fact that the malpractice suit was settled on the assertion that Terri had an undiagnosed eating disorder, the coroner's report showed no evidence of this disorder.

However, it still could be true that 15 years before, she was anorexic. Certainly her low potassium level, and the fact that her weight dropped in a few months over 100 pounds, combined with her drinking large amounts of iced tea, are evidence for this hypothesis.

The autopsy also revealed that Terri Schiavo was not in a minimally conscious state. In fact, she had massive brain damage. "Mrs. Schiavo's brain showed global anoxic-ischemic encephalopathy resulting in massive cerebral atrophy. Her brain weight was approximately half of the expected weight. Of particular importance was the hypoxic damage and neuronal loss in her occipital lobes, which indicates cortical blindness. Her remaining brain regions show severe hypoxic injury and neuronal atrophy/loss. No areas of recent or remote traumatic injury were found."[43]

Finally, without the PEG feeding tube, she would have died. "Oral feedings in quantities sufficient to sustain life would have certainly resulted in aspiration." Aspiration of food in such patients is a serious, even lethal, complication, causing infection, choking, and possible suffocation.

ETHICAL ISSUES

Standards of Brain Death

People have always feared that they might be declared dead prematurely and buried alive. In the eighteenth century, gruesome stories circulated about exhumations that found frantic scratches on the inside lids of coffins. In the nineteenth century, some legislatures required a delay before burial, and in 1882 an undertaker named Kirchbaum attached periscopes to coffins so that a person who woke up after being buried might signal for help.[44] Many people were buried with cowbells which they could ring if they awakened underground.

This whole-body standard became inappropriate when respirators allowed respiration of brain-damaged patients. Before them, heart-lung machines could maintain immobilized patients. As early as 1967, when surgeon Christiaan Barnard transplanted Denise Darvall's heart into a dying patient named Louis Washkansky (discussed in a later chapter), the question arose whether Denise Darvall had really been dead before her heart was removed. She obviously hadn't been declared dead by the whole-body standard since her healthy heart was exactly what was wanted for transplantation. Medicine needed a new standard of death, specifically of *brain death,* to determine when organs could be removed from a still-living body.

Although first described in the medical literature in 1959, brain death did not really become operational until Barnard transplanted a heart in late 1967.[45]

Shortly after that event, an ad hoc committee at Harvard Medical School developed the Harvard criteria of brain death.[46] The Harvard criteria operationally defined brain death as behavior that indicated unawareness of external stimuli, lack of bodily movements, no spontaneous breathing, lack of reflexes, and two isoelectric (nearly flat) electroencephalogram (EEG) readings 24 hours apart. These criteria required loss of virtually all brain activity (including the brain stem, and hence breathing).

The Harvard criteria embody caution: no one declared dead by these criteria has ever regained consciousness. (One could truly say, "If you're Harvard dead, you're really dead.") The extreme conservatism of the Harvard standard disappoints people waiting for organ transplants from donors: during the last 25 years, the standard has covered relatively few patients.

Another standard of brain death is the *cognitive criterion.* This criterion identifies a philosophical core of properties of persons and assumes that without such a core, a human body is no longer a person; the core properties commonly include reason, memory, agency, and self-awareness. For example, neurological disorders such as Alzheimer's or Lewy body disease destroy brain cells at a high rate, so that over a decade, none of the higher person remains.

The cognitive criterion has the greatest potential to generate organs for transplantation. So far, however, this criterion has been too controversial and too vague to be adopted by any state, although countless families in fact act on it when they use it to agree to reduce treatment to speed a patient's death.[47]

A third standard of brain death, the *irreversibility standard*, falls between the Harvard and cognitive criteria. According to this standard, death occurs simply when unconsciousness is irreversible. Operationally, this judgment would be made by a neurologist and by another physician. The irreversibility standard would allow PVS patients to be declared dead after several years (perhaps, in some cases of anoxia, after several months). At the time of the first heart transplant in 1968, this standard was thought to be too broad.

In popular culture, some people believe that a uniform, metaphysical event with physical manifestations, and perhaps as the counterpart of a similar event at the beginning of life, marks death. Some people would have described these metaphysical events as the entrance and departure of a soul. The occurrence of such metaphysical events of course cannot be proven, and even if they do occur, they seem to have no physical manifestations. In medical reality, the definition of death is not so much a discovery as a decision that families and their physicians make. It is not an event, but a process.[48]

As it turns out, the phrase "brain death" misleads us in many ways. Newspapers commonly refer to someone as being "brain dead" for months until "life-support" is removed, after which the patient is said to "expire." Reformers such as North Carolina medical ethicist Lance Stell believe that such terms incorrectly imply that a patient could be dead in two different ways and that there are degrees of being dead. Such equivocation creates confusion about the epistemological criteria for declaring death, and implies that someone might die more than once. Stell thinks a more accurate phrase would be "death by neurological criteria." A being that meets these criteria, he says, "is not a patient but a cadaver."[49]

Proposals to redefine brain death create controversy. On the one hand, reformers want to end public uncertainty over brain death, expand the number of organs available for transplantation, save the medical system money by not maintaining comatose patients, and help families move on after the death of a relative by having a universally accepted, practical definition of brain death. On the other hand, advocates for vulnerable patients want to give them every chance of recovery.

CHANCES OF AWAKENING FROM PVS

Although most patients who have been in PVS for over a year never wake up, on rare occasions, some do. In one well-known study, 7 of 434 adults with traumatic head injuries who were in PVS for more than a year made good recoveries and regained consciousness, some with normal quality of life.[50] These seven recoveries warn against any quick judgment that a patient's condition is irreversible.

Should PVS befall some people, they would want to be given this 7/434ths chance of recovery. Several other studies have shown that, although few patients ever emerge from PVS, some people do within the first year, and once in a thousand times, after three years.[51]

No case exists of anyone emerging from PVS of four years' duration. In Terri Schiavo's case at the end, when activists shouted the contrary at cameras, she had been in PVS for *15 years,* and hence, according to clinical evidence, had no chance of returning to normal consciousness. Physicians who have seen her CT scan said that her brain, instead of being filled with normal brain tissue, then only contained cerebrospinal fluid, an indication of gross neurological damage and vegetative status.[52]

Terri's electroencephalogram (EEG) was flat and her CT scan showed severe atrophy in her cerebral hemispheres. Schindler-friendly physicians suggested vasodilators, but the autopsy showed what professional neurologists had said: nothing would have helped her regain consciousness.

In a more recent study of 19 patients with severe head injuries and persisting post-traumatic unawareness, 58 percent (11 patients) recovered within the first year and 5 percent (1 patient) within the second.[53] In another study of 34 patients with anoxic coma, 2 patients with "malignant EEG's" (the worst classification, where patients were expected to die based on lack of brain-wave activity), eventually made a "good recovery."[54]

Whether anoxia or trauma caused the coma changes the prognosis. More patients seem to emerge, especially in the first few months, after coma caused by trauma than by anoxia. "It's the difference between taking a blow to the brain, which affects a local area—and taking this global, whole-brain hit," asserted New York bioethicist Joseph Fins in explaining the difference.[55] Anoxia probably caused Terri's coma.

Whether or not Terri was really in PVS was very crucial in this case, because several cases have been documented over the last decades where patients have emerged from some kind of deep coma of many years. In other words, patients have on rare occasion emerged out of comas that were not as severe as PVS. Moreover, the rare recovery in PVS warns against any quick judgment that a patient's condition is "irreversible."

Consider four surprising cases of long-term coma. First, after an automobile wreck in Arkansas, Terry Wallis emerged from a coma of exactly *19 years,* and continues to improve three years later."[56] Second, in 1996, ex-police officer Gary Dockery of Tennessee emerged out of his coma of *eight years* to talk for a few hours to his family, after which he lapsed back into a coma and died a year later in April.[57] Third, Patricia White Bull became comatose while giving birth to her fourth child and could not speak, swallow, or move much, but suddenly awoke *16 years later* to full consciousness on Christmas Eve, 1999. Fourth, Sarah Scantlin of Kansas went into a coma after a car accident and emerged *19 years later.*[58] (Note: most of these cases of recovery seem to have been caused by trauma, not anoxia.)

Ethically, the fact that anyone at all comes out of a long-term coma is crucial because it changes the prognosis from a certainty to a probability. Families who want emotional closure on a case prefer to hear physicians say that the patient has "no" chance of recovery. The emotional weight changes when a patient has a "tiny" chance of recovery rather than "no" chance.

A review of these cases reveals an interesting conceptual disagreement among neurologists. Some claim that any patient who emerges from PVS was not really in PVS. But this is a non-falsifiable, circular argument: if you awaken, you weren't in PVS. If you never awaken, you were in PVS.

A NEW CATEGORY OF CONSCIOUSNESS?

The question whether the movements of PVS patients are intentional behavior or merely reflexes raises philosophical as well as medical issues. *Intentional* behavior indicates an organism seeking some goal, such as freedom from pain, and might indicate awareness. As the seventeenth-century philosopher Rene Descartes noted, consciousness (awareness) in others is always an inference from outward behavior; it cannot be directly observed. Unconsciousness, or lack of consciousness, is also an inference. If we claim—as some people do—that flies aren't conscious, this is an inference from flies' behavior and from the comparative anatomy of flies and humans. As far as flies are concerned, we can make such inferences easily. In the case of a human being, however, a lot is at stake if we are wrong.

Although a few neurologists believe that PVS patients experience pain, most do not. In the similar case of Paul Brophy in 1986, the American Academy of Neurology wrote:

> No conscious experience of pain and suffering is possible without the integrated functioning of the brain stem and cerebral cortex. Pain and suffering are attributes of consciousness, and PVS patients like Brophy do not experience them. Noxious stimuli may activate peripherally located nerves, but only a brain with the capacity for consciousness can transfer that neural activity into an experience.[59]

According to the Multi-Society Task Force on PVS, scanning devices show that brain activity of PVS patients falls far below that of patients with locked-in syndrome, and extensive neurological examinations of PVS patients during autopsies reveals deep lesions incompatible with awareness.[60]

Some New York neurologists have recently proposed a new category of *minimally conscious state* (MCS) for patients in long-term coma-like states, a new category between the only two previous ways of classifying them as either *comatose* or *vegetative*.[61] Neurologists Nicholas Schiff, Joy Hirsch, and Joseph Giacino, along with seven other co-authors, proposed this new category after working with brain-damaged patients at several facilities around New York City.[62]

Through an intense program of stimulation, they enabled one or two patients to return to MCS. Using scans of blood flow to the brain, they identified dozens of patients with this potential, and one or two were able to remarkably improve.

Controversy surrounds these claims. Alan Shewmon, a famous pediatric neurologist, calls the new category "an inaccurate name for an invalid concept." Shewmon argues that there is no scientific or philosophical way to distinguish between minimal consciousness and full consciousness, implying that consciousness is something one either has or does not have, like saying you can't be a little bit pregnant.

But maybe that's the wrong analogy. Why can't a light bulb be, not on or off, but bright or dim? Why can't consciousness be a gradient? Terri's defenders retort that people are minimally conscious all the time—in sleep, or after injury—and what is important is the potential for recovery of consciousness. If it's impossible to prove any difference between minimal consciousness and consciousness, it also must be impossible to *disprove* a difference. So if Terri was in MCS, she might at times feel something. After all, the brain does not get injured in neat taxonomic lines.

The potential for recovery of such a patient is probably best when maximal efforts are made *in the first few months* after injury. This potential diminishes as the years increase. At the beginning, physicians should always act as if the brain-damaged person is minimally conscious, but after many years (15 years for Terri), chances of recovery approach zero.

Dartmouth neurologist James Bernat agreed, but understood why laypeople rallied behind Terri. "Just looking at a videotape of someone propped up in bed, with their eyes blinking and so on, it looks like they're aware," he said.[63] They are awake, he said, but not aware. With an intact brain stem, their eyes can still follow things, but only slightly to the left or right. For a diagnosis of persistent vegetative state, "there really has to be zero evidence of any responsiveness that suggests awareness."

But the videotape trumped professional opinion in neurology, even among physician-politicians. So Tom Coburn, a physician and U.S. Senator from Oklahoma said of Terri," All you have to do is look at her on TV. Any doctor with any conscience can look at her and know that she does not have a terminal disease and know that she has some function."[64]

MERCY AND COMPASSION

In cases like Karen Quinlan's or Nancy Cruzan's, the Golden Rule might imply that, "If I ended up in a condition like Karen's or Nancy's, I would want to die, and I hope that those around me would be merciful enough to let me die. If I could somehow possibly be 'conscious' in such a state, I wouldn't want to go on. I wouldn't want to be imprisoned in such a body for months or years, which would be worse than being buried alive. Mercy requires us to make dying humane, not an endless torture."

Such a thought illustrates how the Golden Rule is ambiguous because some people might want a chance to recover, even if it is very slight. Doing whatever someone else wants must take into account that people differ in their personalities and wants.

The Quinlans and the Cruzans did argue that allowing Karen and Nancy to die would be merciful. The issue of mercy is relevant in these and similar cases because we can't know for certain that such patients do not feel—we cannot be certain that they do not experience sensations such as pain and discomfort; we may not even be certain that they do not experience distress, fear, frustration, loss, or other tormenting emotions.

Eventually, the cases of Karen Quinlan and Nancy Cruzan came to symbolize mercy as an issue for both patients and families. These cases seemed to represent an inversion of values in medicine: instead of doing what families wanted, medicine did what bureaucracies required; instead of a dignified death, breathing machines and feeding tubes maintained existence; instead of a quick death, there was slow withering over a decade of an emaciated body. On top of all that, the chance that a shell of a person might still exist in pain was too much for most people. For many people, the long dying of these two patients was merciless.

Would not most people abhor such a life? Abhor the thought of living 15 years inside a body in which they could not scratch an itch, express a wish, or perform any human act? No one knows what might be going on in such a mental remnant. Whatever destroyed the original mind might have left it in disarray, such that Terri's mental life was an endless nightmare.

If Terri Schiavo could have awakened for 15 minutes and could have understood her condition, what she looked like, and what the case was doing to her family, can anyone think that this shy, weight-conscious woman would have wanted her brain-damaged, disfigured body exhibited to the world this way? If emotional revulsion is going to count in ethics, what about *her* revulsion?

Her parents saw this differently. They felt she would have wanted to live, even in such diminished circumstances. This shows the problem with simplistic interpretations of the Golden Rule or substituted judgment.

RELIGIOUS ISSUES

In 1957, Pope Pius XII had told a group of anesthesiologists that they were not obligated to provide extraordinary care to dying patients. As we saw, the Catholic Church opposed withdrawal of a respirator for Karen Quinlan. Over the next 20 years, the Catholic Church softened its opposition to such withdrawals, and Catholic hospitals often appointed patient advocates to assure compassionate care at the end of life rather than "flogging the patient to death with medical technology."

After the *Cruzan* decision, feeding tubes were not considered ordinary but extraordinary care for PVS patients. Prior to John Paul II's comments (see below), feeding tubes had been routinely removed from PVS patients in Catholic hospitals.

As the Schiavo case received greater coverage in the print and visual media, different groups took stands on the case. Within the Christian community, and especially within the Catholic Church, people disagreed about the ethics of removing artificial nutrition and hydration (ANH) from Terri Schiavo.

Perhaps after having seen the videotape of Terri on international television news, and referring to her case, Pope John Paul II said in 2004 that ANH was to be considered ordinary, as opposed to extraordinary care. He specifically said that removal of feeding tubes from patients in PVS was "euthanasia by omission."[65] Although the Pope's comment was not delivered *ex cathedra* as official Catholic dogma, the new remark cast doubt on that practice, as well as on the role of advance directives in Catholic hospitals. Several Protestant leaders and some U.S. Catholic bishops also denounced Michael Schiavo's attempt to have Terri's feeding tube removed, saying it was murder.

In contrast, Father Kevin O'Rourke, one of the leading Catholic medical ethicists in North America, argued that providing ANH was indeed extraordinary care and should not be used to prolong the life of PVS patients. He noted that both

Catholic ethicists working in hospitals, as well as doctors and nurses there, followed a much more liberal standard that allowed removal of life-support from patients in PVS.

Father John Paris, a leading Jesuit bioethicist and professor of ethics at Boston College, noted that the Pope's remarks targeted a specific audience and predicted they would have little impact in America. "I think the best thing to do is ignore it, and it will go away," Paris said. "It's not an authoritative teaching statement," he said.[66]

Catholic hospitals were thrown into confusion by the Pope's remarks about the Schiavo case. They had been removing respirators and feeding tubes for a decade. What were they to do now? Would people fear dying in a Catholic hospital? In the end, they elected to double their efforts to have every patient sign an advanced directive and assign durable power of attorney. Lacking such documents and in such hospitals, young trauma patients could end up like Terri Schiavo.

Bobby Schindler, employed as a science teacher in a Catholic high school, frequently claimed on television that his sister wanted to live. James Dobson's Focus on the Family issued daily news updates on the case. The ultra-conservative Family Research Council emailed its subscribers with headlines such as "Terri Communicates" and solicited donations. Gary McCullough, a Floridian who often escorted Mary Schindler to a microphone, owned Christian News Wire and his service issued daily stories.[67]

Before this case, Catholics and Catholic hospitals had great flexibility about withdrawing feeding tubes. The Schiavo case changed that. Now Catholic patients and their families can ethically remove life-sustaining care under very few conditions.[68] The case also had other effects. A Director of Education for the Catholic Diocese of Birmingham said that the Catholic Church now refuses to recognize the diagnosis of a vegetative state, saying that "a person is never a vegetable."[69]

DISABILITY ISSUES

As interest grew in the Schiavo case, advocates for disabled people began to take notice. While the Quinlan and Cruzan cases had never been conceptualized as involving discrimination against disabled persons, the last decades have witnessed the growing influence of *disability culture,* leading to interest of disability advocates in the Schiavo case.

Advocates for Terri Schiavo claimed that this severely cognitively impaired person was *a victim of discrimination against the disabled.* Since passage of the Americans with Disabilities Act (ADA) in 1990, denial of medical resources to a disabled person because he is disabled violates federal law. However, the ADA has never specified end-of-life cognitive deterioration (which also would include Alzheimer's disease) as a covered disability.

Groups such as Not Dead Yet, the World Association of Persons with Disabilities, the National Spinal Cord Injury Association, and Joni and Friends opposed removal of Terri's feeding tube. Of course, to claim that Terri Schiavo is a victim of discrimination against disabled persons assumes that she is still a person and could emerge from her coma. That is exactly what disability advocates and her parents claimed. Given the increasing acceptance that a patient in PVS for a decade cannot revert back to consciousness, Terri's advocates increasingly *claimed that she is not in PVS at all but in a state of minimal consciousness.*

Charleston disability rights lawyer Harriet McBryde Johnson charged that "Ms. Schiavo has a statutory right under the Americans With Disabilities Act not to be treated differently because of her disability. Obviously, Florida law would not allow a husband to kill a non-disabled wife by denying her nourishment. Because the state is overtly drawing lines based on disability, it has the burden under the ADA of justifying those lines."[70]

Disability advocates say modern culture presents a prejudiced view of life that works against disabled people. This view extols youth, health, beauty, wealth, life-long sexuality, maximal functioning, and intelligence. Such advocates abhor the invidious messages given by television shows emphasizing scantily clad young women and men doing physical feats.

They criticized also the indirect *rationing* that occurs when the medical system does not provide enough financial and medical resources for people with disabilities to function on their own. Such advocates also criticize the idea of encouraging disabled persons to exercise their right to die only when a stingy medical system has made their lives so miserable that the only autonomous decision left for them is to give up and die.

MEDICAL FUTILITY

In December 1991, Helga Wanglie, age 87, had been in PVS for eight months, sustained by a respirator and a feeding tube, at Hennepin County Hospital in Minneapolis, Minnesota.[71] At the hospital the physicians' decision to withdraw treatment opposed the patient's husband, Oliver Wanglie's wishes, who refused his permission for discontinuation of her respirator and feeding tube.

The Wanglie case was unusual for two reasons. First, since Helga Wanglie's medical insurance covered her hospitalization, the hospital would actually lose money by withdrawing artificial life-support. Second, the case involved an ethical and philosophical dispute about whether a medical team could be forced by a family member to continue care it regarded as futile. When Helga Wanglie died, the legal case ended, and the Hennepin County physicians did not continue to seek a precedent in the courts; however, about half a dozen other cases of medical futility were heard by courts and hospital ethics committees.[72]

In Massachusetts in a nasty court suit, physicians were sued in the 1989 *Gilgunn* case for removing medical support they unanimously believed to be futile. Even though the jury agreed that Caroline Gilgunn would have wanted to remain on life-support, the physicians won in 1995 because it agreed that patients could not force physicians to render futile treatment.

During the 1990s, medical futility was widely discussed. The concept is semi-evaluative, but this aspect can be obscured by the desire of clinical physicians for an objective, factual standard for ending care.[73] It is noteworthy that the bioethicists who brought the Wanglie case were mainly physician bioethicists: When bioethics first developed, few physicians entered the field, but this has changed over the last two decades.

In the 1990s, medical futility held out the promise that a descriptive concept could help physicians and families easily make decisions about treatments of minimal benefit at the end of life, but a decade later, most physicians and bioethicists had realized that the promise masked too many ethical and emotional issues.

The Schiavo case is a good example: competent neurologists unanimously agreed that, after three years, further treatment was futile for Terri, yet some staff, her parents, and rogue neurologists disagreed. Today, few bioethicists think medical futility can be invoked as a simple concept to solve end-of-life dilemmas.

Pressure from families for futile care is rare. Most American patients and their families now decline treatment when their physicians advise them that further treatment is hopeless. A study in 1994 that followed over 4,000 patients whose condition was diagnosed as life-threatening or terminal found that only 14 percent of them were resuscitated after being near death. This figure was far less than most physicians predicted and far less than it would have been a decade earlier, when most of those patients would have been resuscitated.[74]

EXTRAORDINARY VERSUS ORDINARY TREATMENT

In the years between the Quinlan case and the Cruzan case, physicians and philosophers debated whether certain levels of medical support had moral significance. The first concerned whether patients could be harmed by not receiving extraordinary, as opposed to ordinary, treatment. In 1957, a group of anesthesiologists asked Pope Pius XII what they owed dying patients. The pope said that they need not take heroic steps to keep such patients alive: patients were owed merely ordinary, but not extraordinary, treatments.

Unfortunately, the word "extraordinary" is equivocal as end points of a continuum that shifts with medical progress. In 1967, when Christiaan Barnard first transplanted a human heart, his heart-lung bypass machine was extraordinary. That machine was the forerunner of the large, bulky respirator which kept Karen Quinlan breathing. Today, miniaturized respirators—some small enough to be used with premature babies—are used everywhere in medicine. Yesterday's extraordinary treatment has become today's ordinary treatment, rendering the distinction much more fluid and unhelpful than it might at first seem.

ARTIFICIAL NUTRITION AND HYDRATION

In the 1980s, some people believed that whatever might be said about extraordinary and ordinary care in the future, providing food and water would always be considered ordinary and humane. They felt that such basic care was morally owed to PVS patients. This issue arose in the Schiavo case.

Artificial feeding is done in three basic ways: (1) by a temporary nasogastric tube run up the nostrils and down into the gastrointestinal tract; (2) by a permanent intravenous feeding line, surgically attached to one of the major veins of the chest; (3) by a surgically implanted gastrostomy tube. With many kinds of feeding tubes, patients must be tied down to avoid dislodging the line. All feeding tubes carry the risk of infection; with many, such a large volume of fluid is needed to supply the nutrients that other problems are caused.

The reality of feeding a chronically vegetative patient is not like spooning chicken soup into the mouth of a patient who is simply weak. Most vegetative patients have no swallowing reflexes, so they cannot be fed by mouth. Therefore, an artificial liquid diet must be mechanically introduced into their bodies.

The chicken-soup image can distort people's impression of a PVS case. Karen Quinlan's sister, for example, thought that her comatose sister would look like Sleeping Beauty and was shocked by the emaciated figure she saw. By the time of Nancy Cruzan's case in 1990, improvements in artificial feeding would create the opposite effect: PVS patients now had rotund "Porky Pig" faces because of retention of fluids.

As said, neither dehydration nor starvation distresses semiconscious, dying patients. Patients near death not on nutritional support seem more comfortable than patients on whom such support is forced. One important national commission noted in 1983 that loss of appetite is "almost the norm in the latter stages of terminal illness" and concluded, "Only rarely should a dying patient be fed by tube or intravenously."[75] Indeed, such feeding may actually make the patient suffer and thus harm her.

Furthermore, artificial feeding also requires medical support. Many physicians involved in caring for PVS patients during the late 1970s decided that artificial nutrition was by no means natural feeding, and that the artificial procedures were not simply "care" but highly sophisticated medical treatment. By the 1990s, most physicians had come to feel that artificial IV feeding lines for PVS patients were comparable to respirators: both were advanced medical technology. The *Cruzan* decision in 1990 agreed with this view.

Arguments abounded in the 1980s for and against withdrawing nutrition and hydration. Some states allowed removal of respirators but not of feeding tubes, and champions of a sanctity-of-life worldview saw removal of feeding and hydration tubes as the immediate cause of death and hence as mercy killing. One such philosopher argued in 1983 that providing food and water to PVS patients is the ordinary care "that all human beings owe each other"; another argued at about the same time that such feeding involves "the most fundamental of all human relationships," and that "to tamper with, or adulterate, so enduring and central a moral emotion" is "a most dangerous business."[76]

On the other side are those who see artificial feeding either as prolonging the inevitable dying or as sustaining the body of a patient who is in fact already dead. People who argued this way gave little weight to the symbolic value of feeding and thought that equating withdrawal of nutrition with murder was conceptually confused. According to this view, the moral question here is simple: Does artificial feeding and hydration benefit or burden the patient?

Not everyone agreed with the emerging idea that artificial nutrition and hydration is just another form of medical treatment, which can ethically be withdrawn for PVS patients. Several physicians and members of the clergy in conservative religions opposed such withdrawal.[77] However, most state courts now allow withdrawal of artificial nutrition and hydration. By 2000, sanctity-of-life champions for the most part had abandoned or changed their views about end-of-life treatment and shifted their attention to embryos, abortion, and stem cell research.

WITHDRAWING AND FORGOING TREATMENT

During the last three decades, a central moral debate has concerned the degree to which a physician may be involved in hastening the death of a dying patient. One cause of this debate was a declaration by AMA in 1973 (two years before Quinlan):

> The intentional termination of the life of one human being by another—mercy killing—is contrary to that for which the medical profession stands and is contrary to the policy of the American Medical Association.[78]

> . . . The cessation of the employment of extraordinary means to prolong the life of the body when there is irrefutable evidence that biological death is imminent is the decision of the patient and/or immediate family.

In this statement, the word "extraordinary" is ambiguous, and AMA policy did not clarify it. Are all patients on respirators receiving extraordinary care? Is a physician who withdraws a dying patient's respirator without the family's consent with the intent of termination of life, guilty of mercy killing? What if the physician withdraws a feeding tube?

Concern about the possibility of being considered guilty of mercy killing led some physicians to forgo the use of respirators and artificial feeding. Since withdrawal of such care might be seen as intentional termination of life (mercy killing), it was far easier to forgo medical support than to withdraw it. This reasoning created an odd situation, in which physicians would forgo the same treatment that they would not withdraw.

To others, it seemed that patients could be harmed both by the AMA's policy and by the interpretation that an extraordinary treatment could be forgone but not withdrawn. They believed that because the outcome is never certain, a patient is morally owed extraordinary treatment—both a respirator and artificial feeding, for example—in order to see if recovery is possible. Also, some people argued that, regardless of whether a respirator or a catheter was ordinary or extraordinary medical support, nobody really thought that a physician who withdrew such a device killed a terminally ill patient. In such a situation, we would say—if the patient had cancer—that cancer killed the patient, not the physician.

In 1975, Karen Quinlan's physicians—Morse and Javed—were upholding the official position of AMA: that withdrawing medical support from a patient was the same as "active euthanasia." In 1986, the AMA changed its policy to reflect a new understanding of chronically comatose patients supported by respirators and artificial nutrition. Now it was ethically possible for a physician, after consulting with the family, to withdraw a respirator and feeding tubes from an irreversibly comatose patient.

This new AMA policy did not say that being irreversibly comatose was equivalent to being brain dead. Criteria for ethical removal of medical support differ from a state's legal standard of brain death. Physicians, under AMA policy, can remove support from patients who are not legally dead under a state's laws.

ADVANCE DIRECTIVES

The Quinlan case caused written advance directives to become popular. Such advance directives can take several forms. A *living will* informs physicians about conditions under which a person would or would not want medical support continued. A *values inventory* specifies what a person values in life and may be useful to a patient's family and physicians if they must make decisions for that person. A *durable power of attorney* assigns to someone else the right to make financial and life-and-death medical decisions if the person becomes incompetent. In those states that allow it to be applied to medical decisions, durable power of attorney is the most powerful device for protecting the rights of dying people; however, not all states have statutes creating powers of attorney for proxy medical decisions. By 1990, 43 states had statutes recognizing some version of advance directives.[79] The decision in the Cruzan case emphasized that such a document would be crucial in meeting the "clear and convincing" standard required by New York and Missouri. After the Schiavo case, many Americans rushed to sign advanced directives.

In December 1991, the Health Care Financing Administration required all American hospitals to ask incoming patients if they had, or wanted to sign, an advance directive. This requirement increased the use of advance directives and has forced hospitals to specify their policies about honoring such directives.

Advance directives contain two major problems. First, most people do not accurately predict how they will feel later when they are actually near death. According to the famous SUPPORT study (Study to Understand Prognoses and Preferences for Outcomes and Risks of Treatment), most competent people change their minds when actually faced with a decision to decline treatment and die, despite having predicted the opposite about themselves many years before.[80]

If this is true for competent patients, what can we infer about the wishes of incompetent patients? Neither the best interests standard nor the substituted judgment standard are decisive: If a patient has a small chance of coming out of a yearlong coma, aren't his best interests in being kept alive? If he had known these odds, would he have wanted to be given the chance? Whose judgment substitutes for his, especially if his choice was made in semi-ignorance?

Worse, evidence has been accumulating that spouses or others designated as legal proxies cannot accurately predict the wishes of previously competent but now incompetent patients.[81] As frequently as they wrongly predict a desire for mere palliative care, they just as frequently wrongly predict desires for aggressive treatment.[82]

Advance directives often do not cover nonterminal, though permanently comatose, patients. Only a few advanced directives are thorough enough and specify whether food and water is included under unwanted medical treatment or name a specific person to be a proxy for the incompetent patient. Because such directives are only requested of patients upon admission to hospitals, most people under 30 do not have one.

SCHIAVO, BIOETHICS, AND POLITICS

Outsiders made things worse in the Schiavo case. Not understanding the history of the false report of abuse and trauma on the 1991 bone scan, outside experts guessed that something malevolent had happened to Terri, making Terri's advocates suspect a cover-up by Terri's husband and the courts. Outside physicians, pushing their own exotic, for-profit schemes, exploited gullible parents and friends. Outlier neurologists, pushing a new category of consciousness not in journals of neurology but on the front pages of the *New York Times* and the *Hastings Center Report*, a bioethics journal, also didn't help any.

When the parents went to national media, especially in an age of fierce competition among cable news stations for sensational topics, the floodgates opened. And because politicians on the national scene love media attention, and as Florida Senator Mel Martinez predicted, U.S. Senators, Congressmen, and even the President got involved.

Since 1997 when scientists announced the cloning of the lamb Dolly, bioethics had become increasingly politicized, with social conservatives extolling the personhood of human embryos and opposing all forms of cloning. The Schiavo case landed on this pedigree and exploded. Whether it's good for bioethics to have its subjects covered all evening on cable news outlets remains to be seen.

FURTHER READING AND RESOURCES

Margaret Battin, *The Least Worst Death: Essays in Bioethics at the End of Life*, Oxford University Press, New York, 1993.

Joanne Lynn, ed., *By No Extraordinary Means: The Choice to Forgo Life-Sustaining Food and Water*, expanded ed., 1989, Indiana University Press, Bloomington, 1989.

Joseph and Julia Quinlan with Phyllis Battelle, *Karen Ann: The Quinlans Tell Their Story*, Doubleday, New York, NY, 1977.

William Colby, *The Long Goodbye: The Deaths of Nancy Cruzan*, Hay House, Carlsbad, CA, 2002.

Robert and Mary Schindler, with Suzanne Schindler Vitadamo and Bobby Schindler, *A Life that Matters: The Legacy of Terri Schiavo*, Time Warner Books, New York, NY, 2006.

Michael Schiavo, and Michael Hirsh, *Terri: The Truth*, Dutton Adult Books, New York, NY, 2006.

Mark Fuhrman *Silent Witness: The Untold Story of the Death of Terri Schiavo*.

Arthur L. Caplan, James J. McCartney, and Dominic Sisti, (eds), *The Case of Terri Schiavo: Ethics at the End of Life*, Buffalo, NY, Prometheus, 2006.

"Between Life and Death: The Terri Schiavo Story," A & E films. $25. This excellent 45-minute summary of the case, made by CBS news, has good pictures of Terri in various stages of her life and pictures of Patricia White Bull and Terry Wallace (coma patients who awakened after many years). http://store.aetv.com/html/search/index.jhtml?search=Terri+Schiavo+Story&x=12&y=6

Downloadable video of Terri Schiavo: http://www.glennbeck.com/news/09092003-1.shtml

Other websites about Schiavo Case: http://www.apfn.org/apfn/Terri_doctor.htm

http://www.pbs.org/newshour/bb/law/july-dec03/lifesupport_10-22.html
Legal Issues about Schiavo Case: http://abstractappeal.com/schiavo/infopage.html
http://www.sptimes.com/2003/11/02/State/How_Terri_s_Law_came_.shtml
Timeline in Schiavo Case: http://www.miami.edu/ethics2/schiavo/timeline.htm
Web Links/Medi Coma Recovery Association, Inc. — ww.comarecovery.org/
Karen Ann Quinlan Hospice, Inc. www.karenannquinlanhospice.org/

CHAPTER 3

Physician-Assisted Dying

Oregon's Legalization

In 1998, a physician legally assisted a terminally ill Oregonian in dying. Oregonians had fought over a decade to make this happen. Twenty-seven years before in 1971, a physician in Holland killed her terminally ill mother, leading Holland to become the world's first ethics laboratory for physician-assisted dying.

Meanwhile in America, Dr. Jack Kevorkian assisted over one hundred patients to die before being finally jailed in 1999 for flouting the law. Critics saw his efforts, as well as developments in Oregon and Holland, as descents into barbarism and as returns to the "euthanasia" of Nazi medicine.

This chapter reviews these developments and arguments about physician-assisted dying.

Voluntary Euthanasia in the Netherlands

The Netherlands began to decriminalize physician-assisted suicide in 1971 when physician Geertruida Postma mercy-killed her mother, who previously had suffered a cerebral hemorrhage that left the elderly woman partially paralyzed, deaf, and with gross speech deficits. Tried and found guilty of murder, Postma received a suspended sentence.

The Dutch Medical Association, in agreement with Dutch legal authorities, in 1973 began guidelines for physician-assisted death. They were that: (1) Only competent patients can request death, (2) Requests must be repeated, unambivalent, unpressured, and documented, (3) Physicians must consult another physician for a second opinion, (4) Patients must be in unbearable pain or suffering, without likelihood of improvement.[1]

Incompetent patients like Terri Schiavo or Karen Quinlan cannot be mercy-killed in Holland.

By 1990, Holland had become an experimental ethics laboratory. The key experimental question was: would its mercy killings lead down the dreaded slippery slope into barbarism?

Its Remmelink Commission studied nearly two decades of data in this experiment and reported in 1990 that another 1,000 deaths occurred in *incompetent* patients, a violation of the guidelines.[2] Virtually 100 percent of the patients killed were terminally ill (most had been given between a week or a month to live), and also, physicians turned down 66 percent of requests for death from competent patients. A follow-up study in 1995 found much the same results.[3] Most of the 1,000 incompetent patients killed had cancer or AIDS and had previously expressed a wish, should they become incompetent, to have physicians help them die painlessly.

Several aspects of the Dutch experience caution against easy generalizations to North America. First, everyone in Holland has free medical care, including long-term nursing home care, and thus no patient, physician, or family needs to decide to die to ease the financial burden of care. Second, the typical Dutch patient has a physician who makes house calls, who has known him for years, whom he trusts, and who will be the one he asks to help him die. To an extent that American physicians would envy, the typical Dutch patient trusts his physician.

Some cases have pushed the limits at the margins, as when a physician killed a woman in her 20s after a decade of severe anorexia. In 1993, a physician killed a severely depressed woman who had been traumatized by the death of her two children and the failure of her marriage.

In 2001, after 30 years of agreements and semi-legalization, Queen Beatrix signed a law making physician-assisted dying totally legal in Holland. After three decades of experimentation, 90 percent of Dutch citizens supported the law. The law lacked a controversial proposal allowing terminal 12- to 15-year olds the same right. The law did include the right of patients in the early stages of dementia, amyotrophic lateral sclerosis, or other progressive diseases to sign advanced directives allowing them to be killed at a later date.

After 35 years, the Dutch embrace their famous experiment. They resent Americans who claim they dispatch their grandparents to save money. The Dutch endure heavy taxes to pay for their national medical system and take pride in how their physicians respect personal autonomy and practice compassionately.

During the 1990s, Dutch physicians still rebuffed about 66 percent of patients who requested death. Patients who had assisted deaths generally had terminal cancer or end-stage AIDS. By 2005, that figure had dropped to 12 percent, with another 13 percent changing their minds and another 13 percent dying before the physician could help them die.[4]

The Vatican and 10 percent of Dutch citizens and physicians condemned the 2001 legalization. In 2002, Belgium legalized the same, and Switzerland legalized some kinds of physician-assisted dying.

The Dutch Parliament in 2002 extended its previous euthanasia legislation to competent adolescents aged 16 to 18 and, with consent of parents, teenagers aged 12 to 16. The *Groningen protocol* began in March 2006 where children under age 12 and especially babies could be killed with parental consent when two physicians agree with parents that the child is terminally ill with no prospect of recovery and suffering great pain.[5] This protocol semi-legalized secret euthanasia in babies reportedly being carried out in Dutch hospitals, especially for babies with spina bifida. Critics saw it as a slippery slope come true.[6] The protocol is expected to soon be expanded to also cover severely retarded adults and those with end-stage dementia.[7]

In America, 55,000 children die each year, and in 2002 the prestigious Institute of Medicine concluded that most such children die badly. "Too often, children with fatal . . . conditions fail to receive competent, compassionate, and consistent care."[8] Children often accept their dying before their parents, who notoriously "flog them to death" in painful experiments in hopes of miracles.

Dr. Jack Kevorkian

In 1990, Dr. Jack Kevorkian, a retired pathologist, helped Oregonian Janet Adkins to die, setting off an ethical firestorm in America.

Adkins, 54 years old, loved music, tennis, and hiking. Around 1988, she became frustrated by her increasing inability to remember things and could no longer read sheet music for her piano. She had the initial phase of Alzheimer's disease, the fourth-largest killer of Americans.

Characterized by progressive loss of memory, Alzheimer's disease results from irreversible degeneration of neural cells. It is incurable. On average and after the onset of symptoms, people with Alzheimer's disease live 10 years. In the final phase, which can last years, patients will not recognize sons and daughters or understand who they are.

According to her husband, Ron Adkins, the diagnosis of Alzheimer's disease hit Janet Adkins "like a bombshell . . . . Her mind was her life." At the urging of her family, she tried the experimental drug Tacrine. According to her son Neil, "The drug didn't work. From then on, her mind was set. Quality of life was everything with her. She wanted to die with dignity intact."

At the time, assisted suicide was not illegal in Michigan, where Kevorkian lived. Adkins flew there with her husband and her three sons. Her family disliked her intention to die and hoped she would change her mind, but in the end, everyone supported her decision.

Jack Kevorkian, then 63, grew up in Michigan, the son of Armenian immigrants, and graduated from medical school in 1953. After finishing his residency, he worked from 1969 to 1978 in Detroit at Sarasota Hospital as director of laboratories. Later, he worked at hospitals in southern California.

In the mid-1980s, he retired from hospital work and lived on his savings and Social Security benefits, $550 a month. He lived simply in a tiny, two-room apartment near his two sisters.

Compassionate assistance to the dying did not originally motivate Dr. Kevorkian. Instead, he wanted to increase organs for transplantation. When first contacted in 1989 by a patient with end-stage lung cancer, he explained his ultimate aim: not to help patients achieve painless, dignified death, but to get terminal people to volunteer for "invaluable experiments" and to transplant their organs to those who needed them.[9] This aim would have constituted a new medical specialty, which he called "obitiary" or "medicide."

Always a loner, he mostly scorned membership in medical societies. "Instinctively, as a student, I thought they were corrupt," he says. "I've been independent all my life."

When Adkins arrived in Michigan, Kevorkian and his two sisters interviewed her and her family for two hours. None of the interviewers thought that she was depressed or ambivalent about her decision to die; nor did they think that she could be helped by medicine. She and her family signed documents and made videotapes to prove that they understood what they were doing.

The next day, June 4, 1990, Adkins met Kevorkian alone and the two drove in his rusty 1968 Volkswagen van to a public park in north Oakland County, Michigan. Kevorkian could not find a better place where he could help her die. He had forthrightly told several clinics, churches, and funeral homes what he intended to do, and none of them would let him use their facilities. In desperation, he had decided on the park and had put a cot and his suicide device in the van.

The simple device in the van that would allow Janet Adkins to kill herself painlessly consisted of three intravenous (IV) bottles hung from an aluminum frame; Kevorkian called it a *Mercitron*. At the park, he connected an IV line to Janet Adkins and started a saline solution for fluid volume. Then she took over and pushed a switch that stopped the saline and released thiopental, a powerful sedative. The switch also started a six-second timer which soon activated a drip of potassium chloride. The thiopental rendered Janet Adkins unconscious, and about one minute later, the potassium chloride killed her. In effect, Kevorkian said, Janet Adkins had "a painless heart attack while in deep sleep." The whole process took less than six minutes.

Neither the Adkins family nor Kevorkian had anticipated the landslide of publicity that ensued. The local district attorney prosecuted Kevorkian for murder. Because no law prohibited assisted suicide in Michigan, a local judge dismissed the case but ordered Kevorkian not to use his Mercitron again (although the judge had no legal basis for issuing such an order).

After 1990, when he assisted at Adkins's death, Kevorkian received hundreds of letters a year from people whose suffering was of biblical proportions. Because he was afraid to fly and hated to drive far, his patients had to come to him. Thus he did not help anyone who was too ill to travel, and that frustrated those who could not get to Michigan. He also accepted no money for helping anyone die.

In the fall of 1991, Kevorkian assisted in the double suicide of two women patients: one with multiple sclerosis and another with chronic vaginal-pelvic pain. Again indicted for murder, the charges were dismissed because no Michigan law prohibited his actions. However, Michigan authorities in 1991 did suspend his medical license.

With his license suspended, he could no longer obtain sodium pentothal and potassium chloride, so he began using carbon monoxide (CO) with his next patients. In May of 1992, he helped another victim of multiple sclerosis to die; this time the patient put on a mask in order to breathe in the CO.

Kevorkian came to believe that CO was a good way to commit suicide: the gas "has no color, taste, or smell; and it's toxic enough to cause rapid unconsciousness in relatively low concentration. Furthermore, in light complexioned people it often produces a rosy color that makes the victim look better as a corpse." After some trial and error, he began to teach patients to attach one end of a plastic tube to a canister of CO and the other to the kind of small plastic mask used in hospitals for oxygen therapy. When the gas is turned on and the patient breathes, death occurs within five minutes.

Most physicians and many medical ethicists denounced him. Asked about criticisms of his actions, he responds, "Why should I care what brainwashed ethicists and non-thinking physicians say?"[10] Nor has he worried about violating the Hippocratic oath: he calls physicians who follow these ancient ideas "hypocritic oafs." He regarded himself as a Socratic gadfly to the sluggish medical profession, saw his struggle in heroic terms, and compared himself to Mahatma Gandhi and Martin Luther King, Jr.

In June 1995, he opened a suicide clinic in Michigan, but was soon evicted by the building's owner. By 1998, he had assisted 100 patients in committing suicide and had been acquitted in three trials involving five of those deaths.

By 1998, the Michigan legislature had passed a law making physician-assisted dying illegal. Afterwards, Kevorkian assisted in the death of ALS patient Thomas Youk. Videotaped, Youk's death appeared on *60 Minutes*. The videotape, shown at the trial, offered irrefutable evidence that Kevorkian had deliberately broken the law. At his trial, Kevorkian clamed that, since his first case of Janet Adkins, he had helped over 130 patients to die.

The then 70-year-old Kevorkian received a 10–25 year sentence. He is scheduled to be paroled in June 2007. He lost two appeals in 2001 and 2002 for new trials. Nothing has been heard from him since he entered prison in Jackson, MI.

Dr. Quill: Another Approach to Dying

In 1990, Timothy Quill, an internist in Rochester, New York, helped a patient named Diane to die. She had terminal, acute myelomonocytic leukemia, and had experienced three tumultuous months, during which her son stayed home from college, and her husband worked from home.

When Dr. Quill knew that her end had come, he gave her the drugs she needed to kill herself. He wrote:

> When we met, it was clear that she [Diane] knew what she was doing, that she was sad and frightened to be leaving, but that she would be even more terrified to stay and suffer. In our tearful goodbye, she promised a reunion in the future at her favorite spot on the edge of Lake Geneva, with dragons swimming in the sunset.[11]

Quill wrote of Diane's death in a medical journal and his district attorney then prosecuted him for murder; however, the grand jury refused to indict him.

Quill's case contrasted in several ways with those of Jack Kevorkian: Quill knew Diane well and had treated her for a long time; he first offered her a course of treatment that might allow her to survive; he helped her die privately and without publicity; he preserved her anonymity; he presented his account in an established medical forum; and he did not desire to specialize in assisted dying. Finally, his actions resembled those of Dutch physicians, for whom assisted death is the end of a spectrum of life-long care of patients.

Oregon's Legalization

After intense battles in the media, Oregonians in 1994 by referendum approved the Oregon Death with Dignity Act. This Act would have legalized assistance in dying from a physician by the prescription of drugs. The Oregon Medical Association opposed legalization, and the Oregon legislature balked, refusing to go along. Another referendum by Oregonians in 1997 approved the measure 60 percent to 40 percent, making the Act into law beginning in 1998.

The Act had draconian restrictions: Patients had to be: (1) clearly competent, (2) have less than six months to live, and (3) to avoid impulsive decisions, wait 15 days before filling prescriptions. Physicians could not administer the fatal dosage, only prescribe it.

In March 1998, a woman suffering from terminal breast cancer with less than two months to live became the first person to kill herself under the new Act.[12] She died about 30 minutes after taking the medication. By July 1998, two more terminal patients had taken lethal drugs. Auguring a future pattern, four terminal patients died during the 15-day waiting period before they could swallow their deadly medications.

Most Oregonians prefer to die at home. Oregon has the lowest in-hospital mortality rate, suggesting many referrals for home health care and respect for advanced directives.[13] Under its ground-breaking Oregon Health Plan, all of the previously uninsured, terminally ill Oregonians can utilize hospice programs.[14] As with Holland's liberalization, we should not generalize Oregon's liberalization to states with poorly funded state Medicaid plans because such generalization may put patients at risk of dying early for lack of money.

What about managed care organizations subtly pushing early death to save money? One misperception is that hospice and palliative care are cheap. A 1998 study showed that physician-assisted death might make a difference in only 1/2 of 1 percent of costs at the end of life.[15]

Doctors cannot be forced to participate in such deaths. They also cannot *abandon* patients. Like abortion, those who object to participating in the death "must transfer care so that the needs of the patient can be met" and "must not hinder the transfer."[16]

Deaths from Physician-Assisted Dying in Oregon[17]

Year	Deaths
1998	16
1999	27
2000	27
2001	21
2002	38
2003	42
2004	37
2005	32

Oregonian physicians write prescriptions for about 50 percent more patients than those who use them. About a third die before the waiting period or die before self-administering the pills. Over eight years, only 246 of about 75,000 dying Oregonians requested terminal drugs.[18] The most frequent diseases causing such requests were ALS, AIDS, and cancer. Physicians most commonly prescribed the barbiturates secobarbital and phenobarbital.

One guidebook for Oregonian physicians encourages them to obtain the drugs for the patient, keep them until the time of death, and be there with the patient in his home as he takes them.[19] Such physicians should insist on an advanced directive specifying a "Do Not Resuscitate" order for emergency-response personnel, counsel the family that the death may not be immediate but may take hours and have complications, be ready to administer antiemetics and analgesics, counsel and support the family during and after the death, sign the death certificate and sign other papers required by the Act, and arrange transfer to a funeral home.

Finally, many terminal Oregonians learned to die simply by not eating. When patients really are dying, the urge to eat disappears. In such a state, fasting is not painful. Although patients must be determined and physicians and family must agree, such dying can be a peaceful alternative to intravenous lines and barbiturates. One dying patient went 11 days without fluids and 51 days without food before succumbing this way. One study in 2003 discovered that more Oregonians die by ceasing food and water than by asking physicians to help them.[20]

Background: Ancient Greece and the Hippocratic Oath

The Hippocratic Oath, considered the origin of medical ethics, forbids physicians to kill patients, and began in ancient Greece at the time of Socrates in fifth century BCE. But did Hippocratic physicians represent most ancient Greek physicians?

Hippocrates was a disciple of the mathematician Pythagoras, who developed the famous theorem, who worshipped numbers as divine, and who held that all life was sacred. As his follower, Hippocrates did not represent most ancient Greek physicians.

The Hippocratic corpus, or body of writings, does not represent the work of one man named "Hippocrates," but was drawn from a number of his followers. The practitioners of the Hippocratic school "possessed no legally recognized professional qualifications" and competed with gymnastic instructors, drug-sellers, herbalists, midwives, and exorcists.[21]

Many people today misunderstand the content of the original Hippocratic oath. Let us see what the original oath makes physicians promise. Here is one translation:

> I swear by Apollo Physician and Asclepius and Hygeia and Panaceia and all the gods and goddesses, making them my witnesses, that I will fulfill according to my ability and judgment this oath and this covenant:
> To hold him who has taught me this art as equal to my parents and to live my life in partnership with him, and if he is in need of money, to give him a share of mine, and to regard his offspring as equal to my brothers in male lineage, and to teach his art—if they desire to learn it—without fee and covenant; to give a share of precepts and oral instruction and all the other learning to my sons and to the sons of him who has instructed me and the pupils who have signed the covenant and have taken this oath according to the medical law, but to no one else.
> I will apply dietetic measures for the benefit of the sick according to my ability and judgment; I will keep them from harm and injustice.
> I will neither give a deadly drug to anybody if asked for it, nor will I make a suggestion to this effect. Similarly I will not give to a woman an abortive remedy. In purity and holiness I will guard my life and my art. I will not use the knife, not

even on sufferers of stone, but will withdraw in favor of such men as are engaged in this work.

Whatever houses I visit, I will come for the benefit of the sick, remaining free of all intentional injustice, of all mischief and in particular of sexual relations with both female and male persons, be they free or slaves.

What I may see or hear in the course of the treatment or even outside of the treatment in regard to the life of men, which on no account one must spread abroad, I will keep to myself holding such things shameful to be spoken about.

If I fulfill this oath and do not violate it, may it be granted to me to enjoy life and art, being honored with fame among all men for all time to come; if I transgress it and swear falsely, may the opposite of all this be my lot.[22]

The original Oath should also be understood in context. By these vows, the Hippocratic school wanted to solidify its membership against competing healers, for example, those who performed surgery or who charged students for teaching them.

Ordinary Greek physicians thought like ordinary Greeks, who thought that life had natural limitations, beyond which only fools tried to extend living. The concept of a *meson* or natural limit infused Greek culture, especially architecture and theater. To attempt to go beyond *meson* was *hubris*, arrogance, and invited the gods to strike one down. So most ancient Greek physicians helped their patients die.

The prohibition against euthanasia by the Hippocratic school thus set its members apart from the majority of physicians in ancient Greece who helped patients die painlessly and with some dignity.

The Nazis and "Euthanasia"

Debates about physician-assisted dying frequently refer to German physicians during the Nazi era, who killed 90,000 patients in the name of "euthanasia" because of mental or physical inferiority. This Nazi argument bears some scrutiny.

Physicians also administered the *Final Solution* to the "problem" of how to cleanse Germany of racially inferior non-Aryan peoples. Physicians kept this program more secret, and under it, killed six million Jews, 600,000 Poles, thousands of Gypsies, and thousands of gay men and lesbians.

Leo Alexander, a New York psychiatrist who observed the Nuremberg trials, famously argued in 1949 that these killing programs by Nazi physicians began with their belief that people are better off dead than alive because their quality of life is poor.[23]

In 1986, another New York psychiatrist, Robert Jay Lifton, argued similarly, although his "first step" differs from Alexander's:

> The Nazis justified direct medical killing by use of the . . . concept of "life unworthy of life," *lebensunwertes Leben*. While this concept predated the Nazis, it was carried to its ultimate racial and "therapeutic" extreme by them.
>
> . . . Of the five identifiable steps by which the Nazis carried out the destruction of "life unworthy of life," coercive sterilization was the first. There followed the killing of "impaired" children in hospitals, and then the killing of "impaired" adults—mostly collected from mental hospitals—in centers especially equipped with carbon monoxide. The same killing centers were then used for the murders of "impaired" inmates of concentration camps. The final step was mass killing, mostly of Jews, in the extermination camps themselves.[24]

People opposed to physician-assisted dying often cite Alexander's and Lifton's work. They emphasize that in Nazi Germany medical professors in elite medical schools took the first step.

J. C. Wilkes argues differently and that the first steps down the Nazi slippery slope were a few cases of merciful deaths for severely handicapped infants.[25] In 1937, a father who killed his mentally retarded child received only a mild rebuke. Two years later, Dr. Karl Brandt examined an infant named Knauer, born blind and missing an arm and leg; Hitler then issued clearance for Dr. Brant to kill Knauer and all similar infants. Wilkes claims these two test cases led to the first phase of deaths in Germany where physicians killed as many as 6,000 (Wilkes's estimate) disabled children.

These cases differ from the so-called Baby Doe cases discussed elsewhere in this book in that the parents usually did not consent to these killings. The babies and children were moved out of the home and away, and the parents never heard from then again.

What about claims by Alexander, Lifton, and Wilkes about the first step that leads down the slippery slope to mass killings?

Many history professors emphasize that Germany had been blatantly anti-Semitic since the time of the Crusades. Instead of a subtle first step propelling them downward, Nazi physicians rode a tsunami that had been building for centuries.

The Nazi "euthanasia" program also misleads people in at least three ways: it had nothing in common with *competent* patients who are *dying* and who *voluntarily* request assistance in dying from physicians. In brief, Nazi "euthanasia" was not "good deaths" but despicable murders.

The Nazi argument also contains many different claims, including:

1. Involuntary killings of people *for medical reasons* led to the Holocaust.
2. Involuntary killings of people *by physicians* led to the Holocaust.
3. Justifying medical killings of people *for reasons of quality of life* led to the Holocaust.
4. *Involuntary sterilization* of retarded, psychotic, and demented people led to the Holocaust.
5. The *killing of impaired children* led to the Holocaust.
6. *Eugenics*, the desire of Nazis to create a Master Race, led to the Holocaust.
7. Deep *cultural racism and anti-Semitism* led to the Holocaust.
8. Acceptance by physicians of a *new role as killers* led to the Holocaust.

Because all its victims died involuntarily, and because no terminal patients died voluntarily by Nazi physicians, "playing the Nazi card" is unfair in modern debates about physicians and terminal patients. The Nazi murders lack relevance to modern debates about competent, terminal patients who request physicians to help them die.

MODERN DEVELOPMENTS

The Hemlock Society/Compassion & Choices

Founded in the United States in 1980 by retired British journalist Derek Humphrey, the Hemlock Society helped people with terminal illness to die with dignity.

After merging in 2005 with other similar organizations, it has been called Compassion & Choices. It advocates legalizing physician-assisted dying.

Americans join such organizations because they fear their physicians will violate their wishes, forcing them to live their final months in pain and undergoing unnecessary procedures.. As the writer and journalist Shana Alexander said about dying in a hospital, "When it comes to following my wishes, I trust my lawyer more than my physician."[26]

The Hospice Movement and Palliative Care

In the 1960s, two physicians—one working in the United States and the other in England—changed medicine to help dying patients. Elisabeth Kübler-Ross, working in Chicago, and Cicely Saunders in Britain, focused on accepting the inevitability of death and making terminal patients comfortable.

Their program began the *hospice movement*. A hospice tries to give dying patients dignity and maximal control over the final months of their lives. Originally, hospices were special separate facilities, but the concept soon evolved to visiting nurses treating patients at home.

Because of the work of these two women, physicians today relieve pain better and attend to the psychological needs of dying patients better than 40 years ago. In the United States, Medicare now pays for six months of hospice care for dying patients.

Around 1986, *palliative care* began. The goal of symptomatic palliative therapy is maximal quality of life during the remaining weeks or months of life, and as such, may rule out full-dose radiation or chemotherapy in cancer patients. Palliative care does not mean giving up on patients but does mean giving up on experimental, often torturous, treatments in seeking a one-in-a-million cure. Palliative care physicians focus on maximal relief of bad symptoms such as nausea, boredom, itching, feelings of suffocation, immobility, depression, and especially pain.

Recent Legal Decisions

In 1994, a federal judge struck down a law in Washington state banning assisted suicide, holding that the equal protection of liberty guaranteed in the 14th Amendment covered not only a woman's right to end a pregnancy but also a terminal patient's right to physician-assisted dying.[27] The liberty guaranteed to Americans by the Constitution included the right to die, she said, and assistance by physicians in so doing.

Over the next three years and in two important decisions, the U.S. Supreme Court disagreed. Although a state such as Oregon *could* legalize physician-assisted dying, no fundamental liberty existed in the Constitution to this assistance such that state laws banning this assistance were unconstitutional.

One case alleged discrimination against dying patients because only some could decide to die by removal of a ventilator or feeding tube, but some others could not. If physicians could legally kill by withdrawing treatment, why not by more direct means? The highest Court answered that "the distinction between assisting suicide and withdrawing life-sustaining treatment, a distinction widely recognized and endorsed in the medical profession and in our legal traditions, is both important and logical; it is certainly rational . . . ."[28]

In the second case, the same Court found that no right to assisted suicide existed in American legal or medical traditions. The Court accepted the AMA's claim that legalization of physician-assisted dying threatened the medical profession's integrity, as well as claims that physician-assisted dying would hurt the disabled and poor. It also found "ample concern" for a slippery slope from increased acceptance of physician killings.

These decisions only said that a fundamental right to die did not already exist in the Constitution, such that state laws banning assisted suicide would violate it. These decisions left open the door for a state to legalize physician-assisted suicide, as Oregon did in 1998. In this way, these decisions mirrored what *Cruzan* said about laws about incompetent patients, i.e., states *could*, but *need not*, pass this kind of law.

When he became Attorney General in 2001, John Ashcroft threatened to void the drug license of Oregonian physicians who prescribed barbiturates to terminal patients. By law, such drugs can only be prescribed for "legitimate medical purposes" and Ashcroft argued that intentionally helping a terminal patient die was not such a purpose.

Oregon challenged Attorney General John Ashcroft's interference with its law, and in 2005 the U.S. Supreme Court decided, 6-3, that physicians and citizens of Oregon, not Ashcroft, would decide what "legitimate medical purpose" meant, and hence, that Ashcroft exceeded his legitimate authority in challenging Oregon's physicians.[29]

ETHICAL ISSUES

Two different kinds of argument occur in ethics. One focuses directly on the morality of acts and argues that they are intrinsically wrong, "just wrong," or wrong without regard to consequences. The other grants that in a few cases, such acts may be justified, but opposes them based on their bad indirect effects. These are *direct* and *indirect* arguments.

The main direct argument against physician-assisted dying is that it is always wrong to kill. Most other arguments against it are indirect and predict slippery slopes.

DIRECT ARGUMENTS ABOUT PHYSICIAN-ASSISTED DYING

Killing Is Always Wrong

The best direct argument against physician-assisted dying is that such actions wrongly kill vulnerable humans. Of course, it is always wrong to kill humans under all circumstances, and just because a human is dying, no exceptions can be made. Evil occurs when one human ends the life of another.

This argument does not claim that what is wrong about killing is that it can become uncontrollable after a few justified cases, for that would be appealing to a slippery slope. Instead, it claims that all killing is *intrinsically wrong*, no matter what the circumstances.

Whether or not an afterlife or God exists, once a person is dead, he's not coming back. Without an afterlife, this life is all a person has, and to take it away is to take away all values because the valu*er* is gone.

For many decisions, such as transplanting a kidney, if mistakes occur, there is backup, for example, hemodialysis. But mistakes in killing have no back-up. Once a person is dead, that's it.

For this reason, killing must not be taken lightly. Life must not be cheapened. The ultimate power on earth is to take away life. All life should be valued, not just human life, but all sentience.

Life is precious, no matter how low in quality. Of all values in medicine, this one must reign supreme.

Killing Is Not Always Wrong

The most ancient justification of the direct argument is based on religious metaphysics: that God exists, that Scripture correctly reveals his laws for humans, and that one such law is for humans never to kill another human. Based on this view, some Christians and some orthodox Jews prefer death to self-defense, refuse war and the draft, and will never kill.

One should note that Scripture really bans "unjustified" killings, and hence, allows just wars and the death penalty for murderers. The question here concerns whether helping terminally ill patients die is "unjustified killing." After all, as God presumably allows the person to have a terminal illness and to be dying, so in one sense, dying for each of us is His Will.

More important, the background conditions need to examined for why the rule against killing has been important throughout the millennia of civilization in the West. Throughout this history, most people have wanted to live as long as possible. That fact is less true today. Why?

Medicine has cured the old, acute diseases that killed swiftly, and left us with chronic diseases, such as cancer and heart disease, that kill slowly. In previous centuries, people tried to live as long as possible because most never experienced the disability and dysfunction that came with chronic diseases.

Now consider the rule against killing and physician-assisted dying. When you help me accomplish what I want to do, you do a good thing, and morality encourages you to help me. When you prevent me from doing what I want to do, you hurt my interests and me, and your actions are probably immoral. Whether or not dying assisted by physicians is good or bad may depend, not on what has been traditionally judged moral or immoral, but on the wishes of the dying patient.

Of course, critics can object that helping me do what I want to do is not a good thing if I want to do something immoral such as steal my neighbor's car. And, they say, helping people die is immoral.

But why should we allow this objection as a good one? Why should we accept the underlying premise that "helping dying people die is immoral" unless some further reason is given? To simply assert this as an objection is to beg the question. It is not an argument against a position to assume that it is wrong.

Killing versus Letting Die

For several decades, bioethicists have debated whether killing differs from letting die. A 1997 survey by the American Hospital Association found that 70 percent of deaths in hospitals involve some decision by a physician or relative to cease treatment.[30] However, intentional termination of a dying patient's life is still considered unethical by the AMA and is illegal in every state except Oregon.

A leading physician in medical ethics once admitted, "I have had occasion to give a patient pain medication we both knew would shorten her life."[31] Does this differ from killing her?

In palliative care, physicians practice *terminal sedation*, which stands on the doctrine of double effect where the physician must not intend death but merely the relief of pain. Does such sedation differ from killing the patient? Is the difference only semantic?

In 1975, in a famous article in the *New England Journal of Medicine*, the philosopher James Rachels attacked the distinction between active and passive euthanasia.[32] Rachels argued that this distinction, though still dominant in modern medicine and law, has no inherent moral value and, when it is erroneously taken for anything more than a shorthand pragmatic rule, leads to decisions about death based on irrelevant factors.

Rachels's logic cuts two ways: first, letting a vegetative patient die is just as bad (or good) as killing him or her; second, killing a vegetative patient is just as good (or bad) as allowing him or her to die. There is nothing moral or immoral in the act of passive or active euthanasia itself; instead, morality or immorality is determined by motives and results in the context of that act. Focusing on whether an act is active or passive, he argued, may confuse our judgments, leading us to think that passively allowing people to die slowly and horribly is morally superior to actively bringing about a quick, painless death.

Rachels caused controversy. Is intending death by removing a respirator equivalent to suffocating a patient with a pillow? If a patient is allowed to die, isn't that patient killed by the disease? But if someone acts directly to bring about dying, isn't that human agent the cause of death? One critic argued:

> What is the difference between merely letting a patient die and killing that patient? Does it depend upon activity or passivity? Does it depend on an agent's intentions? I think that neither of these factors is relevant. What is relevant is the cause of death. When the cause of death is the underlying disease process, the patient is simply allowed to die.[33]

In support of Rachels, it can be argued that in practice the line between active and passive is hard to draw. In some cases, not acting can be considered active; one example might be not giving antibiotics to Karen Quinlan to treat the pneumonia she developed in her final weeks.

This does not entail that killing and assisted dying do not differ; as Jean Davies argues, just as "rape and making love are different, so are killing and assisted suicide."[34]

Relief of Suffering

One of the most persuasive arguments for physician-assisted dying is the appeal to mercy. Observing another human being in untreatable pain howling like a wounded animal can move even the most callous of us to tears. The most natural response is to end such suffering. We do this for our pets; why can't we do the same for humans? Moreover, the suffering of terminal patients is not confined to physical pain, as bad as that is: it also involves helplessness, stress, exhaustion, terror, loss, and other experiences that are difficult to imagine.

A big issue here has to do with relief of pain. Is it possible to relieve all pain and make dying patients completely comfortable? Cicely Saunders, who founded St. Christopher's Hospice in London, says her patients never need suffer pain. She gives them Brompton cocktails, a powerful brew of morphine, heroin, alcohol, and cocaine.

On the other hand, Derek Humphrey of the Hemlock Society argues that "it is generally agreed that ten percent of pain cannot be controlled. That is a lot of people."[35] Margaret Battin and Timothy Quill acknowledge that 2 to 5 percent of terminal patients experience pain that is incontrollable, even with excellent palliative care.[36] It is also true that not everyone experiences pain in the same way, and a condition that would be acceptable to some patients might be intolerable to others.

A second question concerns what the cost of relief might be, and what costs are acceptable. In this context, we are not talking about financial costs: the issue is the cost to the patient's well-being. Powerful narcotics such as Brompton cocktails numb consciousness and can reduce patients to a vegetative state during their last months of life.

Dying patients must make a tradeoff between consciousness and relief of pain, and not every patient considers that tradeoff acceptable. For some patients, being conscious and able to talk to relatives and friends is more important than avoiding pain. Here again, autonomy becomes relevant. What counts as a benefit or a harm must be defined within each patient's own value system, and who else but patients can make judgments about this tradeoff?

Ethics and medicine commonly distinguish between pain and suffering. *Pain* is physical; *suffering* is a broader and more personal matter. Pain is only one aspect of suffering, and relieving a patient's pain does not necessarily relieve suffering.

Peter Admiraal, a physician and one of the leaders of assisted dying in the Netherlands, agrees that uncontrollable pain is rarely the only reason for death:

> There is severe dehydration, uncontrolled itching and fatigue. These patients are completely exhausted. Some of them can't turn around in their beds. They become incontinent. All these factors make a kind of suffering from which they only want to escape. . . .
>
> And of course you are suffering because you have a mind. You are thinking about what is happening to you. You have fears and anxiety and sorrow. In the end, it gives a complete loss of human dignity. You cannot stop that feeling with medical treatment.[37]

In Oregon, uncontrolled pain does not drive most patients to legally kill themselves, but uncontrolled suffering does. Such suffering mostly surrounds tiredness, shortness of breath, vomiting, nausea, open wounds such as those from common pressure sores, and beliefs about the meaninglessness of continuing the slow process of natural dying.[38]

Cries for Help

Joanne Lynn, a physician who has cared for over 1,000 hospice patients, believes that most terminal patients who request physician-assisted death seek attention, control, dignity, relief of symptoms, or relief from depression. Sometimes the request is a plea to see "if anyone really cares whether he or she lives".[39]

Physicians trained in palliative care believe aggressive treatment can ameliorate almost all unpleasant symptoms. With such specialists and good medical coverage, dying need not be undignified or painful.

It is especially important with terminal patients not just to deal with physical symptoms. Terminal patients are often bored and depressed: people avoid them. People who once had important work to do now have nothing to do. People who never watched television now are forced to watch it all day long. Good psychiatrists know how to help.

Dying at home cures some problems. It is empowering to be dying in your own home rather than a hospital, which has its own routine and hierarchy.

Allowing physician-assisted dying would be the easy way out on several fronts. First, physicians don't need to aggressively treat symptoms. Second, the system doesn't need to change to train more people in hospice and palliative care.

In a review of the literature, bioethicist Margaret Pabst Battin, known for her decades of work on dignified death, and physician Timothy Quill conclude that physician-assisted dying should be an option of last resort after all resources of excellent palliative care are exhausted.[40] Even though they defend legalizing physician-assisted dying, they stress that it must be no substitute for lack of great palliative care.

So here is a recipe for physician-assisted dying gone wild: cheap care, poorly trained nurses and physicians, managed care plans that don't pay for palliative medicine or hospice or long-term nursing care, and young people impatient for their elders to "get on with it and die."

Patient Autonomy

Let's be frank: people believe different things about the sanctity of life and the wrongness of killing, but what if you're not religious? Or don't see religion as against helping people die? What are we to do? Fight about it? Kill each other over who's right about killing?

One way to say that each person should decide things himself is to say that the *autonomy* of patients should count most. "Autonomy" means the ability to be self-governing and self-directed. Its opposite is to be treated paternalistically, like an incompetent child.

Autonomy mattered to John Stuart Mill, who argued in his *On Liberty* that "over his own body and mind, the individual is sovereign." Mill's view implies that government should not impose its view of when and how people should die.

Autonomy raises some questions about risks: Who is best qualified to assess the danger of dying too soon? What degree of risk is acceptable? Who should determine acceptability? How does the risk of dying too soon compare with the risks entailed by alternatives?

Physicians usually believe that they are best qualified to assess risk, and they're right as far as statistical risk is concerned. But *acceptable* risk is evaluative as well as statistical, and many patients want the right to make their own judgments about what is acceptable risk.

When terminal patients make such evaluations, their concern is more than just fear of pain. Derek Humphrey of the Hemlock Society has written, "It isn't just a question of pain. It is a question of dignity, self-control, and distress. If you can't eat, sleep, or read, and the quality of life is so bad, and there is a certainty that you are dying, it is a matter of dignity" to be able to end your life.[41]

In order to evaluate acceptable risk, patients need information. Margaret Battin holds that physicians rarely discuss options with dying patients.[42] She believes that patients' informed consent should be sought not only for medical research but also for ways of dying. Especially when experimental drugs and surgery are involved, terminal patients should be informed about different outcomes and different ways of dying so that they can choose the *least worst* death. Alas, few patients get such information and are allowed to make such choices.

INDIRECT ARGUMENTS ABOUT PHYSICIAN-ASSISTED DYING

The Slippery Slope

One of the most famous ideas in ethics is the *slippery slope*, also called the "thin edge of the wedge"—or simply "wedge"—argument. Claims about it figure prominently in debates about physician-assisted dying.

Slippery slope arguments assert that if a preliminary neutral or good step is accepted, a series of other changes then occur, leading to a final terrible result. It metaphorically sees society as teetering like a ball perched atop a steep slope and leaning downward, braced only by chocks or wedges on the ground, preventing it from descending. The chocks are our basic moral principles.

There are two general kinds of claims about slippery slopes: *empirical* and *conceptual*.[43] Claims about *empirical slopes* assert that once you take the first step, something bad in human nature is unleashed, which will be uncontrollable. In the article by Leo Alexander mentioned previously, he refers to an empirical slope: "The destructive principle, once unleashed, is bound to engulf the whole personality and to occupy all its relationships."[44]

A *conceptual* slippery slope asserts that once a small change is made in a moral rule, other changes will soon follow, because of the demands of reason for consistency in treating similar cases similarly. Alexander also refers to this kind of slope:

> The beginnings at first were merely a subtle shift in emphasis in the basic attitude of the physicians. It started with the acceptance of the attitude, basic in the euthanasia movement, that there is such a thing as life not worthy to be lived. This attitude in its early stages concerned itself merely with the severely and chronically

sick. Gradually the sphere of those to be included in this category was enlarged to encompass the socially unproductive, the ideologically unwanted, the racially unwanted and finally all non-Germans. But it is important to realize that the infinitely small wedged-in lever from which this entire trend of mind received its impetus was the attitude of the nonrehabilitable sick.[45]

Once physicians are permitted to kill one kind of patient because quality of life is so low as to make "life not worthy to be lived," they not only can, but *will* use the same reasoning in similar cases.

An *empirical* slope prediction says that once society changes a rule about protecting one class of patient, powerful forces will be unleashed that cannot be restrained and kept contained to the original class. Something like this was unleashed in Dr. Michael Swango when he started to kill: Charged and convicted in 2000 with killing three patients in New York State, Dr. Michel Swango killed at least 60 patients, possibly hundreds, starting in Zimbabwe in the early 1980s and moving around the world (when arrested, he was on his way to Saudi Arabia for a new job).[46] His diary revealed that he killed for the thrill of the power to kill and "the sweet, husky, close smell of an indoor homicide."

It is just such malice in human nature that could be unleashed with legal, physician-assisted deaths. Law professor Yale Kamisar observes that "not all people are kind, understanding, and loving. Yet they will be making decisions about the elderly and helpless.[47]

Consider another example of a conceptual slope: first we will allow abortion of a fetus because of Down syndrome, then we will let a newborn with Down syndrome die. In this kind of slope, as opposed to empirical slopes, *it is always the demand of reason to treat similar cases similarly that expand the initial change.*

This kind of reasoning is seen in the following claims. At the time of the Karen Quinlan case in 1976, disability advocate James Bopp said that if you "accept quality of life as the standard," then "first you withdraw the respirators, then the food and then you actively kill people. It's a straight line from one place to the others."[48] Bioethicist Daniel Callahan then said that the logic of the case for euthanasia will inevitably lead to its extension far beyond terminally ill competent adults. If relief of suffering is critical, Callahan said, "[W]hy should that relief be denied to the demented or the incompetent?"[49] In the claims of these people, what justifies one kind of case will soon justify another.

Contrasts may be made among the two kinds of slope claims. The empirical claim is a prediction about consequences if some moral change occurs, whereas the conceptual claim refers to a linkage in reasoning once particular premises are accepted. Where the empirical slope says one small change will create many others because of something bad in humans, the conceptual slope says the same kind of change can occur because of something higher in humans—reason's need to treat similar cases similarly.

Claims about slippery slopes are difficult to evaluate because the predicted, final bad event is so far away. However, critics predicted that slippery slopes would occur during the Karen Quinlan case, with Holland's changes, and with Oregon's legalization, so we can evaluate such predictions.

In 1975, columnist Nat Hentoff predicted that the *Quinlan* decision would bring on an empirical slippery slope. In 1992, he felt vindicated in describing

Jack Kevorkian's actions and the decriminalization of physician-assisted dying in the Netherlands, all of which he called a "reckless cheapening of life."[50]

What can we say about these claims? First, if the danger of an empirical slippery slope were real, we would have expected the precedent of the Quinlan case to first, make it easy for competent patients to die, and second, to generalize to other kinds of incompetent patients, such as senile, demented patients in nursing homes. Yet neither happened. It took 22 years after the *Quinlan* decision before the first terminal patient legally died with the help of a physician in Oregon in 1998, and the Schiavo case showed us how far we are from readily accepting the deaths of incompetent PVS patients. Hardly empirical slippery slopes.

What about Oregon? Physician-assisted deaths there over the first eight years averaged about 25 to 40 a year. Hardly the thousands and thousands of deaths predicted by critics.

What about Holland? Here a real expansion of cases has occurred. The 1991 Remmelink Report on physician-assisted dying by the Dutch government discovered that about 1,000 patients had died every year who were not competent and hence had not met the guidelines.[51]

What about this? First, almost 99 percent of the patients killed had cancer or AIDS. Second, these patients had a physician who knew them intimately and who had treated them for years, such that when they became unconscious before they could make (and repeat) their request for assisted dying, these physicians knew the wishes of these patients.

But in a sense, claims about slippery slope have come true in Holland. Teenagers, psychiatric patients, and newborns who are suffering and terminal have been killed with their consent or the consent of their proxies. At present, guidelines for killing irreversibly dying infants are being considered.

Callahan's prediction has come true, but the Dutch regard it not as a downward descent but as a moral elevation: if it's justified to kill a consenting, terminal 64-year-old with terminal cancer, why isn't it also to kill a consenting 16-year-old with terminal cancer?

Inefficient Means

Opponents of legalization claim that physician-assisted deaths are botched 25 percent of the time in Holland and therefore should be illegal.[52] This is a strange argument because it complains about the "how to" part of legalization, in other words, physicians at present aren't good enough to guarantee death.

Of course, death for some patients will not be easy. Some AIDS patients who were intravenous drug-users and who attempted suicide at dosages recommended by the Hemlock Society had high tolerances to central-nervous-system depressants, and did not die easily or quickly, sometimes merely ending up in vegetative comas.

To avoid this possibility, the patient needed to ask a friend to be present to possibly help at the end by attaching a large plastic bag over the patient's head and securing it with duct tape, such that the patient could suffocate to death. (This is what critic Nat Hentoff calls the "Exit Bag," sarcastically referring to the efficient, self-administered form of it with velcro straps that once could be ordered from the Hemlock Society.[53]) Use of Exit Bags subjects friends to charges of murder, and leaves dying patients faced with the dilemma of dying alone and botching the attempt or asking a friend to be present, assist, and risk prosecution for assisting in suicide.

This is why Oregonian physicians may attend the deaths of terminal patients. If something goes wrong, they can adjust medications or deal with unexpected complications. In short, this argument is not an argument for no physician-assisted dying, but for *more* of it.

A Financial Empirical Slope?

"Money makes the world go 'round," and some people were shocked when Oregon made it possible for a physician to not only help a patient die, but to be paid for doing so. For them, once we allow physicians to make money on assisted death, Pandora's Box is really open and great evil will occur.

In fee-for-service medicine, the more procedures a physician does on a dying patient, the more money the physician makes. New systems of managed care give the physician all his money at the beginning of the year, and if he goes over that allotment, he loses money, whereas if he is under, he gets a bonus. In the old, fee-for-service system, physicians had a financial motive to keep a dying patient alive as long as possible. In the new system, the motives are reversed.

The claim about an empirical slope here is that the cheapness of families and the avarice of physicians will conspire to speed sick patients to an early grave.

Is this claim true? The honest answer is that we don't know. Hard times have not tested American physicians this way. They are used to aggressively treating patients and being well-paid to do so, especially in oncology, cardiac surgery, and cancer surgery.

One nagging worry is that some historians think that the ultimate reason for the rise of Nazi Germany was economic. After losing World War II, the Germans were made to pay huge war reparations, which caused great harm to the German economy and created much ill-will. Since World War II, and especially in the last two decades, North America has experienced an unparalleled economic boom. What will happen when times turn bad again and families must choose between grandma's care in a long-term nursing home and a child's college tuition?

It is odd that in formal discussions of ethical issues in medicine, money plays only a small role. One emergency room physician, Norman Paradis, raised this issue publicly in connection with the death of his own father, a surgeon, who was diagnosed with pancreatic cancer, the most lethal and swift of all cancers.[54] Paradis's father told him that he had seen "physicians torture dying patients" and insisted that he wanted neither surgery nor chemotherapy. Paradis assured his father that, as a physician, he knew what to do. He was sure that his strong, direct, professional-to-professional communication with his father's physicians was unequivocal: Make my father comfortable; do no more.

As soon as he left, however, his father was taken to surgery. Why? Because, Paradis says, "consulting surgeons get paid thousands of dollars an hour when they 'decide' to operate." When the younger Paradis called to refuse his consent for further surgery, he was told that his decision was "mistaken." His father underwent further, massive surgery and died the next day. Medicare paid more than $150,000 for these operations. When Paradis objected to Medicare officials, claiming that his father's physicians had proceeded without consent and had violated proper procedures, he was told that there were so many cases of fraud over $1 million that they could not be bothered with his case. Paradis concludes, "Our health system is structured to meet reimbursement rather than patients' needs."

Perhaps the surgeons in this case were genuinely convinced that surgery was an acceptable risk and in the patient's best interest, but perhaps they were guilty of a conflict of interest. If it is fair to argue against physician-assisted dying by pointing out that some families and institutions may seize the advantage to save money, it is also fair to note that some physicians and institutions make millions by maintaining the status quo. Isn't it possible that some specialists could lose enormous amounts of money if assisted dying were practiced? And if so, might they not have a conflict of interest in opposing assisted dying?

In most areas of life, we assume that people work for money, and we give them monetary incentives to work harder. When it comes to physicians, we assume that they will be moral and will not recommend treatments only to make money. Perhaps most of them don't. However, when a reasonable case can be made for denying treatment, treatment is often administered anyway—and the physician makes more money. Is this just a coincidence, or is there some connection?

In sum, this argument cuts both ways. If money motivates everything, then patients are kept alive and "tortured" so physicians can make more money. Which is worse? Such torture or early deaths?

The Roles of Physicians

Some physicians argue that "Physicians should not kill" and should always be healers. This statement assumes incorrectly that physicians can always heal. That is false. The mortality rate is 100 percent among humans. No human has ever been "healed" of death. So eventually, each human must confront death with his or her physician.

Second, to simplistically assert that, "Physicians should not kill" begs the key question of this chapter. It is like saying that, "Physicians should not do what is wrong," while assuming without argument that such-and-such is wrong.

It should be noted about roles of physicians that in Oregon where the law allowed physician-assisted dying, no physician in the United States must assist a patient who wants to die. As with abortion, only a small percentage of physicians help terminal patients die and it is voluntary.

Lastly, the controversy about the role of physicians in assisted suicide has focused too much on Jack Kevorkian and not enough on the larger picture. Every year, over two million Americans die. Most of us will die of cancer, coronary artery disease, stroke, or one of the degenerative diseases. Despite all the newest drugs and all the medical advances, and according to the detailed descriptions of

Yale surgeon Sherwin Nuland's *How We Die*, almost every American over age 60 will die a miserable death.[55] Is this progress? Every day, hundreds of people are spending their last six months of life in misery. Again, is this progress?

Mistakes and Abuses

Physicians make mistakes. Surgeon Christiaan Barnard recalled a young woman with ovarian cancer who repeatedly begged him to kill her painlessly with morphine.[56] Aware that she was terminal—and hearing her screams at night—Barnard decided to help her. When he came into her room with a syringe loaded with morphine, she was quiet, and he thought at first that she was in too much pain even to scream. Then he realized that she was semiconscious, beyond pain, and he changed his mind. The next morning, she felt better; soon she was in remission, and then lived another few months. Stories like this abound in medicine.

In Holland, some critics claim that physicians often misdiagnosis "intractable and unbearable" suffering. In Janet Adkins's case, many people were quick to say that physicians aren't infallible diagnosticians and that patients sometimes defy a dire prognosis.

Let us put this point differently. In bioethics, many discussions begin with a phrase like, "If a patient has a terminal illness. . . ." Notice the word "if." In presumably terminal illnesses, few claims are absolute until the patient's last days. Before then, how "terminal"—how close to death—the patient is may depend on many factors that are not easy to assess: the patient's attitude, the family's attitude, the attitude of staff members, the quality and level of care, and so on. Moreover, some terminal patients were misdiagnosed and recovered. Physician-assisted dying allows a mistaken diagnosis to become a death sentence. Once physician-assisted death occurs, there is no appeal.

Israeli physician Seymour Glick also reveals a dirty little secret of medicine: every physician has some patients that he or she really hates. Some deaths are messy, some families are intolerable, and sometimes, physicians make mistakes and harm patients. In all these cases, physicians want the cases to "go away." The easiest way to make them go away is for them to die. But we should never open this door.

Conclusions

Since Karen Quinlan's court decisions in 1976, critics have predicted that euthanasia would sweep North America. It hasn't. Only one state legalized physician-assisted dying, and since 1998, it has had remarkably few patients use the new law—fewer than two hundred. Holland continues to be happy with its liberalization, and several European countries have liberalized their laws, too.

Nevertheless, physician-assisted dying remains contentious in America and in American medicine. Perhaps the most heartfelt concern is among disability advocates, who fear that lack of resources will push families and the disabled themselves to accept too-early deaths.

FURTHER READING AND RESOURCES

Sherwin B. Nuland, *How We Die: Reflections on Life's Final Chapter,* Vintage Books, 1995.

Kathleen M. Foley and Herbert Hendin, eds., *The Case Against Assisted Suicide: for the Right to End-of-Life Care,* Johns Hopkins University Press, 2002.

Derek Humphry, *Final Exit: The Practicalities of Self-Deliverance and Assisted Suicide for the Dying,* 2nd rev. ed., DTP, 1997.

Sherwin B. Nuland, *How We Die: Reflections on Life's Final Chapter*, Vintage Books, 1995.

The Case Against Assisted Suicide: For the Right to End-of-Life Care, (eds) Kathleen M. Foley, Herbert Hendin, Johns Hopkins University Press, 2002.

Derek Humphry, *Final Exit: The Practicalities of Self-Deliverance and Assisted Suicide for the Dying,* 2nd Rev. ed. DTP, 1997.

Timothy Quill and Margaret Pabst Battin, eds. *Physician-Assisted Dying: The Case for Palliative Care and Patient Choice,* Baltimore, Md.: Johns Hopkins Press, 20.

CHAPTER 4

Abortion

The Trial of Kenneth Edelin

This chapter discusses abortion and its history prior to its legalization by the U. S. Supreme Court in 1973, the trial of Kenneth Edelin for the death of a late-term fetus, subsequent legal developments, and ethical issues about abortion. It also discusses the 1973 *Roe* v. *Wade* decision and its fine-tuning, controversial fetal experiments in the 1970s, fetal and fetal-tissue research, the killings of physicians who perform abortions, and emergency contraception (Plan B).

Kenneth Edelin and Alice Roe

The case of Kenneth Edelin began in Boston in October 1973. To understand it, we must understand events that happened several months earlier, just after the U. S. Supreme Court announced *Roe* v. *Wade* in January 1973.

One earlier event involved an experiment that had been performed on aborted fetuses at Boston City Hospital, where Edelin was a resident. Some physicians reasoned this way: Since aborted fetuses were going to die anyway, why not use them in experiments to help other fetuses?

This research studied substances ingested by the mother that might harm the fetus. To determine which drugs crossed the placenta, physicians gave women undergoing abortions the antibiotics clindamycin and erythromycin and examined aborted fetuses. They discovered that these antibiotics cross the placenta and concentrate in fetal livers.

In another study in 1973, researchers tried to develop an artificial placenta. They obtained eight fetuses by hysterotomy weighing between 300 and 1,000 grams. When researchers placed the largest of them in a warm saline solution that mimicked the amniotic sac, it gasped frantically and moved its limbs as it died.[1] In another experiment on lack of glucose to the brain, researchers severed heads of 12 nonviable fetuses after stopping their hearts but before anoxia damaged their brains. The researchers successfully maintained the fetal brains with artificial replacements for glucose.[2]

An article describing the first experiment appeared in June 1973 in the *New England Journal of Medicine*, a publication edited in Boston.[3] Boston Catholics got copies of it in the mail.

74

Protestant theologian Paul Ramsey called such experimentation "unconsented-to research on unborn babies" and exploitation of a "tragical case of dying" babies.[4] These experiments outraged Americans. After publicity about them in 1975, Congress banned all federally funded research involving fetuses or embryos.

A councilman held a hearing in September 1973 to investigate fetal experimentation at Boston City Hospital. During it, antiabortionists packed the auditorium and heard Mildred Jefferson, an assistant professor of surgery at Boston University, who not only opposed abortion but who also was African-American. At his trial, she testified against Edelin.

Jefferson testified, perhaps correctly, that some women undergoing abortion in a study at Boston City Hospital were too young to consent legally and had not consented in writing. If the researchers had failed to obtain legal consent, they could be charged with "grave robbing," illegally procuring bodies for medical experimentation.

As a result of these hearings, nothing happened to the researchers or to Boston City Hospital, which continued to experiment. But the city of Boston, overwhelmingly Catholic, festered about legalized abortion. In this milieu in late 1973, Edelin performed a controversial abortion at Boston City Hospital.

In 1973, Kenneth Edelin was 35 years old. The son of a postman, he grew up poor in Washington, D.C. He did his undergraduate work at Columbia University, received his M.D. from Meharry Medical College, interned in Ohio, and then served for three years as a U.S. Air Force physician. In 1971, he began his residency at Boston City Hospital, known as a public hospital for poor people and the model for the television show, *St. Elsewhere*. Edeline was also African-American.

Alice Roe is a pseudonym for a 17-year-old black West Indian student, who remained otherwise anonymous. Edelin's faculty supervisor, Hugh Holtrop, examined Alice, estimating her to be 22 weeks pregnant. Enrique Giminez, a first-year resident from Mexico, estimated her to be 24 weeks pregnant (Giminez later testified against Edelin); a third-year medical student, Steve Teich, who assisted during the abortion, agreed with Giminez's estimate. At the time, the underfunded hospital had no ultrasound machine and could not make the estimate more precise.

Even though Holtrop had admitted Alice Roe, and even though he intended to abort a late second-trimester fetus, he delegated third-year resident Edelin to perform the abortion. Like most attending physicians at this hospital, Holtrop had a private practice and spent little time there, so third-year residents normally did this kind of surgery.

To complicate matters, Holtrop had obtained Alice's and her mother's permission for another fetal experiment, this time to see if aminoglutethamide increased the hormone output of the placenta. Accordingly, Holtrop gave Alice aminoglutethamide intravenously and analyzed her urine over the next 24 hours. His study took place on October 1-2, 1973.

Edelin planned to abort the fetus by injecting saline solution into the amniotic sac, but the next day, when he inserted a needle to sample her amniotic fluid, he drew blood. This indicated that Alice had an anterior placenta, one attached to the front wall of her uterus. Saline injected into the placenta could travel into her bloodstream, where it could be lethal.

So Edelin rescheduled the abortion as a hysterotomy for the next day. A hysterotomy is abortion by caesarean surgery; and involves cutting through the lower abdominal wall. Instead of Giminez, Edelin chose as his assistant the third-year medical student. However, Giminez watched the hysterotomy anyway, uninvited, from a distance.

What happened next is controversial. Giminez later testified that Edelin made the cesarean section, reached in, cut the placenta from the abdominal wall, waited three minutes, and then removed a dead fetus. If such a wait took place, that is important, because a baby cannot breathe on its own inside the uterus: it only begins breathing when it is brought outside. Edelin would soon be charged with neglecting the baby by not removing it immediately, causing it to suffocate.

Afterwards, someone took the fetus to the morgue, and—as required by hospital policy for aborted fetuses weighing more than 600 grams—preserved it in formalin. This meant that the district attorney had a body for the crime and photographs of it to show a jury.

One fact about this case merits emphasis. Edelin had originally intended to abort the fetus by saline injection, and if the position of the placenta had been different, he would have been able to do so, and legally. For the safety of the mother, he performed the abortion by hysterotomy; this left him vulnerable to a charge of manslaughter.

The Case in the Courts

A grand jury decided that enough evidence existed to indict Edelin. Some legal strategists believe that Edelin erred by testifying at his pretrial hearing and by not invoking his Fifth Amendment right against self-incrimination. In contrast, Holtrop invoked this right, did not testify, and was not indicted. After the hearing, Edelin changed lawyers.

The principal participants in the trial were Newman Flanagan, the prosecuting district attorney, known as competent, tough, and a showman; Edelin's trial lawyer, William Perkins Homans, Jr., a rich Boston lawyer who often defended unpopular causes; and the presiding judge, James McGuire. The jurors—selected after much wrangling between the lawyers—were mostly white; three were women and 13 were men; 10 were Catholic. A study had predicted that jurors likely to convict Edelin would be blue-collar Catholics over 50 years old, who had dropped out of Catholic high school and who read Catholic newspapers.

The district attorney charged Edelin with manslaughter, defined in Massachusetts as "wanton, reckless" omission or commission of an act which causes death; Massachusetts law further defined "wanton, reckless" conduct as "the legal equivalent of intentional conduct" and as "disregard of the probable consequences to the rights of others." The trial judge gave the jury the following description: "The essence of wanton or reckless conduct is the doing of an act or the omission to act where there is a duty to act, which commission or omission involves a high degree of likelihood that substantial harm will result to another."[5]

Massachusetts did not pass an abortion law until August 1974 (19 months after *Roe* v. *Wade*), and in the absence of a specific state law, Judge McGuire instructed the jury that *Roe* v. *Wade* was "absolutely controlling." Since *Roe* v. *Wade* equated personhood with viability, this meant that the jury had to determine whether Alice's fetus had been viable.

The Supreme Court had said only that viability is "usually" placed at 24 to 28 weeks, not that viability necessarily falls within that range. It had not specified how to determine whether a late-term fetus was viable. In Alice Roe's case, if the fetus was not viable, no person had been killed; and if no person had been killed, a manslaughter charge could not be brought.

Edelin testified that the procedure he performed on Roe had seemed long to Giminez because at this stage of pregnancy the thick abdominal wall had not yet stretched enough to be easily cut. Because he considered it safer than a vertical incision and because it would leave less of a scar, Edelin said he had made a Pfannenstiel ("bikini") incision. One surgeon commenting on the case wrote that making such an incision would take a while, especially for a resident who had never done one before, but not three minutes.[6] Edelin testified that Giminez had confused the initial abdominal incision with the second incision detaching the placenta.

Over the angry objection of the defense attorney Homans, the prosecution introduced a picture of the fetus as evidence. Homans argued that the picture would be inflammatory and would tell laypersons nothing about fetal viability. Judge McGuire allowed one picture to be shown, but charged the jury with not viewing it "from any emotional point of view."[7]

When district attorney Flanagan summed up, he argued that when Edelin cut the placenta, the fetus had been a person; that Edelin had waited three minutes; that this delay constituted "wanton, reckless conduct"; that legal abortion was not intended to produce a dead fetus, but merely to end a pregnancy, and therefore that Edelin should have saved the fetus (which Flanagan said had been live-born) before cutting its placenta.

Judge McGuire instructed the jury that an unborn fetus was not a person and could not be the subject of a manslaughter indictment. Such an indictment could refer only to a person, which Massachusetts law defined as a fetus that has been born, *a baby*. Birth was the key event, and the judge instructed the jury: "You must be satisfied beyond a reasonable doubt . . . that the defendant caused the death of a person who had been alive outside the body of his or her mother."

So the jury had to decide: (1) Had Alice Roe's fetus been alive outside Alice's body? (2) If so, did the baby die as a result of "wanton, reckless conduct" by Edelin? The jurors said, "yes" to both points and convicted Edelin of manslaughter.

Judge McGuire sentenced Edelin to a year of probation. If this conviction and sentence had stuck, he would have lost his medical license.

National media intensely followed Edelin's trial. Pro-abortion groups supported Edelin, as did some antiabortion physicians who hated prosecution of physicians more than legalization of abortion. Medical journals supported Edelin.

Antiabortion groups saw Flanagan as their white knight. Edelin had stepped over a legal line separating persons from nonpersons and killed a person; he had to be punished. A few months later, as they contemplated crossing a similar line, Karen Quinlan's physicians took notice.

After the verdict, liberal media implied that a black man in an abortion case in Catholic Boston couldn't get a fair trial. Even the conservative William Buckley said, "The case can be presented as the lynching of a black Marcus Welby by a big-oted community."[8] The foreman of the jury retorted that the aborted fetus was black and that he had also been concerned about its life.

Edelin appealed, and the Massachusetts Supreme Court heard his case on direct review. Almost immediately, Boston City Hospital gave him a vote of confidence by offering him a permanent position.

In 1976, more than three years after Edelin had aborted Alice's fetus, the Massachusetts Supreme Judicial Court overturned his conviction, declaring that no evidence of criminal negligence had been presented at his trial. The higher court said, "In the comparative calm of appellate review, the essential proposition emerges that the defendant had no evil frame of mind, was actuated by no criminal purpose, and committed no wanton or reckless act in carrying out the medical procedures on Oct. 3, 1973."[9] Because its judges split about abortion and the case, the Court did not require a new trial but simply acquitted Edelin.

Upon hearing of his acquittal, Edelin was "jubilant." He said, "It's great to be able to smile again after 2 1/2 years."[10] In his television news program that evening, anchor Walter Cronkite triumphantly announced that Edelin had been acquitted of "manslaughter by abortion."[11]

William Nolen, a surgeon-writer who carefully examined the evidence in the case, concluded that the fetus had not been outside the womb, had not been born and thus there should have been no manslaughter charge.[12] Nolen concluded so not only as a surgeon but also as someone who opposed abortion.

Nolen believed that Edelin had intended to abort a late, second-trimester, or early third-trimester, fetus but once he had opened Alice, had been surprised to find her fetus viable. Nolen doesn't say that Edelin suffocated the fetus, but he does say that whether a newborn has a will to live can be known only if the physician takes it out of the womb, slaps it, and helps it to breathe:

> What is disturbing in the Roe case is that, by his own admission, Edelin made no attempt to see if the child had that spark. As [Jeffrey] Gould [another physician who testified] said, the will to live isn't always immediately apparent; it becomes obvious only if "the physician will try to stimulate, will try to give a little bit of oxygen, and look for a favorable response." . . .
>
> The Roe baby wasn't given this bit of provocation that might—just might—have shown it had the will to live. Why? The answer is distressingly simple. No one wanted the Roe baby to live.[13]

Newman Flanagan went on to become one of the longest serving district attorneys in America, working in one capacity or another in the Boston DA's office for decades. Kenneth Edelin practiced medicine around Boston for a decade and later became associate dean for students at Boston University Medical School.

BACKGROUND: PERSPECTIVES ON ABORTION

The Language of Abortion

This book will use medically accepted terms for the stages of a human life, so after sperm meets egg and conception occurs, an *embryo* results, which after nine weeks until birth is called a *fetus*, which at birth is called a *baby*.

Definitions of these terms have legal and ethical consequences. For example, a baby can be the subject of a homicide charge, but not a fetus. Critics of abortion object to the connotation of "fetus" as a being containing less value than a baby and refer to the growing fetus as a "baby."

Abortion and the Bible

Many Christians and Jews believe that the Bible or the Torah forbids abortion. In this regard, Paul Badham, a British professor of church history writes:

> The Bible certainly teaches the value of human life, and forbids the murder of any human being (Psalm 8). But life, in biblical terms, commences only when the breath enters the nostrils and the man or woman becomes a "living being" (Genesis 2:7). . . . Consequently in biblical terms the fetus is not a person. This is brought out clearly in the laws relating to murder. For though the Ten Commandments in Exodus state clearly, "You shall not murder," the text goes on, in the following chapter, to differentiate between causing the death of an adult human being and causing the death of an unborn human fetus. For whereas "whoever hits a man and kills him shall be put to death" (Exodus 21; 12), " . . . if some men are fighting and hurt a woman so that she loses her child, but is not injured in any other way, the one who hurt her is to be fined." There is no suggestion in the Old Testament law, as there is in a comparable Assyrian one, that "he who struck her shall compensate for the fetus with a life." Indeed, the biblical text does not ever regard the loss of her fetus as causing the woman "harm," for it goes on to specify what should happen "if any harm follows." At no point is any consideration given to the notion that the fetus itself might have rights. And this absence of concern for the fetus is also implied by the imposition of the death penalty on women who conceive out of wedlock, without any consideration being given to the fact that this killed both the fetus and the woman (Deuteronomy 22:21, Leviticus 21:9, Genesis 38:24). . . .
>
> Turning to the issue of abortion as such, I am somewhat puzzled that biblical fundamentalists, who oppose abortion so strongly, should pay so little heed to the silence of the Bible on this issue . . . Whether this silence is significant or not, the fact ought to be faced that whatever views one may hold about abortion, no straightforward appeal can be made to the teaching of the Bible, for the Bible simply does not discuss it.[14]

Nor does Jesus speak against abortion anywhere in the Gospels.[15]

If abortion is not condemned in the Old Testament or the Gospels, why do so many Christians reject it? An answer will be given in historical stages.

The Old Testament took its final form during the fifth century before the Common Era (B.C.E.) and the New Testament was finalized around the year 200 of the Common Era (C.E.)—when Christianity began as an organized religion. As an organized religion, Christianity has always opposed abortion, but its view of what constitutes an abortion has changed over two thousand years.

By the fourth century C.E., Christian teaching about sex was in crisis. Christianity idealized celibacy, but if too many Christians took it seriously, Christianity would die out (as the later Christian Shakers did die out). Practically, most people could not uphold lifelong celibacy. Consequently, Augustine revised Christian teaching to allow sexual intercourse in marriage, but only if the couple intended to have children.[16] It follows for Augustine that abortion is sinful because it thwarts the only justification for having sex: to produce a child.

In the 12th century, Christian doctrine began to separate abortion from homicide by distinguishing between "formed" and "unformed" embryos. The concept had to do with the soul rather than with physical development.

In the 13th century, St. Thomas Aquinas held that God ensouled male embryos at 40 days of gestation, female embryos at 90 days. Aborting a male embryo at 40 days was punished more severely than aborting a female embryo at the same age, since the male was formed but the female was not. Although abortion at any time was sinful, penalties increased when the fetus was formed.[17]

During the 19th century, scientific evidence discredited the Thomistic concept of ensoulment. Microscopes revealed life at tiny stages, including human life.

In 1870, Pope Pius IX resisted the growing power of science by convening the First Vatican Council. It declared that his edicts and those of future popes would be infallible.[18] From 1869 to 1900, the Church encouraged veneration of Mary (which had been neglected), supported Creationism against geological explanations of the origins of the universe, emphasized miracles, and vigorously attacked Darwinism.

Around 1850, popes denounced abortion in increasingly absolutistic terms. During this time, Catholicism came close to teaching that personhood began at conception, a view called immediate animation.[19]

The Catholic *doctrine of double effect* allowed two exceptions: ectopic pregnancy and uterine cancer (in which uterus and fetus must be removed together). According to this doctrine, an action having two effects, one good and the other evil, is morally permissible under four conditions: (1) if the action is good in itself or not evil, (2) if the good follows as immediately from the cause as from the evil effect, (3) if only the good effect is intended, and (4) if there is a proportionately grave cause for performing the action as for allowing the evil effect.

Historical Catholic doctrine was stricter than the law. During the 17th century, European common law did not indict women for aborting even a quickened fetus. Finally, in 1803, an English statute made abortion of a quickened fetus a capital crime.

From the 17th through the 19th centuries, American law followed English common law: Abortion before quickening was only a misdemeanor. In 1973 in its *Roe v. Wade* decision, the United States Supreme Court reviewed the legal background of abortion and concluded:

> It is thus apparent that at common law, at the time of the adopting of our Constitution, and throughout the major portion of the 19th century, abortion was viewed with less disfavor than under most American statutes currently in effect. Phrasing it another way, a woman enjoyed a substantially broader right to terminate a pregnancy than she does in most States today. At least with respect to the early stage of pregnancy, and very possibly without such a limitation, the opportunity to make this choice was present in this country well into the 19th century. Even later, the law continued for some time to treat less punitively an abortion procured in early pregnancy.[20]

In America, this leniency changed after the Civil War, when most states criminalized abortion. From 1870 to 1970, the American medical profession opposed abortion.

Feminist historians argue that this opposition stemmed from paternalism, misogyny, and protecting professional turf:

> Anti-abortion legislation was part of an anti-feminist backlash to the growing movement for suffrage, voluntary motherhood, and other women's rights in the nineteenth century. The prevailing public prudery and anti-sexual moralism condemned feminism and considered sex for pleasure evil, with pregnancy as punishment.[21]

Before the Civil War, midwives delivered most babies, and in doing so, competed with physicians over birth. After this war, physicians took over birth, and most physicians were men. So bans on abortions helped men drive midwives out of obstetrics and helped medicalize birth.

Modern Developments

Before the Supreme Court legalized abortion in 1973, women who had abortions often had horrible experiences. Physicians who performed abortions often did so only for the money, and some demanded sex. Others lectured women on their promiscuity.

Though abortion is painful, abortionists didn't use anesthesia. Beforehand, physicians didn't explain to women what would happen or why. If damage occurred, women had no legal recourse. Women frequently did not know the name of the abortionist, who forbade them to contact him again. Illegal abortions cost a lot and were beyond the reach of poor women and teenagers.

Despite these conditions, during the 1950s and 1960s, hundreds of thousands of American women had illegal abortions. Some died as a result: 193 died in 1965 alone, and during the 1960s, over 1,000.[22]

Because what they had done was illegal, victims of botched abortions came into emergency rooms only at the last moment. Some died of widespread abdominal infection, and those who recovered often were sterile. Poor women of color ran the greatest risks; in 1965, 55 percent of abortion-related deaths were among them.

1962: Sherri Finkbine

In 1962, Sherri Finkbine, living with her husband and their four children in Phoenix, Arizona, became pregnant with a fifth child.[23] During her fifth month of pregnancy, she took thalidomide, an antinausea drug. It was just becoming apparent then that thalidomide is a teratogen ("monster former") that produces babies with missing arms or legs.

Thalidomide had been tested on animals, but not on *pregnant* animals. The tragedies it caused made the FDA test all future drugs on pregnant animals.

Sherri Finkbine requested an abortion at a local hospital, ostensibly for her health, but really to abort a fetus that would be born missing its arms and legs. However, if she had the abortion, the district attorney threatened to prosecute her, so the Finkbines flew to Sweden, where therapeutic abortion had been legal since 1940. Swedish physicians then aborted her severely deformed fetus.

1968: *Humanae Vitae*

In 1968, five years before *Roe* v. *Wade*, Pope Paul VI issued his encyclical *Humanae Vitae* that declared use of birth control to be a sin. The edict startled liberal Catholics and drove them to defy church teachings. A quarter of a century later in 1993, Pope John Paul II vigorously defended *Humanae Vitae* and its ban on birth control.[24]

The 1968 encyclical had an unintended effect: when they were not allowed to teach both sides of the moral issues about contraception at Catholic University in Washington, D. C., Catholic priests such as Warren Reich, Albert Jonsen, William Curren, and Paul Tong left the priesthood and Catholic universities. These apostates became founders of the new field of bioethics, a field that tries to teach all sides of moral issues in medicine.

1968–1973: Steps Toward *Roe v. Wade*

In the years preceding *Roe* v. *Wade*, 18 states liberalized laws about abortion. Hawaii began in 1970, followed by Colorado, North Carolina, and California. Governor of California, Ronald Reagan, signed its bill into law.

If *Roe* v. *Wade* had not eliminated the need, more states would have followed suit. If the Supreme Court ever made abortion an issue of states' rights, and because these state laws are still on the books, most American women could still have legal abortions in these states.

By legalizing abortion, *Roe* v. *Wade* did not force people to change their views. Many Americans had already changed their views, and *Roe* v. *Wade* in 1973 simply reflected that change.

1973: *Roe* v. *Wade*

The decision of the United States Supreme Court in *Roe* v. *Wade* (1973) concerned Jane Roe, a woman from Dallas, Texas, whose real name was Norma McCorvey. Wade was Henry Wade, district attorney of Dallas County. When this case began in 1970, Texas criminalized all abortions. Norma McCorvey wanted a safe, legal abortion and challenged the Texas law.[25] (She later recanted and became an antiabortion advocate.)

The Supreme Court had already decided in *Griswold* v. *Connecticut* (1965) that the Constitution's implied right to privacy or liberty allowed couples to receive birth control pills. In *Roe* v. *Wade*, it decided that the same liberty included the right of a woman to decide whether she wanted to stay pregnant or to abort her fetus.

This right was not unqualified. A woman's right to abort her fetus was balanced against the rights of the fetus to live, which increased as its gestational age increased. The Court's decision over time has been regarded as well-reasoned. It defended a *gradient view of personhood*, that the fetus becomes more of a person as it develops, such that personhood is not all-or-nothing but admits of degrees.

For legal purposes, the Court drew the line at viability. After but not before viability, states could ban abortions. The Court defined viability as the point when a fetus is able to live outside the mother's womb. It placed viability between

24 and 28 weeks. The Court summarized its trimester system, in which viability divides the second and third trimesters, as follows:

> (a) For the stage prior to approximately the end of the first trimester, the abortion decision and its effectuation must be left to the medical judgment of the pregnant woman's attending physician.
> (b) For the stage subsequent to approximately the end of the first trimester, the State, in promoting its interest in the health of the mother, may, if it chooses, regulate the abortion procedure in ways that are reasonably related to maternal health.
> (c) For the stage subsequent to viability, the State in promoting its interest in the potentiality of human life may, if it chooses, regulate, and even proscribe, abortion except where it is necessary, in appropriate medical judgment, for the preservation of the life or health of the mother.

Note that a state "may" forbid abortion, but need not. A state could legalize abortion at any time up to birth. Note that a state may pass a law allowing abortions in the third trimester not only to preserve the *life* of a mother but also to protect her *health*.

Antiabortionists argue that this permission constitutes a loophole justifying any abortion. Two physicians can almost always be found who will say that continuing the pregnancy would endanger the mother's health.

After abortion became legal, American women had about 1.5 million abortions per year, a figure that remained steady for a decade.[26] During the last decades, the number steadily dropped. In 2006, it dropped to about half the original number, around 800,000 a year.

ETHICAL ISSUES

Personhood

What is a person? With abortion, some philosophers draw a distinction between a person and a human being. They argue that although a fetus is human, it does not meet certain criteria of personhood; and that since a fetus is not a person, it does not have a right to life. In this sense, *human* is a factual term, whereas *person* is an evaluative term.

Mary Ann Warren famously defends *a cognitive criterion of personhood* and holds that a fetus does not meet this criterion.[27] According to her, to be a person is to be able to think, to be capable of cognition. What separates a person from a rat is certain capacities—for reasoning, reflective self-awareness, communication, agency, and consciousness of the external world. Warren does not think that any one of these capacities alone is sufficient for cognition; rather, these capacities define as a group the core criterion. A being lacking *all* of these capacities fails to meet the cognitive criterion and cannot be a person

Let us examine some issues concerning this cognitive criterion. To begin, the definition may be both too broad and too narrow, because it includes some nonpersons and excludes some persons. The cognitive criterion does seem to admit to personhood some beings that we don't traditionally regard as persons; for instance, apes communicate, are conscious, may reason and may be self-aware, yet we don't ordinarily consider them persons.

The cognitive criterion may imply that society should not protect human beings whose cognitive capacities are absent, have been lost, or that are merely potential, such as patients in the late stages of Alzheimer's disease, permanently comatose patients, or newborn babies. If a fetus can be aborted because it fails to meet the cognitive criterion, is it permissible to kill these others? The cognitive criterion seems to say it is.

Personhood as a Gradient

Why does personhood have to be all-or-nothing? Why does the moral status associated with personhood have to be all-or-nothing? In practical reasoning, the all-or-nothing fallacy consists of treating complex issues as if they have only two simplistic, extreme answers when in fact there are many compromises in between. Often, practical solutions reside not on black or white poles but in gray areas in the middle.

Biologically, we know that the human embryo develops by degrees during the first trimester into a fetus, and then over the next trimester, the fetus grows into viability, and finally, during the last trimester, into a baby. Just as no one event or day along this nine-month journey marks *the* day of personhood, so no one day at the end or beginning marks *the* day. The most accurate view is that personhood accumulates by degrees over time.

On this view, a 2-year old is more of a person than a newborn baby, and a 26-year-old at the height of his powers and health is more of a person than a 2-year-old. If personhood depends in part on capacities, then a human at maximal capacities is more of a person than a human with few capacities.

At the end of life, people lose personhood by degrees, especially with diseases that rob them of their minds. A person who once had a great memory and an I. Q. of 140 is only "half the man he once was" at age 90 with initial Alzheimer's and an I. Q. of 80.

We think of personhood as all-or-nothing for two reasons. First, some people believe that a metaphysical event occurs in which human bodies get ensouled or where a soul departs. Before ensoulment, there is no personhood and no moral value, and after that event, there is.

Second, people confuse personhood with moral concern. If granddad with Alzheimer's at 90 is only half the person he once was, that does not mean that his caretakers only owe him half the concern of a full person. Just the opposite: humans who have lost their former capacities need *more* concern and care than persons at maximal capacity. Who is a full person differs from whom we care about.

That's true for nonhuman animals, too. Some of them may be half-persons, especially as they function in our family. Some family pets may be as high on its scale of concern as its children.

In biology, the gradient view expresses human evolution by degrees from other primates, and primates in turn from lesser organisms. All life is an evolving continuum, connected by common ancestors and by degrees, not huge leaps.

Marquis and Quinn on Potentiality

If we accept the cognitive criterion, a problem arises. If what makes people valuable is cognition, is it wrong to deprive beings of potential cognition? And wouldn't deprivation of potential cognition make abortion wrong? Philosophers Don Marquis and Warren Quinn offer two premises: first, what is wrong about killing a person—a college student, for example—is depriving him or her of future cognitive experiences; second, what is wrong about killing an adult person is also what is wrong about killing a human fetus.[28]

Their argument is an interesting one, and many people accept their first premise. Other explanations of why it is wrong to kill a person—that killing violates a person's rights, for instance, or that killing is against God's will—beg the question: phrases such as "violation of rights" and "against the will of God" are simply other ways of saying that an act is wrong.

Marquis's and Quinn's second premise may be more vulnerable. A being without an already existing self or personal identity cannot have a personal future of which to be deprived. Consider an analogy: Imagine an omnipotent deity—God—who creates a universe, then considers creating a second parallel universe, but then decides against it. Now imagine a powerful evil force—Satan—who wants to destroy the existing universe. It seems that destruction of the existing world by Satan would be wrong; but it does not seem wrong for God to refrain from creating a second world. Although God has disallowed a vast amount of cognitive experiences in the parallel universe, he has neither done any wrong nor wronged any person in not creating it. In the same way, failing to allow the potential cognition of a human fetus to come into existence wrongs no existing person.

This attack on Marquis's and Quinn's position appeals to the idea of a baseline and harm, discussed in the next chapter. The basic idea is that without some baseline of existence, no person can be harmed.

What about contraception or masturbation? As either of these prevents potential persons from coming into existence, are they wrong? Probably not. They seem to be a straw man—a false opponent, too easily refuted. No antiabortionist wants to produce billions of extra people.

Instead, antiabortionists see each particular person as valuable from conception. Federal judge John Noonan advocates a genetic criterion, and argues that when sperm and egg meet and merge genes, a genetically unique individual is created. The resulting embryo has all the potential in its DNA to be a full person, provided that it finds a nurturing uterus.[29]

But *potential* to become a person is not being a normal person, as we realize when we consider the thousands of frozen embryos stored around the world. Another problem with the genetic criterion is that it collapses the distinction between being human and being a person—as we realize when we consider that a dead human has a unique set of genes. These implications seem to be a *reductio ad absurdum* of the genetic criterion.

A third possible criterion for personhood might be called the *neurological criterion*. This minimal version of the cognitive criterion defines a person as a human being with a detectable brain wave. This simple standard applies to many issues of medical ethics; it recognizes as persons both quasi-anencephalic babies and adults in persistent vegetative states. With regard to abortion, the neurological criterion would consider a fetus a person when it developed brain waves, but not before.

Viability

The concept of viability is vague. A vague concept is one with no sharp boundaries, e.g., "baldness." When does viability begin? In *Roe* v. *Wade*, the Supreme Court said only that viability is "usually placed" at about 28 weeks, but "may occur earlier, even at 24 weeks."

In Edelin's trial, district attorney Newman Flanagan seized on this vagueness and tried to establish that Alice Roe's fetus had been viable. One antiabortion physician testified that a baby could live outside the womb after as little as 12 weeks of gestation. But for how long? Only a few minutes, the physician testified, though maybe for longer. However, the defense attorney, William Homans, counterpunched by asking the physician how he defined viability; the physician said that viability was "capacity to survive [outside the womb] even for a second after birth." As Homans questioned several other physicians who were testifying as expert witnesses for the prosecution, he got each of them to admit that he had never known a fetus to survive for even a few days outside the womb before 24 weeks of gestation.

Edelin's critics knew exactly what was meant by viability: ability to survive independently of the mother. In reality, some fetuses that are born early are not viable: They will die no matter how hard physicians try to keep them alive. Others will survive, and will only do so if given the chance.

To Edelin's opponents, the point was that he had never tried to determine viability. His supporters replied that of course he had not tried because *the whole point* of abortion is to kill a fetus. The point is not to look inside the uterus, see if the fetus is viable, and if it is, rescue it. No, the goal of abortion is to produce a dead fetus.

The Argument from Marginal Cases

In the Edelin case, one question that arose was, "Where do you draw the line?"—that is, the line between fetuses which may and may not be aborted. Reasoning based on this kind of question is called the *argument from marginal cases*, and it is one of the most widely used ideas in ethics. With regard to an issue like abortion, the argument from marginal cases is as follows: Beings at the margins of personhood cannot be nonarbitrarily distinguished from those at the core.

This argument also appeals to a gradient of personhood, only this argument flips the conclusion. Where pro-choice advocates say an embryo is not a baby, antiabortionists point to the smooth continuum and say there is no place to draw the line.

So there is no identifiable point of ensoulment, personhood, or even viability. No matter what week of gestation we consider, it is arbitrary to make that week the marker of personhood, because the fetus of a week earlier has almost the same qualities. Whatever time or marker is chosen, someone can always ask: Why not choose a day before?

The argument from marginal cases is related to the problem of jumping the fact-value gap, since another way of expressing this argument is to say that when marginal cases exist, there is no factual point or marker that could serve as a nonarbitrary connecting premise between facts and values. That is, the question "Where do you draw the line?" implies that in certain moral issues, any candidate for a fact-value connecting premise will inevitably jump the fact-value gap. Consider the argument about abortion that was used as an example above:

Premise I: A human with a brain wave is a person.

Premise II: Killing a person is morally wrong.

Conclusion: Therefore, killing a human with a brain wave is morally wrong.

In this argument, premise I—which combined the evaluative definition of a person with a factual statement about fetal brain waves—connects facts (brain wave) and values (personhood); but according to the argument from marginal cases, that premise is arbitrary. Why? Because any other event in fetal development might equally be chosen as the factual marker. Any other marker we could choose (human form, sentience, neural development) would also be arbitrary, because fetal development is a continuum.

Is the argument from marginal cases a good one? Consider an analogy with the color spectrum: although each shade in the spectrum resembles the shades next to it, we can distinguish widely separated colors. Similarly, a full-grown oak tree differs from an acorn, even though an acorn becomes an oak by continuous growth. Similarly, we can distinguish a eight-cell human embryo from a newborn baby. Marginal cases do not make distinctions impossible.

Thomson: A Limited Pro-Choice View

Suppose we admit that the fetus in the Edelin case was a person. Does it follow that killing it was immoral? Philosopher Judith Jarvis Thomson argues that it does not.[30]

Imagine you have been admitted to a hospital for an operation, and awaken to find yourself hooked up to a famous violinist. His kidneys have failed and his blood is entering and leaving your body through tubes. Without your permission, your kidneys have been used to keep the violinist alive.

Thomson argues that it is immoral for the hospital to force you to keep the violinist alive. Although it would be saintly of you to agree to stay, you are not *obligated* to do so. Why? Because you did not consent to have your body used this way and no one else has a right to make you use your body to keep another person alive.

Just as the violinist cannot demand as a right that you keep him alive by allowing your kidneys to be used, so a fetus has no right that a woman keep it alive. For Thomson, the most telling case is rape, because a rape victim has not consented to sexual intercourse or conceiving a child. She thinks a similar argument applies when a woman has used contraception responsibly but it fails.

Thomson's argument is an example of reasoning by analogy. The violinist's dependence on the other patient is analogous to the fetus's dependence on the

mother. In analogical reasoning, the closer the fit between the two things compared, the stronger the inferred conclusion is supported.

Thomson's critics object to her analogy. They argue that the patient who is
being involuntarily used can simply unhook herself, and that detaching tubes
from your body is not like killing a fetus. Since something active must be done to
end a fetus's life, for a proper analogy, the violinist would have to blocking the
patient's way out of the room, so that the patient could escape only by cutting up
the violinist.[31] (Better: imagine a gigantic baby blocking the way out.)

The above arguments suggest abortion as self-defense. In the 16th century, theologian Thomas Sanchez used Augustine's doctrine of just war to identify an embryo
growing in a fallopian tube as an unjust aggressor against the mother's life. So
Sanchez maintained that a mother could kill such a lethal embryo in self-defense.[32]

Feminist Views

One feminist writer argues that the key question about abortion is whether
women should be forced to bear children in a way in which men are not. If an
embryo is a person who has a right to life at the mother's expense, then women
will always be potential slaves of biological reproduction:

> With all the imperfections of our present-day attitudes, I'm still a lot better off in
> terms of the sexual choices I have than women of my mother's generation. I was
> a lot better off after the sixties than I was before them. What sexual freedom I now
> have has been very hard-won. I wouldn't give it up for anything. . . . There is
> larger crisis, one that has to do with the tensions between feminism and the back-
> lash against it. On the one hand, society is encouraging sexual freedom; on the
> other hand, it's punishing people for indulging in it and not emotionally prepar-
> ing them for it. Both women in general and teenagers in particular are caught in
> the middle.[33]

Conservative Religious Views

Some people believe that each human pregnancy happens for a reason. Each
human embryo that has been conceived and survived to implant itself in the uterine wall was meant by God to have been created at this place and time. Any interference with the growth of that embryo would thwart God's plans. As one
sometimes hears, "God must mean for me to be pregnant, else I wouldn't be."

Two replies can be made to this view. First, how does a woman know God's
will about a particular pregnancy? Unless God speaks to her directly, how can she
just assume that *planning* when to have children is not God's will for her? How
does she know that God does not want her to do what she believes will be best for
her, now and in the future?

Second, such a view is fatalistic in one's personal relation to God. It seems
reasonable to ask, "Why must I accept everything that happens? If everything
comes from God, doesn't the choice to have an abortion also come from Him?
Why make the fatalistic assumption that one can follow God's will only by
accepting pregnancy? Why can't a reasoned choice to have an abortion also
reflect God's will?"

Abortion as a Three-Sided Issue

Many people living in a tolerant democracy, where individual liberties are respected, fail to understand how they got where they are or to understand the larger, worldwide picture. In the United States, they forget that our modern policy of individual rights and personal liberty represents a hard-won victory that citizens of many other countries never achieved.

For instance, if they became pregnant before their mid-20s or after they already had a child, millions of women in China were forced to undergo abortions (the Chinese government imposed a limit of one child per family). In Romania under the long dictatorship of Nicolae Ceaucescau, millions of women were denied contraception or abortions because this dictator wanted a larger population and forced women to have as many children as possible.

Perhaps this ignorance explains why the media frame abortion as an issue with only two sides: antiabortion versus pro-choice. In fact, the global picture of abortion is three-sided, with two extremes and a compromise: *forced birth* versus *forced abortion*, with individual choice as the middle ground.

Antiabortion Violence

Efforts to overturn *Roe* v. *Wade* took various paths since 1973. Some involved legislation, but the most prominent involved protests and violence.

During the 1980s, protesters bombed many abortion clinics. Two men from Texas who attacked several abortion clinics in Florida were sentenced to 30 years in prison; among other crimes, they had kidnapped a physician who performed abortions. In 1984 alone, there were 24 arson or bombing attacks on abortion clinics. One bombing, in Pensacola, Florida, took place on Christmas morning and was described by one of the conspirators as a "birthday present to Jesus."[34] A few weeks earlier, a bomb at a clinic near Washington, D. C., almost killed a guard.

By 1990, public opinion had turned against antiabortion violence. As a result, the vast majority of the antiabortion movement turned to the kind of nonviolent protest mounted by Operation Rescue, an organization founded by Randall Terry in 1988. Modeling themselves on the nonviolent demonstrations in the South during the civil rights movement, protesters practiced civil disobedience in front of abortion clinics, hoping to arouse the conscience of the nation. Some leaders were fined and jailed for blocking traffic and other minor infractions of the law.

During the 1990s, the protest movement targeted physicians who performed abortions as the weak link in the chain; these physicians sometimes found protesters outside their homes on Saturday mornings. Such harassment led in 1993 to the murder of physician David Gunn as he was leaving an abortion clinic in Pensacola, Florida. Dr. Gunn, who lived in Birmingham, Alabama, with his two teenagers, had been performing abortions once a week there. His picture had been posted across northern Florida by antiabortionists with a "WANTED" sign on it. Spokespersons for Rescue America and Missionaries to the Unborn announced that Dr. Gunn's death had saved numerous babies from abortion; later, one of these spokespersons "rejoiced" when the Pensacola clinic found it difficult to replace Dr. Gunn.

In 1994, physician John Britton and his security escort James Barrett were killed for performing abortions at another abortion clinic in Pensacola, Florida. The assailant, a former minister, Paul Hill, also wounded Barrett's wife. Although Britton wore a bulletproof vest, Hill fired at his head at point-blank range. In 2003, the state of Florida executed Hill for the murder.

In January 1998, an explosion rocked the campus one peaceful morning at the University of Alabama at Birmingham. Across the street at Ronald McDonald House and a block away at a dorm, windows shook from the blast. When he touched the package outside the small abortion clinic, Robert Sanderson, an off-duty Birmingham policeman, was killed. When the dynamite exploded inside the package, a steel plate ricocheted hundreds of nails into the face, torso, and legs of Emily Lyons, a nurse at the clinic, and into Sanderson. Due to intense efforts a few blocks away at UAB hospital, Lyons survived.

An alert UAB student spotted Eric Rudolph leaving the scene and police searched for him for five years in the hills of North Carolina. Arrested in 2003, he confessed in 2005 to bombing abortion clinics in Birmingham and Atlanta, gay/lesbian nightclubs, and the Centennial Olympic Park bombing during the 1996 Olympics, where he killed three people and injured 111.

In 1998, a New York physician who performed abortions was killed by a sniper after he returned home with his wife and four sons from synagogue. During the previous four years, snipers shot and wounded three Canadian physicians and a physician practicing near Rochester, NY. Dr. Barnett Slepian was shot and killed in his kitchen by a gunman firing through a window and crouching behind his backyard fence. Slepian had been targeted by antiabortion groups since the 1980s and had vowed not to let the groups deter him from providing abortions.

At abortion clinics between 1977 and 2006, seven physicians and nurses were killed, 17 attempted murders occurred, 41 bombings occurred, and 173 bombings/arson attempts were foiled. Antiabortionists retort that, in the decades since abortion has been legalized in America, 30 million human fetuses were killed, five times the number of humans killed in the Holocaust.

Access to abortion continued to be an issue in rural states such as North Dakota and Nebraska, where abortion clinics have been closed because of lack of support of the medical community.

Attempted Abortions Resulting in Live Births

Attempts to abort late-term fetuses have sometimes resulted in live births. In 1977, physician Ronald Cornelson testified in a California criminal court that after a botched saline abortion resulted in a live-born 2 1/2-pound baby, his colleague William Waddill had choked the infant and suggested injecting it with potassium chloride to kill it.[35] Waddill was tried twice for murder, but both juries deadlocked. In 1979, at the University of Nebraska Medical Center, after an attempted abortion, another 2 1/2-pound baby was born alive; it was purposefully left unattended and died after a few hours.

Because of such cases, physicians today rarely abort a fetus after 23 weeks. Today, physicians doing abortions rarely use prostaglandins to induce abortion because, although safer than suction or surgical techniques, they result in 30 times more live births.

For first-trimester abortions, the most typical technique was formerly injection of saline or urea, followed by dilatation and curettage (scraping, a technique called D & C); but D & C has been replaced by suction curettage or uterine aspiration. For late-term abortions, dilatation and evacuation (D & E) is used: The fetus is cut into parts and removed piecewise. To ensure that all the pieces have been removed—since any fragments left behind would produce infection in the mother—the dismembered fetus must be reassembled outside the womb. Late second-trimester or third-trimester abortions use hysterotomy, as in the Edelin case.

Because abortion is controversial, residency programs in obstetrics sometimes offer no training in performing abortion. Some residents in obstetrics have demanded such training.[36]

In 2005, a review of several hundred scientific papers concluded that nerve connections in the fetal brain are not developed enough before 29 weeks for the fetus to feel pain.[37] As such, the authors concluded, aborting a fetus before this point caused it no pain and no anesthesia need be used to spare the fetus pain.

Fetal Tissue Research

Tissue from aborted fetuses may help patients with neurological disorders such as Parkinson's disease. The tissue required for such neurological research must be adrenal tissue producing dopamine; and it must be obtained from fetuses whose gestational age is eight to 11 weeks, since after 12 weeks the tissue begins to differentiate into the normal cells of the brain and loses its elasticity. Treatment consists of dopamine delivered as fetal cells: In the operation, a small hole is drilled through the patient's skull and fetal cells are dripped directly into the devastated area of the brain.

A panel of the National Institutes of Health studied this issue and concluded that even if abortion were immoral, fetal tissue obtained from abortions could be used for research if the woman's decision to donate tissue was separated from, and came after, her decision to abort.[38] In 1993, President Clinton lifted the four-year ban on fetal tissue research.

Emergency Contraception

In America, the traditional approach to preventing pregnancy has been either abstinence or contraception, with abortion as a backup for failures. A middle ground exists between these extremes.

Emergency contraception (EC) has been used without publicity for 35 years in America. It consists of taking a double dose of birth-control pills within 72 hours of an act of unprotected sex, followed by a second dose 12 hours later.[39] When the first dose is taken within 72 hours of sex, EC reduces the risk of pregnancy by 75–90 percent.

Such pills contain estrogen and/or progesterone and block the release of the egg from the ovary, block the movement of the embryo down the fallopian tube, or prevent implantation of the embryo in the endometrium.

This method is a days-after and just-in-case strategy. If Plan A is not to get pregnant, Plan B is how to prevent pregnancy developing.

EC requires either a woman to have birth control pills on hand, or to be able to obtain them 72 hours after unprotected sex. A woman cannot wait for a pregnancy test because her urine changes chemically only after embryonic implantation.

RU-486 (mifepristone), another form of EC, became controversial in the 1990s. Because it was expensive, required visits to medical clinics, and caused extensive bleeding, it has been replaced by other forms of EC.

Advocates for family planning today promote Plan B, a progestin-only form of emergency contraception available over the Internet (www.go2planb.com/) without seeing a physician (and directly, in some pharmacies in the Northwest).[40] Another drug, Previn, which contains both estrogens and progestins, has been used for years in Canada, Africa, Asia, and South America. According to a decision by the Food and Drug Administration in August 2006, a woman can get Previn or Plan B without a prescription at pharmacies in the United States.

In 2005, pharmacists in Illinois at a Walgreens refused to fill prescriptions for Plan B, as did the national Wal-Mart chain of pharmacies. Suits against both by women physicians were successful. Wal-Mart made Plan B available by prescription at all its pharmacies, and Walgreens fired pharmacists who refused to fill prescriptions for it, igniting a debate about conscientious refusal of pharmacists to fill prescriptions.

Maternal versus Fetal Rights

Nancy Klein was in her 20s in 1989 when she went into a coma at an early stage of her pregnancy. Her physicians wanted to abort her fetus to increase her cerebral blood volume and to awaken her. They were also reluctant to give Nancy certain drugs that might injure a fetus brought to term. Antiabortionists went to court to block the abortion, while Nancy Klein's husband, Martin, pressed for it. Martin prevailed and the abortion was performed while people protested outside. After 11 months, Nancy emerged from the coma and now lives a normal life.

Another case of maternal-child conflict concerned Angela Carder and her 26-week-old fetus in Washington, D. C. In 1985, Angela was dying of a rare form of cancer and had requested chemotherapy and resisted a cesarean section to save her baby. The baby was delivered alive but died two hours later, and Angela died two days later.[41]

Both cases raised the issue of who the patient was, the mother or the fetus. Legally, the answer is clear. A fetus inside the womb is not a baby and not a person, but the mother is, so her wishes and her health trump the good of the fetus. But ethically, things become murky *if* either the mother is going to die or *if* the fetus is going to be born. But both cases above show that these "ifs" are often difficult to know.

A flashpoint for maternal-child conflict concerns pregnant mothers using alcohol or illegal drugs. Fetal alcohol syndrome causes the most mental retardation in children.[42] Between 1987 and 1992, 160 women in 24 states were charged with injuring a fetus during pregnancy by taking drugs such as cocaine.[43]

In *Whitner v. South Carolina* in 1993, the South Carolina Supreme Court upheld a law making pregnant mothers on drugs choose between mandatory drug rehabilitation and jail. The law forced the mother to stop using drugs for the good of her fetus.

Critics said that pregnant black women using cocaine were prosecuted but not pregnant white women drinking alcohol, and that harm to the fetus during gestation from cocaine was exaggerated. Defenders of the law estimated that 70,000 American women used cocaine while pregnant and agreed that pregnant women abusing alcohol, white or black, should also be prosecuted. Some also wanted to prosecute women who smoked during pregnancy.

The Supreme Court Fine-tunes *Roe* v. *Wade*

In the three decades since *Roe* v. *Wade*, abortion-rights advocates have pressed for broader protection and antiabortion forces have mounted legal challenges to the original decision. All of this came to a head in 1992 with the Supreme Court's decision in *Planned Parenthood* v. *Casey*. The Court reaffirmed the "essential holding" of *Roe* v. *Wade*, including "the right of a woman to choose to have an abortion before viability and to obtain it without undue interference from the State."[44] However, *Casey* rejected the trimester framework, which the Court decided was too rigid, and removed rights of pregnant women from the legal analysis, replacing them with liberty interests, leaving open the door to protect fetal rights more before viability.

However, over the last decades, it fine-tuned *Roe* v. *Wade*. To this, we now turn.

Viability

In 1983, Justice Sandra Day O'Connor predicted that medicine would push viability "further back toward conception" and that the trimester system established in *Roe* v. *Wade* would be on a collision course with itself. Her prediction has not come true.

Although medicine has made intense efforts to treat premature babies more effectively, the consensus in neonatology is that "before 23 or 24 weeks, [the fetus] simply cannot survive. And nothing that medical science can do will budge that boundary in the foreseeable future."[45] The unsolvable problem is that even with a respirator, the lungs are too immature to function earlier than 23 or 24 weeks of gestation, and certain essential organs, such as the kidneys, do not develop early in pregnancy.

This recently acknowledged fact weakens one argument against abortion. Clearly, the argument from marginal cases must lose some of its force, since lung viability has served for over 30 years as a practical indicator of viability and as a mark of personhood.

In 1979, in *Colautti* v. *Franklin*, the Supreme Court made its major decision about viability. It said that "the determination of whether a particular fetus is viable is, and must be, a matter for the judgment of the responsible attending physician," thus precluding another case like Kenneth Edelin's.

Informed Consent

In *Planned Parenthood* v. *Casey* in 1992, the Court ruled that informed consent and a 24-hour waiting period did not constitute "undue burdens" on women seeking abortions. Antiabortionists said this change brought abortion into line with

informed-consent requirements for other surgical procedures. Pro-choice advocates pointed out that many surgical procedures would not occur if hospitals
enforced a similar 24-hour waiting period.

Consent of Fathers

In 1976, in *Planned Parenthood* v. *Danforth*, the Court invalidated state laws requiring a woman to get consent for an abortion from either a matrimonial or a biological father. The Court held that such consent amounted to giving these men a veto
over the woman's decision. Because the woman "is the more directly and immediately affected by the pregnancy," she should not be subject to any such veto.

Consent or Notification of Parents

The *Danforth* decision also said that a state cannot pass a law giving parents of
teenage girls an absolute veto over a decision to have an abortion. Two later decisions allowed a state, before a teenager's abortion, to require the minor to obtain the
consent of one or both parents, or required the clinic to *notify* one or both parents.

By 2006, 44 states had laws requiring a parent's consent or notification when
minors sought abortions, although nine of those states did not enforce their laws.[46]
Such laws had to have an escape clause where the minor could appeal to a judge
for an exception for parental notification or consent (for cases of incest).

Government Support

Several Court decisions concerned whether the federal government or state governments could be required to fund abortions for women who are unable to pay
for them. In *Harris* v. *McRae* (1980), the Court held that, although a woman has a
right to an abortion, she does not have a right to one at government expense. Congress passed laws banning use of public funds for abortions for women unable to
afford them, and many states followed suit. *Webster* (1989) said that states may
ban public employees or public hospitals from performing abortions.

Partial-Birth Abortions

On the gradient view of personhood, aborting a fetus just before birth is to kill a
being 90 percent a person, and hence is a serious matter. Opponents of abortion
rejecting the gradient view want such fetuses legally recognized as full persons.

The two areas where this concern arises are in murders of pregnant mothers
(Lacy Peterson) and abortions in the late third trimester. Killing a pregnant woman
and her child is a heinous crime, and to inflict greater punishments, people push
for a charge of double homicide. Similarly, few reasons justify killing a fetus after
eight months of gestation, and the methods to do so are grim and surgical.

Opponents of abortion hope that everyone can agree to protect fetuses from
such acts and push for changes in the law to do so. Pro-choice advocates oppose
such legal changes, fearing a slippery slope to protecting the fetus from abortion
at earlier stages.

State legislatures frequently have passed bills making such changes, but federal courts have struck them down 18 out of 19 times.[47] Why? Because a long legal tradition has defined legal personhood as beginning at birth, with the fetus being a baby, and courts have been reluctant to overturn that tradition. To do so would be to go into territory where there is no logical stopping point until viability.

FURTHER READING AND RESOURCES

Francis M. Kamm, *Creation and Abortion*, Oxford University Press, New York, 1992.
Don Marquis, "Why Abortion Is Immoral," *Journal of Philosophy*, vol. 86, 1989, pp. 183–202.
Warren Quinn, "Abortion: Identity and Loss," *Philosophy and Public Affairs*, vol. 13, 1984.
Michael Tooley, *Abortion and Infanticide*, Oxford University Press, Oxford, 1983.
Mary Ann Warren, "On the Moral and Legal Status of the Fetus," *The Monist*, vol. 57, 1973.

CHAPTER 5

Assisted Reproduction:

Louise Brown, the McCaughey Septuplets, Paid Egg Donors, and Elderly Parents

During the last three decades, assisted reproduction has been one of the most exciting fields in medicine, raising many ethical issues.

This chapter discusses the controversy surrounding the birth of Louise Brown, the first "test tube baby," surrogate mothers and the case of Mary Beth Whitehead, buying eggs of younger women, the McCaughey case of septuplets, older parents having children, and related ethical issues.

"Test tube" conception is called in vitro fertilization (IVF). ("In vitro" means "in glass.") It involves fertilization outside the womb, in a Petri dish. Before IVF, people knew how to have sex without making babies; now they have discovered how to make babies without having sex.

Louise Brown: The First "Test-Tube" Baby

Lesley Brown, the mother of the first child conceived in vitro, had damaged fallopian tubes from ectopic pregnancies. For a living, she worked in a cheese factory and her husband, John, drove a truck.

With in vitro fertilization, an egg from the woman is removed and put in a Petri dish, where sperm from a man is mixed in to form an embryo. The embryo is then returned to the woman's womb and, like a normal conception, she then gestates the fetus to birth.

Of relevance to human cloning, the first conception of a human by in vitro fertilization did not happen without years of preparatory work and controversy. Two decades of research by Robert Edwards, a physiologist at Cambridge University, preceded this conception.

Edwards worked with mice in the 1950s and by trial-and-error, learned how to control ovulation. He learned to precisely balance hormones, resulting in the Fowler-Edwards method for induced superovulation.

In 1965, 13 years before the birth of Louise Brown, Edwards tried to fertilize a human egg. Interestingly, Edwards faced barriers so enormous that many scientists thought a birth through in vitro fertilization was impossible, much the same way that human reproductive cloning is thought so today. As with human cloning, Edwards also faced the task of achieving his goal without harming the mother or the fetus.

96

In cloning the lamb Dolly in 1996, Steed Willadsen had to overthrow known "laws" of physiology about cellular differentiation. Similarly, Edwards needed to overthrow "laws" and facts of his time, such as the view that gonadotrophic hormones could not make a mammalian ovary release eggs. Having learned to do so first with mice, Edwards balanced progesterone and estrogen in women, which thickened the lining of the uterus to receive a fertilized egg.

Human sperm had to be "capacitated" for conception by removing chemicals that inhibited penetration of an egg from the head of a sperm. Most scientists believed that capacitation occurred only by exposure to uterine secretions, but Edwards found another way.

Next comes an amazing story. After adding his own semen one night to a ripe human egg in a Petri dish, the next morning Edwards unexpectedly discovered that he had created a human embryo in a test tube.

Did Edwards know that he had thereby unleashed some of the greatest fears of ordinary people about science? The image is from a scary science fiction movie: Lone scientist late at night in lab artificially creates human life, stealing mystery from Life itself.

Perhaps Edwards realized people would be frightened by his feat, so he destroyed the embryo. Later, he tried to repeat his accomplishment, but could not. Nor did he announce what he had done, partly because he could not repeat it and partly to avoid publicity.

Whatever way we look at it, this was truly a seminal experiment.

His next goal was to get enough eggs for his research. Edwards needed lots of eggs, such that sperm could be introduced to many eggs, and he could return only the healthiest embryos to the uterus. To do so, eggs had to be removed, which was a problem in the mid-1960s.

Enter Patrick Steptoe, an obscure gynecologic surgeon practicing in a small hospital near the industrial city of Manchester. Steptoe became Edwards's key partner.

In the mid-1960s, scientists in France and Germany used newly developed fiber optics to create a *laparascope,* a long thin tube containing a lens with a light. Steptoe published a paper describing how he made an incision near the navel and with it could see the reproductive organs and eggs.

Edwards realized its potential for removing eggs and proposed a partnership. Interestingly, Edwards's colleagues frowned upon this partnership. As Joseph Goldstein remarked in 2001 in awarding Edwards the Lasker Award, one of the most prestigious awards in medical research,

> Edwards' colleagues in Cambridge raised their academic eyebrows, thinking he was mad to hook up with a non-academic surgeon in private practice in a backwater hospital who was fiddling around with a dangerous foreign device that should never have been allowed into England in the first place.[1]

Edwards's collaboration with Steptoe began in 1968, but it took a decade of failed attempts to produce Louise Brown. Amazingly, roads were so poor on the east side of England that the trip between Cambridge and Manchester took eight hours, and Edwards worked in a lab at Cambridge that lacked running hot water. In 1969 and 1970, the duo successfully harvested eggs from infertile women and created embryos under glass.

The next decade saw Olympian attempts by the two to achieve an IVF pregnancy, attempts indicative of much medical research today, where one breakthrough comes on the backs of a thousand failures. In the first phase, only after 41 tries did they get an embryo to implant, but then it failed to travel down to the uterus and begin to grow in a fallopian tube.

Over the next decade, they recruited over a hundred infertile women, who volunteered for their experiments in quests to have a baby. They changed from implanting the embryo in the fallopian tube to implanting it directly in the uterus, where they finally succeeded on the 102nd attempt.

The key to success? The same as with the mice: getting the hormone balance right. That "102nd attempt" resulted in Louise Brown.

With Lesley Brown, Steptoe slipped the laparascope through a small slit at her bikini line and guided it into her ovaries, where he searched among the hundreds of eggs for the one being primed for ovulation. Searching for it was difficult enough; but when he found it, he had to insert another thin tube and suction it out. Without Steptoe's perfection of this delicate procedure, IVF would have been impossible.

Then John Brown's semen was introduced to Lesley's egg in a Petri dish containing a culture fluid of salt, potassium chloride, glucose, and a bit of protein. Examination by microscope revealed that a sperm had penetrated the ovum. After being cultured for two days, the resulting embryo was mixed with supportive fluids, put in a syringe that had attached a tiny, flexible tube (like the thinnest strand of spaghetti), and eased it through Lesley's dilated cervix into her uterus.

In 1977, Dr. Steptoe told Lesley she was pregnant. Now a long wait began to see if Lesley would lose her fetus. Before this, many women had eggs successfully fertilized in vitro; a smaller number had eggs implanted with a resulting pregnancy. But of the few who had become pregnant, each had lost the embryo or fetus. Lesley made it to five months, when amniocentesis showed a normal pregnancy.

Lesley developed minor problems during pregnancy: She had a mild case of septicemia (a metabolic disturbance caused by absorption of bacteria at the laparascopy site); also, the fetus was small (today we know this is both normal for IVF babies and a risk to their health). She spent the last month of her pregnancy at Oldham Hospital, by then under siege by the media.

The baby, a girl, was delivered by cesarean section on July 25, 1978. In order to avoid reporters, the delivery took place around midnight with only a few people present.

The Browns called their baby "Louise Joy." She weighed 5 lbs. 12 oz., was entirely normal, and was described as "beautiful, with a marvelous complexion, not red and wrinkly at all."[2] Immediately after the birth, John Brown said, "For a person who's been told he and his wife can never have children, the pregnancy was 'like a miracle.' I felt 12 feet high."

The day after Louise Brown's birth, the London newspapers had huge banner headlines, "IT'S A GIRL!" "THE LOVELY LOUISE!" "BABY OF THE CENTURY! JOY TO THE WORLD!" and the *New York Times* gave the story front-page coverage for three days.

Media coverage exploded. An American reporter telephoned a fake bomb threat to the hospital, hoping to force Lesley outside; in the ensuing evacuation, a pregnant woman went into labor. Another disguised himself as a priest and approached John Brown, asking to be admitted to comfort Lesley. Throngs of Japanese photographers photographed anyone—man or woman—who left Oldham Hospital, on the off chance that one was Lesley.

When someone at the hospital revealed that the birth was imminent, six reporters for the *National Enquirer* left Florida and within 24 hours were at Oldham Hospital trying to buy worldwide rights to the Browns' story from Steptoe; a bidding war started among English tabloids. The *Enquirer* tried to bribe an administrator, offering $100,000 for details about the birth. Before the birth, headlines spread rumors ("TEST TUBE BABY ALMOST DIES").

Steptoe and Edwards refused to be interviewed by reporters. Although everybody wanted to know the Browns' identity and background, Steptoe initially protected their anonymity. He did not want Lesley Brown to be upset; he also wanted to act as a go-between to get the Browns a trust fund for their baby, as he eventually did—reportedly $100,000—for an exclusive story.

This silence on the part of Steptoe and Edwards frustrated reporters, some of whom took liberties in their stories or simply guessed at the facts. *Newsweek* said, for instance: "Steptoe, 65, is a flamboyant and somewhat mysterious figure; he declines to discuss his origins (reported to be in Eastern Europe)."[3] In fact, Steptoe was born near Oxford, had been educated in London, was married, and had two children. The "flamboyant" physician lived the life of an overworked obstetrician at a county hospital in an English industrial city.

Amusingly, *Newsweek* also wrote that Edwards often commuted "in the company of a rabbit that was serving as traveling receptacle for an egg under study." But Edwards wrote that:

> We transferred some fertilized human eggs into rabbits to see if they would grow there, but they didn't. This brief episode with rabbits led to all sorts of rumors in the press and elsewhere, and to a description of me taking hundreds of embryos to Cambridge, and of Patrick driving his Mercedes through Oldham with a rabbit in the seat next to him![4]

Brief Background: In Vitro Fertilization

Conception takes place when a sperm fertilizes an egg. Some people mistakenly believe conception happens in the woman's vagina or uterus, but conception occurs in the upper third of a fallopian tube, when the first sperm penetrates the egg. Sperm move up the vagina, through the uterus, and into one of the narrow fallopian tubes. The two tubes, the size of the lead in a mechanical pencil, normally carry one egg a month from an ovary to the uterus.

In human embryology, a successful union of sperm and egg is called a *zygote*. After conception, a zygote immediately begins dividing. After three days, when this organism travels down the fallopian tubes to try to implant on the uterine wall, it is called an embryo.

In an ectopic pregnancy, the embryo does not reach the uterus but grows in one of the two fallopian tubes; for the mother, this is a life-threatening condition.

Surgery usually must remove the threatening embryo. This is a paradigm where the doctrine of double effect allows an abortion to save the mother's life.

A woman has all her eggs at birth, but only one egg is normally primed each month for conception. Drugs such as Clomid and Pergonal stimulate the ovaries to release more than one egg (a process called *superovulation*).

In at least 40 percent of pregnancies, and possibly as many as 70 percent, the embryo fails to implant on the wall of the uterus, often because of genetic irregularities. More commonly, the mix of hormones is not quite correct that month for gestation.

From nine weeks of gestation until birth, the organism is called a *fetus*. A newborn human being, alive outside the womb, is by custom and law called a *baby*.

About one married couple in 12 cannot conceive a child after two years of trying. Infertility stems from many factors, including the woman's age at the first attempt to conceive, damage from pelvic inflammatory disease, previous abortions, uterine abnormalities, and a man's low sperm count or low sperm motility. Infertility is often blamed on the woman, but men account for 50 percent of it.

Women today anguish as popular reports emphasize that only 7.8 percent at age 42 will be able to have children because 90 percent of their eggs will be abnormal. Because of assisted conceptions to celebrities such as singer Celine Dion and model Cindy Margolis, young women often believe falsely that they have decades to become mothers, when in fact their fertility declines markedly at age 27.

Scientific Reaction to the Birth

Not all medical researchers greeted Louise Brown's birth with jubilation. Two contradictory forms of criticism were that IVF was trivial and it was dangerous.

One director of a fertility program characterized Steptoe's achievement as merely "a cookbook thing." Another critic called the birth a "cheap stunt." Richard Blandau, a well-known fertility researcher and a competitor to achieve this breakthrough, criticized Steptoe for not revealing how many failures had preceded his success and for giving "false hope to millions of women."[5] Blandau claimed Steptoe had violated medical ethics by selling his story to the *National Enquirer* instead of publishing it in a medical journal.

Researchers such as Blandau resented Steptoe because this self-described "county doc" in a small city hospital with poor research facilities had surpassed institutions with enormous budgets. Some of their criticisms were unfair. For instance, Steptoe had sold the story to the *Enquirer* not for himself, but for the Browns. Moreover, Blandau missed the point: Louise's birth mattered not because of its probability or improbability, but because it could be done at all.

Blandau's skepticism was understandable in the light of earlier claims. In a scenario that presaged later scandals about human cloning 50 years later, in the 1940s, physician John Rock had announced a successful IVF but had been unable to prove it. The Italian researcher Petrucci also then claimed to have fertilized a human egg in vitro, grown it for 29 days, and then destroyed it because it was "monstrous." Petrucci's story later fueled fears about monsters, though he had never provided any evidence for his claims.[6]

As events in recent years have shown, fraud can be committed in assisted reproduction. To counter skepticism, Steptoe needed to prove that Lesley Brown's fallopian tubes had indeed been irreparably damaged, otherwise, many critics would say that an egg had "sneaked down" and been fertilized the normal way. This explains why he delivered Louise by cesarean section and why he filmed Lesley Brown's damaged tubes.

Harm to Research from Alarmist Media

In previous years, Edwards had worked on infertility at the National Institute for Medical Research in London, experimenting with surgically excised ovaries, which he bathed in hormones in an attempt to induce the release of eggs. After an alarmist television show on IVF that opened with pictures of an exploding atomic bomb, the institute had suspended his funding. Edwards claims that his scientific supervisor, who had also frozen sperm, flatly told him his work was "unethical"; when asked "Why?" she would say only, "Because it is."[7]

Edwards left for Cambridge University, where he worked on a Ford Foundation grant to study population control and fertility. In 1974, this Foundation stopped funding Edwards because his work offended people.

The press incorrectly called Louise Brown a "test tube baby." This term implied something bizarre—that a baby had been created without egg or sperm. When Lesley later took her baby outside, neighbors expected to see a little monster.

From the beginning of its coverage, the press equated means of overcoming infertility with genetic manipulation and, as with cloning later, predicted creation of mindless slaves or dangerous superhumans. Mindlessly, the chief editor at the *London Times* equated in vitro fertilization with state-controlled eugenics.

In contrast, John Brown saw in vitro fertilization merely as "helping nature along a bit."

Newspapers and television reported constantly about genetic manipulation citing Aldous Huxley's 1932 novel *Brave New World*. Yet such citation was muddled: The controls Huxley had imagined were based on psychological conditioning and worries then about behaviorism, a school of psychology which was then as misunderstood as IVF was in 1978. The extension of Huxley's fictional ideas about psychological manipulation to "genetic manipulation," and then to IVF misled people. Ironically, *Brave New World* described the devastating consequences of loss of choice by individuals, yet media citations of it questioned whether couples should be able to choose IVF to create a baby!

The media and journalists often consider themselves guardians of the public interest, but in the case of Louise Brown, their reporting was misleading. *Quis custodiet ipsos custodes?* (Who guards the guardians?)

Later Developments in Assisted Reproduction

Patrick Steptoe died at age 74 in 1988, just a week before he was to have been knighted at Buckingham Place by Queen Elizabeth II. The same week, Robert Edwards became a Fellow of the Royal Society, one of the greatest awards of the English scientific community.

Edwards today champions greater public support for assisted reproduction and urges England and America to follow the example of Australia, Germany, and France, which fund cycles of in vitro fertilization. He believes that children will be safely created one day by cloning and that such origination poses no deep moral problems.

Louise Brown's mother chose to have a second child, Natalie, by IVF in 1982. In 1993, the three female Browns appeared on American television shows to support research in assisted reproduction. At age 15, Louise was a chubby girl whose friends teased, "How did you ever fit into a test tube?"

On July 25, 1998, Louise celebrated her 20th birthday in London at the House of Commons, along with other adults conceived through IVF. Louise today works in a day care center in Bristol and enjoys going to pubs, playing darts, and swimming. Although she understands the media's interest in her, she now says she just wants to fade into the background and enjoy the life of any 30ish woman at the local pub.

The first IVF baby in America, Elizabeth Carr, was born in 1981. Between then and 2002, over 50,000 babies were born in America through assisted reproduction.[8]

Only 5 percent of babies conceived by assisted reproductive technology (ART) are a result of IVF. Most babies are created by less dramatic techniques such as egg stimulation and injection of concentrated sperm.

In the United Kingdom, one industry source says 50,000 babies have been created by assisted reproduction.[9] In Germany, France, and Australia, where national medical services pay physicians for ART, probably another 100,000 babies have been born. Adding ART births from Scandinavia, Mediterranean countries, and others, the worldwide total is well over a million babies.

Unfortunately, in most of the 1990s and today, about 75 percent of couples who tried IVF and who spent from $10,000 to $100,000 still go home without a baby. In 2002, fertility clinics claimed that about 23 percent of attempts at IVF allowed couples to take home a baby, although the actual figure may be more like 20 percent.[10] Chances worsen for women over 40, and drop with each unsuccessful attempt, from 13 percent on the first to 4 percent on the fourth.[11]

Egg Transfer

Australia's Carl Woods in 1983 created the first human pregnancy from an egg transfer. In the same decade, scientists began gamete intrafallopian transfer (GIFT), which unites sperm and egg not in a Petri dish but inside a fallopian tube, approximately where normal conception takes place.

By the 1990s, egg retrieval no longer required surgery; it could be done by tubal aspiration using ultrasound imaging. Researchers now try to insert embryos not in the uterus but in one of the fallopian tubes. In the 15 years between Carl Woods's first egg transfer in 1983 and 1998, about six thousand middle-aged women gave birth using eggs from young women.[12]

Older men are luckier than older women. A Belgian group in 1993 succeeded in using a single sperm to fertilize an egg, a process called *intracytoplasmic sperm injection (ICSI)* making it possible for the sperm of older men to be used.[13]

Women over 40 can still gestate embryos created from eggs of other, younger women, giving the gestational mother a biological connection to the child. About

10 percent of IVF attempts today use eggs of younger women. This is therapeutic for women who have many genetic diseases in their families, who have eggs damaged by chemotherapy or poisoning, who have had several miscarriages, or who suffer from premature menopause.

Previously, age of the sperm or the age of the gestational mother were thought to cause infertility. However, these two factors can be overcome. The absolute barrier to successful gestation is age of the egg, with rapid drop-offs as eggs deteriorate in women over age 27.

Young eggs in older surrogates make a big difference. Using egg transfer, the success rate for taking a baby home was higher, about 30 percent, and more important, it was 30 percent *regardless of the age of the female gestator*, making egg donation the hope of last resort for many infertile couples. This explains why fertility doctors need the eggs of young women.

Freezing Gametic Material

In October 1997, the first birth occurred using previously frozen human embryos at an Atlanta clinic run by Bruce Tucker.[14] In 1990, two embryos were created from different eggs at a California clinic.[15] One was implanted and became a baby; the other remained frozen. Seven-and-a-half years later, the second embryo was implanted and became a male fraternal twin to his 7-year-old brother. In 2006 in Britain, Emma Davis was an IVF baby born in 1989; her sister, Niamh, also created as an embryo the same year, was born 16 years later.[16] The record for such siblings created together by IVF is 21 years.

In 2002, a California clinic began to freeze eggs of young women about to undergo hysterectomy but who wanted to later become pregnant.[17] Whether these eggs will be viable after unthawing is questionable.

Embryos are screened (selected for good and bad qualities) during assisted reproduction in several ways. As with freezing and thawing of sperm for insemination, freezing and thawing of embryos screens embryos because those incapable of successful implantation do not survive this process. Normal sexual reproduction also screens embryos because 40 to 60 percent of embryos fail to implant because of abnormalities.

When embryos and sperm are stored and frozen, mishaps occur. In the 1990s, a white Dutch couple had non-identical twins, one of which was black (the black couple who created the embryo decided to adopt the baby). In 2002, a white couple in London had black twins because the wrong embryos had been implanted.

On the criminal side, IVF pioneer physician Cecil Jacobsen, who practiced in Fairfax, Va., went to jail for mixing his own sperm to create embryos for implantation in dozens of cases. In southern California, physician Ricardo Asch fled to South America when he was charged with increasing his rates of success by using embryos of other couples without their consent.

Historical Background: Transferring Sperm

The history of helping infertile couples by artificially inseminating sperm of the husband (AIH) is instructive. Around 1850, physician J. Marion Sims, while practicing in Montgomery, Alabama, artificially inseminated 55 infertile women with their husbands' sperm.[18] He produced one pregnancy, though it later miscarried. He was forced to stop because of strident condemnation of his work.

Later in the 1890s in America, Dr. Robert Latou Dickinson was vilified for practicing AIH, although he persevered. Dickinson was accused of abetting "adultery."[19] Indeed, it took nearly a hundred years after Sims's first inseminations for people to accept artificial insemination of donor sperm (AID). That is not progressive. Had Sims *paid* his first sperm donors, his critics would have been legion.

The net result? Hundreds, maybe thousands, of couples in America and Europe remained infertile, blaming each other for being barren, going childless not by choice but by fate, and not having heirs. Thousands of children might have been born, who today might have had hundreds of thousands of descendants.

At the end of the 20th century, insemination of sperm has mostly been accepted. Indeed, Americans have gone from accepting (1) injection of a husband's sperm into the wife's womb, to (2) injection of another man's sperm into a wife's womb, to (3) paying a man for use of his sperm to create a pregnancy, and finally to (4) injection of anonymous donor sperm (AID) into unmarried women wishing to become pregnant. Today, couples and single women can select sperm from men at about 400 sperm banks, where donors receive between $50 and $75 per visit.

Notice that for decades, the media's radar screen rarely noted that men were paid to donate sperm, even though genetically, sperm do not differ as gametes from eggs. Do the issues really differ just because women are now paid for *their* gametes?

ETHICAL ISSUES

Ethical issues about assisted reproduction can be sorted in various ways. As usual, we can ask whether someone is saying that a form of assisted reproduction is intrinsically wrong or merely that it has bad effects now associated with it. In the remainder of this chapter, we sort these issues differently by asking, first, whether some forms of assisted reproduction (AR) are wrong (intrinsically or extrinsically), and second, whether it's wrong (for intrinsic or extrinsic reasons) to pay people who work in AR.

ARE SOME FORMS OF ASSISTED REPRODUCTION WRONG?

IVF as a Religious Issue

Some people feel that infertility is a punishment for sin, imposed by God. Abortions and sexually transmitted diseases contribute to infertility, as do professional women who delay first attempts at conception into their 30s. From these facts, some people claim that God is punishing infertile women and men for their aberrant behavior.

Catholic Views: The Vatican and Augustine

In 1978, the year of Louise Brown's birth, the Vatican condemned in vitro fertilization; one Catholic priest in New York feared that humanity had slipped from "doctoring the patient to doctoring the race." Lest that condemnation be thought of as merely the hasty reaction of just one clergyman, note that after nine years of study, the Vatican *Instructions* of 1987 equated IVF with "domination" and "manipulation of nature."[20] One bishop said: "The Christian morality has insisted on the importance of protecting the process by which human life is transmitted. The fact that science now has the ability to alter this process significantly does not mean that, morally speaking, it has the right to do so."[21] The official position of the Vatican in 2006 is that sexual intercourse between husband and wife is necessary for moral conception; IVF is condemned because it takes place without intercourse.

Nevertheless, many American Catholics reject this condemnation. They see nothing immoral in helping infertile couples have the children they want. Ironically, these Catholics may be closer to historical Church doctrine than the modern Vatican.

For 1,500 years, Christian theology accepted the views of Augustine, a fourth-century philosopher and theologian who taught that *concupiscence,* the desire for intercourse, was evil. Augustine specified that original sin expressed itself in lust, and that sin was transferred through intercourse from generation to generation, and thereafter, Christian doctrine followed his views.

To Augustine, marriage was the only context in which this desire could be fulfilled, and even then, only for the purpose of having children. For Augustine, having children within a marriage was a license to sin; and once a marriage had produced enough children, that license was revoked.

All of which is to say that there is a certain irony in the claim by the Catholic Church that its theological teachings build directly on the teachings of patriarchs such as Augustine. The modern Church says IVF is wrong because no sex act was involved in creating a child, but Augustine said that such a sex act was inherently evil and, if possible, to be avoided at all costs.

Two Protestant Views: Fletcher and Ramsey

During the 1970s, then Episcopal priest Joseph Fletcher defended IVF as permissible for Christians:

> It is depressing, not comforting, to realize that most people are accidents. Their conception was at best unintended, at worst unwanted. There are those who are so bemused and befuddled by a fatalist mystique about nature with a capital N (or "God's will") that they want us to accept passively whatever comes along. Talk of "not tinkering" and "not playing God" and snide remarks about "artificial" and "technological" policies is a vote against both humanness and humaneness.[22]

For Fletcher, each kind of case should be considered on its own merits to see if it would help or hurt humanity; society must not be locked into antiquated religious prohibitions that take no account of consequences. Religion is best when it is "pro people," not when it worships abstract "thou shall not's":

> The real choice is between accidental or random reproduction and rationally willed or chosen reproduction . . . Laboratory reproduction is radically human compared to conception by ordinary heterosexual intercourse. It is willed, chosen, purposed and controlled, and surely those are among the traits that distinguish Homo sapiens from others in the animal genus, from the primates down.[23]

Later, in part because he disagreed so much with the conservative views of Christianity, Fletcher gave up the priesthood and became a secular bioethicist.

Paul Ramsey, a socially conservative Protestant theologian at Princeton University, equated IVF with genetic manipulation and predicted societal horrors from it. In 1970, he implied that if physicians could find a tiny egg and fertilize it, why couldn't they alter its genes?[24] He predicted that if they could, they would; and he held that if they did, it would be sinful.

Ramsey came up with some provocative phrases suggesting vague but disturbing harms to society: "test tube babies," "dial-a-baby," "playing God." He was especially good at creating neologisms for rhetorical effect: "mercenary gestation," "supermarket of embryos," "spare-parts man" (a hypothetical cloned twin grown for this purpose and kept unconscious), "celebrity seed" (sperm banks), "human species suicide" (eliminating genetic diseases).

When Lesley Brown was several months pregnant, at the invitation of Sargent Shriver, Robert Edwards attended a symposium on the ethics of IVF at Washington's Kennedy Institute for Bioethics. While senators, national columnists, and other scientists listened, Ramsey condemned IVF and Edwards. As Edwards described it:

> He had to be seen and heard to be believed. I had to endure a denunciation of our work as if from some nineteenth-century pulpit. It was delivered with a Gale 8 force, and written in a similar vein a year later in the *Journal of the American Medical Association*. He doubted that our patients had given their fully understanding consent. We ignored the sanctity of life. We carried out immoral experiments on the unborn. Our work was, he thundered, "unethical medical experimentation on possible future human beings and therefore it is subject to absolute moral prohibition." I was as much surprised as made wrathful by this impertinent scorching attack. He abused everything I stood for.[25]

Ramsey's view of IVF was not based on its presumed consequences to the child, to the parents, or even to society. Rather, in a view that resurfaced 20 years later in debates about research on embryos, it stemmed from the idea of an embryo as a person. IVF is wrong in itself, Ramsey held, because it is "unconsented-to experimentation" on a person, the embryo."[26]

IVF and Harm to Louise Brown

Many critics predicted that the first baby born after in vitro fertilization might be defective. One obstetrician emphasized that severely defective babies could be created, and that "the potential is there for serious anomalies should an unqualified scientist mishandle an embryo."[27] Another obstetrician said, "What if we got a cyclops? Who is responsible? The parents? Is the government obligated to take care of it?"[28]

Leon Kass, who would later be appointed by President George W. Bush in 2002 as chair of his bioethics commission, argued strenuously that babies created by artificial fertilization might be deformed. "It doesn't matter how many times the baby is tested while in the mother's womb," he averred, "they will never be certain the baby won't be born without defect."[29] Without the certainty of a normal baby, Kass implied that experimental modes of conception were unethical.

Nobel Prize winners were surprisingly afraid to condone experimental methods of assisted reproduction. James Watson feared that deformed babies would be born and that they would have to be raised in custodial homes or killed.[30] (Watson later recanted this view, saying he had been incorrect.) Nobelist Max Perutz, who was a colleague then of Edwards's at Cambridge, also condemned IVF research:

> I agree entirely with Dr. Watson that this is far too great a risk. Even if only a single abnormal baby is born and has to be kept alive as an invalid for the rest of its life, Dr. Edwards would have a terrible guilt upon his shoulders. The idea that this might happen on a larger scale—new thalidomide catastrophe—is horrifying.[31]

In 1977, in *Who Shall Play God?* the alarmist writer Jeremy Rifkin began three decades of self-serving opposition to new reproductive techniques. Rifkin decried any kind of assisted reproduction as evil, as "genetic engineering," which he defined as "artificial manipulation of life." Before Louise Brown's birth, he revved up fears that Louise might be psychologically traumatized:

> What are the psychological implications of growing up as a specimen, sheltered not by a warm womb but by steel and glass, belonging to no one but the lab technician who joined together sperm and egg? In a world already populated with people with identity crises, what's the personal identity of a test-tube baby?[32]

Socially conservative, pioneering bioethicist Dan Callahan argued that the first case of IVF was "probably unethical" because there was no possible guarantee that Louise Brown would be normal, though it would be ethical to proceed with IVF after this first healthy birth. He added that many medical breakthroughs are actually "unethical" because we cannot know that the first patient will not be harmed.[33]

These arguments do not seem compelling. What these critics overlooked was that no reasonable approach to life can avoid risks. Moreover, they demonstrate a psychologically normal but nevertheless illogical tendency to magnify the risk of a harmful but unlikely event. A highly unlikely result, even if that result is bad, still represents a small risk. For instance, an anencephalic baby is an extremely bad but unlikely result, so that possible result shouldn't deter people from having kids.

Paradoxes about Harm and Reproduction

Whether children can be harmed by in vitro conception is a philosophically interesting consideration. The theologian Hans Tiefel writes, "No one has the moral right to endanger a child while there is yet the option of whether the child shall come into existence.[34] But can a "being" be harmed who may or may not exist?

This is an example of what we will call the *paradox of harm,* the seemingly self-contradictory idea that someone can be harmed by being born. This idea appears to be morally paradoxical because, first, it seems queer to say that we can harm a being by bringing it into existence; but second, it seems equally odd to say that a mother who could have prevented harm to her child but did not, did no wrong by that omission.

A *paradox* results when two different meanings of a key term are used simultaneously. Paradoxes can be dissolved by carefully specifying the different meanings in each part of the paradox and deciding which meaning applies best to each. With the paradox of harm, any approach to dissolving it must distinguish between different meanings of the word "harm." Like the concept of good, the concept of harm covers a broad range of meanings. In law school, such meanings are covered in one of the major courses, *torts.*

We will distinguish two ways of thinking about harm. In the first, both a baseline and a temporal component are necessary, so that a change occurs which makes someone worse off. In this *baseline harm,* harm requires an adverse change in someone's condition. With the baseline concept, someone who doesn't yet exist cannot be harmed, because there is no baseline from which change can occur. (Consider the old Yiddish joke: 1st—Life is so terrible! Better to have never existed." 2nd—"True, but who is so lucky? Not one in a thousand.")

In the second way of defining harm, harm involves comparing a present deficient condition with what normally would have been. In this *abnormal harm,* someone can be harmed by being brought into existence with some defect that could have been avoided by taking reasonable precautions. With abnormal harm, the event or omission that causes the defect is the cause of harm. The abnormal concept underlies the belief that women should do everything possible to have healthy, unimpaired babies, that anything less than the maximal effort is blameworthy, and that it is wrong for a woman to take risks with a future person's intelligence or health. To sum up these two concepts of harm:

Baseline harm. Requires a starting point (baseline) from which an adverse change is plotted; that is, it requires an existing being who is made worse off.

Abnormal harm. Requires a norm of development that is not met, for example, because of a woman's actions or omissions while carrying a fetus.

In *wrongful life* cases in the courts, it is claimed that the lives of some children are so miserable that their very existence is a tort. In *wrongful birth* cases, the claim is not that the child's life is totally miserable but simply that the child has been damaged by being born less than normal. Wrongful birth suits appeal to the abnormal concept. The courts have rejected wrongful life suites by assuming the baseline concept; that is, they have assumed that preventing a birth or killing a baby cannot possibly be a benefit, even to prevent or end a life of total harm.

These two concepts of harm can be applied to IVF. According to baseline harm, a person created by IVF cannot thereby be harmed because otherwise that person wouldn't have existed. According to abnormal harm, IVF could harm a baby if it caused some defect or deficiency that a normal baby would not have had.

Wronging versus Harming

For utilitarians or consequentialists, what matters about new kinds of human creation is that babies are not harmed. On the other hand, virtue theories or Kantians focus on the motives of prospective parents. Whether it is AID, IVF, surrogacy, or cloning, they ask, "What would a good mother do? What kinds of risk would she take?"

This approach emphasizes that, even though a child might not be harmed by being brought into existence, a mother can still be wrong in bringing the child into existence. That's because "wrong" here is divorced from consequences to the child and instead married to the motives of the mother in conceiving a child. To take a mundane example, if a mother conceives a child not because she wants a child but to try to force a wealthy man to marry her, then the child who comes into existence is not harmed, but the mother is wrong to bring the child into existence for this motive.

In a Scottish study in 2005 of women trying to conceive at an infertility clinic, most of the 81 women would, if given an either-or choice, rather have a child with cerebral palsy or partially blind than no child at all.[35] But is this the right motive for approaching child-bearing? This issue intensifies with dilemmas raised by implanting multiple embryos (see below), where couples face choices between risks of no child and risks of several children, with one or more having major disabilities.

Harm by Not Knowing One's Biological Parents?

Can a child be harmed by not knowing his genetic ancestors? One compromise solves this problem: allowing gametic donors or surrogates to be *confidential* but not *anonymous*. In this practice, names and identities of donors are kept from children created from gametes of men and women, but these men and women are allowed (or encouraged) to update their files every five to ten years, so that their biological children can know about genetic diseases and their lives. This practice protects the desire of some donors and some surrogates not to have contact with children created from their gametes, while also giving them the chance to change their minds.

It is mainly the parents who adopt the donated sperm, egg, embryo, or child who object to children knowing such donors.[36] Surprisingly, many sperm and egg donors, or surrogates, do not mind maintaining such records and express a desire to know about the lives of such children.[37] Pediatrician/internist Matthew Neidner registered online in 2006 with the Donor Sibling Registry and discovered that his sperm over the last 10 years had created at least nine children, who can see his handsome picture online and follow his career.[38] Single women in San Diego originally selected his sperm from his profile at the Fertility Center of California.

Harm to the Family?

Many of the criticisms against new forms of assisted reproduction, or of paying for reproductive assistance, assume that the ideal nuclear family is the one pictured in old television comedies such as "Leave it to Beaver" or "The Donna Reed Show." Although students know that such perfect families rarely exist today, most falsely believe that something like these nuclear families actually did exist in the past. They think that only recently did the nuclear family decline, due to working mothers, high rates of divorce, feminism, or lack of religious schooling.

In her surveys of American family life over the last centuries, historian Stephanie Coontz contradicts these widespread beliefs. In *The Way We Never Were*, she writes,

> . . . the middle-class Victorian family depended for its existence on the multiplica-
> tion of other families who were too poor and powerless to retreat into their own lit-
> tle oases and who therefore had to provision the oases of others. . . . . For every
> nineteenth-century middle-class family that protected its wife and child within the
> family circle, then, there was an Irish or a German girl scrubbing the floors in that
> middle-class home, a Welsh boy mining coal to keep the home-baked goodies
> warm, a black girl doing the family laundry, a black mother and child picking cot-
> ton to be made into clothes for the family, and Jewish or an Italian daughter in a
> sweatshop making "ladies" dresses or artificial flowers for the family to purchase.[39]

The family pictured on "Leave it to Beaver" did not exist for most Americans at most times in history.

Professor Coontz also describes a study where researchers tracked kids to adolescence and predicted, based on their childhoods and parenting, which kids would be happy, which unhappy. The predictions were *wrong two-thirds of the time*, worse than if they had guessed randomly. They vastly overestimated the trauma resulting from the typical stresses of childhood, while they underestimated the lack of maturity that resulted from having a protected, stress-free adolescence.

Today, it is taboo to acknowledge any evidence that contradicts the prevailing wisdom about the family and child development. In 1999, family values conser-vatives attacked psychological studies showing that sexual abuse of adolescents and children does not universally damage kids and that some adults emerge unscathed.[40] Similar studies in 1999 showed that most children do fine in homes without live-in fathers. Rather than being seen as good news about the resilience of children, or the effectiveness of therapy, conservatives attacked the messengers, vowing to revoke federal funding of the studies.

Little empirical research exists about what forms of child raising harm chil-dren, in part because we cannot experiment on children or put them in controlled studies. This point is important when people claim that new forms of child-creation harm children. Being raised on a kibbutz, in day-care, or being gestated by a surrogate, may not harm children at all. Speculation about harm to teenagers when they later discover their unique origin is just that, speculation.

Only Perfect Babies?

At some clinics, researchers store extra eggs for later use with infertile couples. Pictures of the women from whom the eggs were taken are available to be shown to prospective parents, and indeed, private egg brokers may arrange a meeting between prospective buyers and sellers.[41]

Some critics argue that allowing any selection by prospective parents is wrong, and that such parents should be forced to accept the first available embryo, or that embryos should be randomly assigned. A similar argument once was used to attack in vitro fertilization, where critics said all adoptable babies should be placed before new reproductive techniques are allowed.

Such restrictions would be unacceptable to many prospective couples, who want to maintain the semblance of an ordinary pregnancy and childhood. They want an embryo from parents who will be ethnically as close to them as possible. Also, people who want a child of their own may not be willing or able to adopt a special needs baby. Also, many infertile foreign couples come to American physicians for assistance either because their countries do not offer such services or because there are few suitable egg and sperm donors in their countries. They are only interested in a specific kind of donor, e.g., Japanese-American for prospective Japanese parents.

In some American clinics, couples may select embryos at a cost ($2,750) much less than what it would cost ($16,000) to create an embryo from people selected in advance. These extra embryos can be created when one couple changes its mind after contracting for an egg donor. When that happens, the young woman has already taken fertility drugs for a month and her ovaries are full of ripe eggs, so the clinics remove the eggs and fertilize them with a variety of different sperm, keeping records of each embryo created. Couples may then select an embryo from this woman's eggs (seeing a picture and description of her) that will be fertilized by sperm from a man whose picture they see and whose life they read about.

Will such choices lead to desires for only perfect babies? This is a large question, connected in part to questions about eugenics and controls on biotechnology. Note that many people believe that it is permissible to use such techniques to let infertile couples choose *against* diseases that embryos might carry. Sensationalistic stories imply that allowing preimplantation diagnosis will lead to a society that encourages eugenics. Is this fear realistic?

One reason it is not is the cost of screening: for a single disease, it can be as much as $20,000, which most insurance companies will not pay.[42] It is unlikely that a couple will screen out hundreds of embryos and only implant the perfect ones because few couples have the millions of dollars to pay for so many screening tests. Should a cheap screening test be available where a couple could screen an embryo for hundreds of genetic diseases, and then for a batch of selected traits, this objection would carry some moral weight.

What worries critics is that if couples already want to try to influence traits of their future babies, and if there is market for sperm and egg sellers, then couples will select traits in ways the critics don't like. That is, they will select traits of men and women that the purchasing couple deems desirable. As one such critic put it in discussing a market for egg donors, "this approach is harmful not only because it serves to reinforce social prejudice but also because it fragments women as persons by commodifying their characteristics, which seems at least as harmful as commodifying their eggs."[43]

The view's implications for denial of personal choice are staggering. The dangers to personal reproductive liberty come from both choice-restricting liberals and social conservatives. The same critics who decry selection of traits in embryos always ignore adoption. Why is selection by ethnicity or race bad in one case but permissible in the other? Why are both selection by ethnicity and race plus large payment permissible for adoption but not for eggs or embryos or surrogates?

Finally, the critic forgets that there is a whole range of choice in life where people make selections based on what they value in others: in fraternities and sororities, in country clubs, in hiring and firing, in dating, in choosing a person to marry and have children with, in making friends, in deciding where to live, and in choosing whom to hire. Many of these choices reinforce existing attitudes and the government does not ban them.

Older Parents

One of the consequences of using eggs of younger women, and ICSI, is that more older people can create their own children. In 1980, an Australian team led by Carl Woods was criticized for accepting a 42-year-old woman as their first IVF candidate because of her increased chances of birth defects. Her baby was born without defects. In 1993, a 59 year-old Englishwoman gestated twins from embryos fertilized by her husband's sperm and eggs donated by a young woman. In 2006, American Lauren Cohen did the same.[44]

In 1990, one-third of American AR clinics excluded women over 40. By 1998, the practice of using eggs of younger women has removed such limits, especially as elderly infertile couples willingly paid extra for donors' eggs. Soon cases popped up everywhere of women over age 55 gestating and giving birth to babies.

Several births pushed this debate into public consciousness. In 1997, 63-year-old Arceh Keh gave birth to a healthy baby girl. That same year, actor Tony Randall fathered a daughter at age 77 (he died at age 89 in 2005). In 2005, 66-year-old Adriana Iliescu gave birth to a healthy baby daughter in Bucharest, Romania.

Should society encourage older people to have children when they may be senile or dead when their children are in college? In answering, note that no limits have historically been placed on men. In 1968, Senator Strom Thurmond at age 66 married a 22 year-old former Miss South Carolina and had four children with her (he died in 2003 at the age 100). Should fertility clinics place restrictions on women that aren't placed on men?

The Ethics of Gender Selection

Gender selection has brought about a new problem in countries such as China, the Republic of Korea, and India. For centuries in these societies, females have often been neglected and seen as inferior to males. The strong preference for a male child leads many families to abort females after determining the sex of a fetus by the use of a sonogram. Thus, high rates of female abortions have led to an extreme shortage of females and a highly unbalanced male to female ratio.

Women are in demand in China, where 20- to 44-year-old never-married men outnumber two to one their female counterparts, who are often kidnapped and sold into marriage. *Science* magazine predicts that in the year 2020, one million "excess" Chinese males will enter the matrimony market.[45] Despite laws that ban sex-determining testing in India and China, at least 60 million females are "missing."

A new technology, Microsort, can distinguish sperm by gender. Because X chromosomes are heavier than Y chromosomes and because they carry more DNA, a modified flow cytometer instrument can separate heavier from lighter sperm, producing accurate results 90 percent of the time.[46] Although intended for use in preimplantation genetic diagnosis, Microsort may be used by people in China and India to select male babies, making gender selection there cheap and easy.

Multiple Births: The McCaughey Septuplets

The number of multiple births worldwide has soared as a result of implantation of multiple embryos through IVF, and as a result of the introduction of Clomid and Pergonal, drugs that induce superovulation.

The multiple pregnancies that frequently result from assisted reproduction have created ethical issues as well. In a multiple pregnancy, nutrients and oxygenated blood in the womb become a scarce resource. To prevent disabilities resulting from deprivation in utero, physicians recommend "selective reduction" (abortion) of all but one or two fetuses. In 1985, a Mormon couple, Patti and Sam Frustaci, conceived septuplets but refused to have such a reduction performed. Four of their seven babies died, and the three survivors had severe disabilities, including cerebral palsy. The Frustacis sued.

Multiple birth babies are often premature (they may weigh less than two pounds), are three times as likely as single babies to be severely handicapped at birth, six times as likely to have cerebral palsy (which may not show up for a year or more), and may have to spend many months in neonatal intensive-care units (NICUs). Nevertheless, in France, where pregnancy is sometimes pursued with an almost religious zeal, and where each new baby means a bonus from the government, the number of triplets has increased 10-fold since 1982 and the number of quadruplets has increased 30-fold.

In 1996 in England, after taking the fertility drugs Merton and Pregnyl for two days, Mandy Allwood released seven eggs (unknown to her) before she had sex with her lover. All of them were fertilized. Four months later, she was offered a large cash bonus by a London tabloid for exclusive rights if all made it to term. So Mandy announced she would not reduce any and would go for maximal births. As a result, she lost all seven. In 1997, Denise Amen and her husband were offered the chance to reduce five growing embryos but refused. One of their quintuplets was born blind and others are "developmentally slow."[47]

Ten years before in 1987, Ron and Roz Helms of Peoria, Illinois, had quintuplets with the help of a fertility drug Pergonal, after taking Clomid to no effect for five years. Though warned that Pergonal might produce multiple births, they went ahead. One child spent a year in a NICU, another has seizures, and a third has mild cerebral palsy. The quints' medical bills for their first decade topped $3 million.

In 1997, an Iowa couple, Bobbi and Kenny McCaughey, used Pergonal to conceive seven embryos, refused to reduce any, and chose to risk having disabled babies. They said that any results were God's will.

The appeal to God and the role of human choice in multiple pregnancies has become a national controversy. To say "it's up to God" how many babies come about is misleading since humans took drugs to artificially stimulate release of many eggs, something that wouldn't have happened naturally. (Another problem with attributing so much to God is seen in the case of a Pentecostal woman named Jane Simeone who prayed that all her triplets would survive like the McCaugheys but who felt like a failure in God's eyes when two of her babies immediately died.)

Couples who desperately want to conceive often pray intensely for pregnancy and consider any reduction to be a violation of that prayer. Even though they are often given a choice of how many embryos to implant, they often maximize the number implanted to maximize chances of success, taking multiples as a bonus. They do not perceive this to be choosing to risk having a disabled child in order to maximize their own chances of having any children. (It appears that the McCaugheys were not given a choice by their two physicians, i.e., after seven eggs were released, they were not told, "Since you don't believe in reduction, it might be better to wait until next month when so many eggs aren't released.")

Critics of the decision by the McCaugheys said that if God was clear about anything in this case, it was that the McCaugheys were not intended to have kids. They also said that if a couple takes a fertility drug, and it results in too many conceived eggs, they should be willing to reduce the embryos for the good of the children born. In other words, a couple shouldn't run the risk of severely disabled kids and say it's "God's will" if it happens.

Going back, the year 1996 set a record for births of multiples with 6,000 babies born in groups of three, four, or more, a 20 percent jump from the previous year. Why did that happen then?

For most couples without reimbursement for in vitro fertilization, the easiest way to overcome infertility was to first take the drug Clomid, and if that didn't work, Pergonal or Metrodin to stimulate the ovaries to release many eggs at the same time. The problem is that introduction of sperm can create one, two, or eight embryos. In vitro fertilization, in contrast, allows physicians to control how many embryos are introduced.

At their fourth birthday in 2001, the McCaughey septuplets lagged in development behind normal children (true for all preemies) and were not all potty trained.[48] Joel has suffered seizures, for which he is on medication. Nathan has a form of cerebral palsy called spastic diplegia that requires botox injections (to paralyze spastic muscles) and orthopedic braces. Alexis has a different form of cerebral palsy, hypotonic quadriplegia, which results in weak muscles. Alexis also has had trouble walking and learning to talk. In addition, for four years she has had an indwelling feeding tube. Another child, Natalie, also has required a feeding tube during these years. Although Bobbi and Kenny McCaughey are homeschoolers, the task of homeschooling Nathan and Alexis, who are developmentally delayed, was too great, and the two children attend a public school for such children.

By 2002, the American Society for Reproductive Medicine (ASRM) had still not reached a consensus on how many embryos to implant to reduce the risk of creating damaged children. The probability of an impaired baby varies directly with the number of embryos allowed to gestate. In other words, if six are implanted, one is almost certain to be born with cerebral palsy or blind.

Unfortunately, the chance of having any baby at all also varies directly with the number of embryos implanted (hence, the ethical dilemma of how many embryos *should* be implanted). The ASRM suggests implanting no more than two embryos for women with good prognoses, no more than three for women with above-average prognoses, and no more than five "good-quality embryos" for women with below-average prognoses.[49]

ART physicians are torn between wanting to achieve high rates of pregnancy per number of couples versus low rates of multiple births and impaired newborns.

Gladys White, a bioethicist specializing in reproductive ethics, suggests clinics may be biased in favor of the first.[50]

Risks to Children from IVF Conception

Babies conceived through IVF have approximately twice the normal rate of birth defects, around 4 percent overall instead of 2 percent.[51] They have increased risk of Beckwith-Wiedemann syndrome, which causes enlarged organs and cancer in children, and are five to seven times more likely to develop retinoblastoma, a rare cancer of the eye.[52] Another Australian study found that 9 percent of babies conceived through IVF or ICSI had birth defects versus 4.2 percent of those naturally conceived. Another American study found that babies conceived through IVF were almost three times more likely to be born underweight and premature than babies naturally conceived.

What's going on here? Researchers point to four possible causes: IVF or ICSI, age of gametic donors and gestators, adverse selection of couples already having problems, or implantation of too many embryos in the womb.[53] Although it is tempting to impute all problems to the latter, a study by the Centers for Disease Control found that even singleton IVF babies are twice as likely to be born at very low birth weight than other children.[54] Researchers have suggested an IVF registry to track problems.[55] Others suggest that men with fertility problems have chromosomally abnormal sperm, so all the problems with IVF kids may due to this or another underlying cause of the couple's infertility. Others point to aggressive marketing of IVF and to couples turning more quickly to IVF to solve problems as the practice has become accepted.

A Need for Regulation?

Faced with the many innovations and problems of assisted reproduction, some critics such as Leon Kass want to regulate medical clinics and research in assisted reproduction. They emphasize that infertile couples are experimental subjects, vulnerable, and often do not fully understand the risks ahead.

Given that the ART industry performs over a hundred thousand procedures a year and generates $1 billion in fees, this is what critics call "the wild west of medicine," where almost anything goes.[56] These critics would subject ART to wise consensus before new conceptions are attempted, especially animal–human hybrids or cloning-to-children.

ETHICAL ISSUE: IS IT WRONG TO PAY FOR ASSISTED REPRODUCTION?

Historical Background: Paying for IVF

For reasons described in the last chapter, during the 1970s, the United States instituted a ban on federal funds for experimentation on embryos. Since 90 percent of experimentation in the United States is federally funded, this ban hoped to stop research on assisted reproduction.

So if assisted reproduction was going to flourish in America, it would have to be in private clinics that accepted no federal funds. Because few states required insurance companies to cover ART, clinics had to subsidize any research they did from fees paid by clients.

At the time, critics doubted that couples would pay much for such services, especially if their chances of achieving a baby were low. The last two decades have proved such critics wrong, with over a million American couples paying for some form of assistance in ART clinics.

An unintended but foreseeable by-product of the federal funding ban on human embryo research in such clinics, with the resulting reliance on funds generated from their paying patients, is that research in these clinics is not regulated by the NIH or IRBs. For better or worse, new forms of ART can be attempted without going through the cumbersome process of NIH or FDA approval.

Surprisingly, this process has created one of the fastest growing and most controversial areas of medicine with some stupendous breakthroughs, fueled in part by competition between ART clinics for success in creating babies.

Payment for Adoption

Because roughly one out of 12 couples in North America is infertile after two years of trying to conceive, and because in vitro fertilization only works for 20 couples out of 100, demand is high for healthy, adoptable babies. Because most couples in North America are white and want a child of the same ethnic background, demand for healthy, white babies has skyrocketed.

Such demand lets many adoption agencies charge substantial fees for their services, and the average couple in 2002 seeking to adopt a baby paid agencies nearly $20,000. Some couples pay over $100,000 in their quest for a healthy toddler.

Like transfer of eggs or organs, agencies do not technically sell babies, which is illegal. But a new industry has sprung up that connects couples to pregnant women and that recruits women who might carry their fetuses and later put their babies up for adoption. According to one investigative journalist, "That has left only the thinnest line between buying a child and buying adoption services that lead to a child."[57] The doubling of licensed child placement has increased adoptions in North America in the last few years to nearly 2,000.

Some agencies spend half a million dollars a year just on advertising. Their fees vary according to where the baby comes from and its ethnicity: $20,000 or more for a healthy, white baby, $22,000 for a Vietnamese baby, $17,000 for a Chinese baby, and $8,000 or less for a black baby.[58] Agencies that specialize in "closed adoptions" (where the mother never knows the adopting couple) of white babies charge over $100,000 for a successful adoption. Louisiana allows agencies to fly in pregnant women from out-of-state and house them during pregnancies, and allows large payments to facilitating agencies (and some charge surreptitious payments to the young women).

In 1993, Russia had no foreign adoptions, but in 1997, it placed more children in America than any other country. Many adoptions also come from Romania, the Balkans, Vietnam, and China.

Although black critics have recently decried the differential payments that seem to demean black babies, virtually no one has condemned payment. Virtually no one has criticized "pregnancy counseling centers" that encourage pregnant girls not to abort and to give up their babies for adoption, while charging lucrative fees to couples who adopt the same babies.

Paid Surrogacy: The Baby M Case and Its Aftermath

Fertilization of embryos outside the womb made it possible for another woman to gestate that embryo to birth, creating so-called "surrogate mothers," either for pay or altruistically.

Several hundred women had helped infertile women create babies when in 1986 biochemist Bill Stern and pediatrician Elizabeth Stern hired Mary Beth Whitehead for $10,000 to bear a child created by his sperm and Whitehead's egg through artificial insemination. At birth on March 27, 1986, in Monmouth County Medical Center in Long Branch, New Jersey, Mrs. Whitehead claimed to have bonded with the Baby M, whose real name was Melissa Stern, and refused to give her to the Sterns. When Mr. Stern threatened legal action, Mrs. Whitehead fled to Florida with the baby, but was discovered and returned to New Jersey.

At the lower court trial in 1987, Judge Harvey Sorkow upheld the legality of the contract, said it did not constitute baby selling, required Whitehead to hand over the baby, awarded Whitehead $10,000 and decided it would be best for the baby never to see Mrs. Whitehead again. On appeal in 1998, the New Jersey Supreme Court unanimously reversed his decision, declared Mrs. Whitehead the legal mother with full visiting rights, and invalidated surrogacy contracts. Mrs. Whitehead later became a well-known critic of surrogacy.

Feminists supported Mrs. Whitehead, who believed not only in bonding but that women were naturally superior to men in nurturing children. Such *social feminists* opposed *merit feminists* who sided with Elizabeth Stern and who thought women should be held accountable for contracts they signed. Ironically, merit feminists saw social feminists as sexist.

Several states (Michigan, New York, Washington, Utah, Arizona, and New Mexico) reacted to the Baby M case by criminalizing commercial surrogacy, laws still in effect in 2006. Arkansas, Florida, Ohio, Virginia, Nevada, and New Hampshire legally recognized paid surrogacy. At least 26 states have no law about surrogacy. California, which has many paid surrogates, recognizes a series of decisions in case law as regulating paid surrogacy.[59]

Controversial cases make news; successful cases do not. Jaycee Buzzanca, aka "the child with five parents," was born in March 1995 from a paid surrogate and became embroiled in a divorce between the parents who hired the surrogate. Jaycee was conceived from sperm and egg other than from the parents who hired the surrogate. A California Appeals court ruled in 1998 that the parents who had hired the surrogate were legally responsible for her.

A common objection to paid surrogacy is that it's not best for the child. This objection holds that it is wrong to deliberately bring a child into the world where the rearing mother does not do the gestational work. Paying for gestation is inherently wrong because having a confused identity with at least three, and maybe five, parents harms a child.

As time passes, this objection may be seen the same as saying that it's wrong for a woman to have a child whom she doesn't rear or educate herself and instead uses day care, public schools, or baby-sitters. In past centuries in wealthy families, children had nannies and au pair girls who did much of the work of day-to-day childraising. Long ago, we handed over home schooling to professional teachers. Whether such arrangements are best for the child largely depend on the details of the case and the motives of the parties. Properly done, such arrangements need not be bad for the child, whether it be a method of reproduction or a method of rearing a child.

Paying Egg Donors

Because so many women in North America are childless, and because eggs of young women increase chances of successful in vitro fertilization with a husband's sperm, it has become necessary to pay young women for transfer of their eggs. Originally, volunteers supplied eggs, but altruism doesn't come close to meeting the demand. The whole practice is called "egg donation," and donors receive variable amounts of money. In 1993, the American Society for Reproductive Medicine (ASRM) suggested a flat fee of $2,500, but by 2006, a good egg donor could make over $10,000 in Birmingham, AL, for several cycles.

Women get paid more than men because egg retrieval is more complicated than obtaining sperm. A woman takes drugs daily for a month or more to induce superovulation, after which eggs are aspirated with a long thin needle inserted through the vagina into an ovary and guided by ultrasound imaging. Some people claim that the drugs increase risk of some cancers over the life of the woman, but no long-term data support this claim.

Europeans find the argument against sales compelling. Mark Sauer, a leading American researcher in AR, relates, "While attending the World Congress [in 1996] of in-vitro fertilization in Vienna, I was impressed by the almost universal criticism leveled at practitioners in the USA by colleagues abroad with respect to the payment of egg donors. Allegations of 'pimping' for patients in need of eggs seemed a rather cruel accusation. . . ."[60] Yvon Englert, a Belgian researcher, was convinced that "U.S. ooycte donors come from the middle and poor classes of American society" (in reality, most are middle class) and that with payment, "the risks for both donors and receivers not to observe sanitary norms are much higher, oocyte donors being interested in hiding possible health problems."[61] Yet European researchers lament their lack of altruistic egg donors.

In the winter of 1998, a New Jersey AR clinic advertised that it would pay young women $5,000 for a month's worth of eggs. This was double the approved rate of $2,500. A year later, an ad ran in a newspaper at Princeton University and at other Ivy League Universities, stating that an anonymous couple was offering $50,000 for a "woman over six feet tall and with SAT scores over 1450 who was willing to sell her eggs."[62]

Typical, breathless prose describing these ads (not actions!) began an article in *Boston* magazine:

Ivy League women have been offered as much as $50,000 to "donate" their eggs to infertile women. When one desperate couple bought another woman's eggs, they entered a brave new world of egg harvesting, where biology, technology, and the marketplace collide, raising disturbing questions about breeding for perfection and profit.[63]

In a process like the coverage of the birth of Louise Brown, sensational media reports left the impression that paying elite women for their eggs was an out-of-control juggernaut, when in truth it had hardly begun.

Is Commercialization Intrinsically or Indirectly Wrong?

Some critics believe that such sale of eggs is either intrinsically or indirectly wrong. The first belief stems from religious or Kantian premises about the inherent value of humans being incompatible with being priced in the market. It may also look at the larger structure of society and claim that reproductive relationships between people should not be subjected to money.

The other kind of objection is that commercialization creates bad consequences. This is an empirical claim, capable of falsification. One bad consequence is the slippery slope, where critics say that commercialization of sperm, eggs, and gestation will spread to other areas, such as selling of organs or sexual favors in prostitution.

Defenders of payment retort that the wrong assumption here is the simplistic either-or categorization. Indeed, perhaps the really exploitive argument is to say that only good, unpaid, altruistic women should be allowed to be surrogates—what is often called the *compassion trap*. This is the false first step of casting all surrogates as either whores or Madonnas: A woman must either be a bad surrogate and earn money, or be a good surrogate and earn no money. The compassion trap insidiously implies that women who bear children for others in return for money aren't compassionate, just greedy.

Defenders of payment also ask whether enough young women will go through egg donation for altruistic reasons. Altruism hasn't worked in other areas of medicine. Voluntary donation has failed to meet the need for blood for operations, organs for transplantation, or bone marrow for leukemia patients.

So if we don't permit compensation, we will not get enough eggs from young women and hence, infertile couples will not get the babies they want. If we permit compensation but not a market, many other problems arise, such as trying to set the right fee (see below). Finally, if payment for assisted reproduction is wrong, why isn't payment for adoption? If payment for assisted reproduction is not for babies but merely for services, why isn't this true of adoption, too?

Payment as Exploitive and Coercive

The New York State Task Force on Life and Law attempted in 1988 to set a standard fee to egg donors for their services.[64] Its approach mirrored the central planning in socialist countries like Cuba and China.

In practice, a regulated fee may not satisfy anyone. The Task Force wanted the fee neither to exploit nor to coerce poor women. To do so, it had to gaze into its crystal ball and guess at the motives of women who do reproductive work.

But whether it's worth $10,000 or $30,000 for a woman be a nanny, surrogate mother, or assembly-line worker depends on factors about each woman that may change from year to year.

Sometimes, objections about payment to women imply that men are exploiting women. From reading interviews with paid surrogates, nothing could be further from the truth.[65] Paid surrogacy empowers many women who do it, making them special and contributing to their family's income. A surprisingly large number do it despite objections from husbands, or battle husbands who want to keep the gestated baby.

Conclusions

American society now permits payment for adoption, sperm donation, surrogacy, and egg transfer. Europeans regard such practices as rampant American commercialism. England bans most of them.

At the least, we should have a consistent policy of payment for services leading to creation of human life. If payment is banned for egg donation, it should be banned to facilitate adoption. If payment is allowed to a pregnant woman to support her gestation for later adoption, similar payment should be allowed when a couple contracts with a woman for surrogate gestation.

Assisted reproduction is a new frontier of medicine, wrapped in joys of created, wanted babies, a profitable field of medicine, but rife with ethical controversy and increasing concerns about premature babies or babies with disabilities from their new modes of creation. As older women create and bear such babies, and more embryos are implanted, issues of harm and wrong to babies arise, and the lives of these children need to be studied over decades to access the risks of their unique origins.

FURTHER READING AND RESOURCES

Cynthia Cohen, ed., *Oocyte Donation*, Baltimore, Md.: Johns Hopkins University Press, 1997.

Joseph Fletcher, *Ethics of Genetic Control: Enduring Reproductive Roulette*, Doubleday Anchor, New York; reprinted by Prometheus, Buffalo, NY, 1984.

Elaine Tyler, *Barren in the Promised Land: Childless Americans and the Pursuit of Happiness*, Harvard University Press, Cambridge, Mass., 1995.

Paul Ramsey, *The Ethics of Fetal Experimentation*, Yale University Press, New Haven, CT, 1975.

Stephanie Coontz, *The Way We Never Were*, New York: Basic Books, 1992.

RESOLVE: The National Infertility Association http://www.resolve.org/main/national/advocacy/insurance/facts/history.jsp?name=advocacy&tag=insurance

CHAPTER 6

Battles over Human Embryos and Stem Cells

This chapter discusses research on human embryos and creating stem cells from them, activities called *embryonic cloning* or *therapeutic cloning*. It also discusses adult stem cells (cells created without creation of human embryos), and controversies about embryos in medical research, including one of the greatest frauds in scientific history.

The next chapter focuses on cloning to produce children, or *reproductive cloning*. Since the announcement of the cloning of the sheep Dolly in February 1997, controversy has surrounded cloning anything human. Since then, measures to promote embryonic cloning have been contentious.

Before Dolly's announcement, many issues in bioethics had enjoyed a consensus among liberals and conservatives, but cloning shattered that peaceful co-existence. In the decade since, bioethics has become politicized. In that politicization, medical research on embryos has become a flashpoint. This chapter also describes that politicization.

HISTORICAL BACKGROUND
OF EMBRYONIC RESEARCH

In 1973, *Roe* v. *Wade* made abortion legal in all states. This judicial decision circumvented democratic consensus and legislation, which in 32 states had not yet permitted abortion.

As discussed in Chapter 4, between 1973 and 1975, the public became aware of experiments in 1973 that had studied an artificial womb and the effect of deprivation of glucose on the fetal brain by experimenting on 20 live-born, but dying, human fetuses.[1] What shocked people then was that, as soon as abortions were permitted in January 1973, researchers had *legally* experimented on live-born fetuses. Such research seemed to substantiate predictions about a slippery slope from legalizing abortion to trivializing nascent human life.

Five years after *Roe* v. *Wade*, "test-tube" baby Louise Brown was born, again without agreement, approval of an ethics committee, or cultural preparation of laypeople. As discussed in the last chapter, Steptoe and Edwards created and destroyed about a hundred human embryos to perfect their techniques of in vitro fertilization (IVF). Then, as of today, the creation of babies by IVF had the foreseen but unintended byproduct of sacrificing human embryos that did not implant. Again, human life at its beginnings seemed under attack by technicians, far removed from the natural wombs of motherhood.

In 1979, obstetricians Howard and Georgeanna Jones established the first American IVF clinic at Eastern Virginia Medical School (EVMS). In 1981, they achieved the first American baby born with IVF, Elizabeth Carr. While the embryo that became Elizabeth Carr was being created, opponents protested outside. The Catholic Church and conservative Christian groups saw IVF as alien, suspect, and at war with nature. Followers of such religions came to believe that scientists were attacking natural conception.

So began the politics of the embryo, which have intensified over the last 25 years. In 1977, partly in response to protests at EVMS and elsewhere, Congress created the *Ethics Advisory Board* (EAB) to decide which federally funded research on embryos and fetuses should be done. At the time, Congress thought that creation of the EAB would allow funding of such research and would mute criticisms from antiabortion groups, which had equated research on human embryos with abortion.

The EAB concluded that some research with embryos should be permitted, but as we shall see, Congress never accepted its conclusions. As a separate issue, the EAB never took up what kinds of research with embryos could be federally funded.

The Rios Case

In 1981 Mario and Elsa Rios, a wealthy American couple, died childless while their IVF-created embryos existed in a frozen limbo. Because neither the Rios nor the infertility clinic in Australia they used had provided for this contingency, their story made headlines.

Several questions arose. Could their embryos be destroyed? If they were implanted in surrogate mothers and carried to term, could the children later sue for an inheritance from the estate? Should the anonymous donor, whose sperm had been used with Elsa's egg, be consulted about his wishes?

An ad hoc committee of the Australian government required that the embryos be preserved until each of them could be adopted. They never were, and over the years, freezing made them deteriorate, making the issue moot.

The Demise of the EAB

Before the EAB could take up issues of what kinds of research with embryos could be federally funded, the Reagan administration in 1981 came to Washington, D.C. Believing that destruction of embryos did not differ from destruction of fetuses in abortion, Reagan refused to renew the EAB's charter. Hence, no federally funded research involving human embryos was ever approved.

In England and Australia, governments allowed public monies to fund medical research using embryos up to day 14 of the embryo's life. Australian infertility companies soon began to license their breakthroughs to American physicians.

The nonrenewal of the EAB was the first salvo in the coming political war in bioethics. The next salvo came two years later with the Baby Doe Rules and their investigative squads. Gradually, issues in bioethics left the previous harmony where parties worked toward consensus and did not use rhetoric for ideological gain.

The Davis Case, 1990

In 1990, Mary Sue and Junior Davis of Tennessee divorced and fought for custody of seven embryos frozen in an IVF clinic. Both had remarried. After her remarriage, Mary Sue Davis wanted to donate their embryos to an infertile couple. In 1992, the Tennessee Supreme Court decided that Junior did not have to become a father against his will, and after that, a lower Tennessee court ruled that he could destroy the embryos, which he did.[2]

The Human Embryo Research Panel, 1994

In 1993, the Clinton administration (1993–2001) revoked the regulations requiring EAB approval of embryo research. It also allowed federal funds for research in experiments using tissue derived from aborted fetuses.

In 1994, skeptical about its new freedom and wary of the growing clout of antiabortion politicians in Congress, the National Institutes of Health (NIH) formed a new oversight committee, the Human Embryo Research Panel. This panel consisted of four bioethicists, two lawyers, seven scientists, and six other members.

The panel was charged with dividing possible research with human embryos into three categories: acceptable for federal funding, unacceptable, and warranting further review. When antiabortionists targeted the panel's public meetings and mailed members graphic pictures of decapitated fetuses, members of the panel realized that some organized Americans felt passionately about human embryos.[3]

Under these circumstances, the panel concluded that federal funding of research with embryos would improve the success and safety of procedures to reduce infertility, and that prohibiting federal funding would harm the quality of such research. It also concluded that such research would help physicians understand pediatric cancers. (In 2006, a cancer geneticist at the Whitehead Institute in Massachusetts confirmed that cancer stem cells exist in a variety of tumors, making the study of stem cells one key to curing cancer.[4])

Embryos created specifically for research are called *research embryos*. Embryos left over after successful IVF are called *spare embryos*. The panel rejected the compromise that research could proceed on spare embryos. Why? It said that embryos from unsuccessful couples attempting IVF had higher rates of genetic abnormalities, so basic research needed to be also done on their embryos.

Politically savvy members of the panel thought Congress would accept their modest recommendations, but, preoccupied with partial-birth abortions in 1995, Congress rejected them.

The Dickey-Warner Amendment, 1996

In 1996, conservative Congressmen added a clause to NIH's appropriations bill: "None of the funds made available in this act may be used for . . . research in which a human embryo or embryos are destroyed, discarded, or knowingly subjected to risk of injury or death greater than allowed for research on fetuses in utero." This political power of champions of the embryo surprised scientists and NIH officials.

NIH saw the writing on the wall. Previously, it had gotten around the federal ban on embryo experimentation by interpreting some medical research, such as genetic screening of embryos for hereditary disease, as not putting embryos at risk. But what about the embryos found to carry genetic disease and thus not implanted? They would be destroyed (after all, that was the whole point of screening!), and Congress did not want to defend that.

The Hughes Incident, 1997

The Dickey-Warner Amendment nixed the research of geneticist Mark Hughes. In 1992, Hughes had made *Science* magazine's list of top breakthroughs for his technique of taking DNA from a single cell of a human embryo and testing it for cystic fibrosis. Taking the cell did not damage healthy embryos, but such testing did mean that embryos with cystic fibrosis would be destroyed.

Although the ban on federal funds had stayed in effect, scientists such as Hughes could work on embryos that were *privately funded*, such as those which Hughes obtained from Planned Parenthood. In 1997, Hughes had private funds to pursue embryonic screening and much larger federal funds to pursue other genetic research that did not involve human embryos. Yet Hughes lost all federal funding because such funds had paid for a small refrigerator mistakenly placed in the private lab where he stored his embryos.

Advances in Assisted Reproduction, 1978–1997

The two decades between the births of Louise Brown in 1978 and the announcement of the lamb Dolly's birth in 1997 saw dramatic breakthroughs in assisted reproduction, which the media hyped. As the last chapter discussed, among them were conception of a child from a frozen embryo, birth of a child by a hired surrogate, birth of a child from an embryo created from the egg of a (younger) woman other than the gestating or adopting mother, gestation of a child created through IVF by a woman over age 55, and creation of children from a "genius" sperm bank where characteristics of anonymous sperm donors could be selected by prospective mothers.

Several conservative critics consistently and loudly decried each departure from conception by heterosexual married couples: physician-biochemist turned bioethicist Leon Kass, philosopher and bioethicist Daniel Callahan, and leftist, best-selling author/speaker Jeremy Rifkin. At first quietly against IVF as unnatural and a minor sin, the Catholic Church gradually stiffened its stand against assisted reproduction.

As the previous chapter described, these critics lost these battles because private IVF clinics funded their research out of patient fees rather than government funds, and hence were unregulated by federal or state governments. On the backs of legalized abortion, new forms of assisted reproduction made conservative critics feel that medical technology was a lethal force destroying traditional forms of creation, parenting, and biological bonds.

Dolly Is Announced, 1997

On February 24, 1997, every newspaper in the world screamed that a lamb named Dolly had been created by cloning (she was actually born on the previous July 5th, 1996, but patents on the techniques came through in February). Cloning, a technique previously thought to be impossible for use in mammals, conjured scary scenarios from science fiction. Everyone wondered if humans would be cloned next. Dolly's birth also galvanized interest in cloned human *embryos,* especially embryos that might be created through cloning, implanted in a woman, and gestated to a human baby.

While they had been ambushed by *Roe* v. *Wade,* the birth of Louise Brown, and the unanticipated success of IVF clinics, social conservatives vowed this time not to accept cloning. It is as if they said to scientists, "Here we draw the line and beyond, 'You shall not pass!'"

Immortalized Human Stem Cell Lines Created, 1998

What are stem cells and why are they important? Found in embryos and the umbilical cord, stem cells help the body, when it is injured, to grow new cells. If the body is hurt and loses blood, stem cells are activated to make new blood. Stem cells are primordial cells that can develop into any kind of differentiated cellular tissue: bone, muscle, nerve, etc. In theory these primordial cells could be directed to form new bones, neural cells, cardiac tissue, and hence, to cure many diseases.

Physicians already knew that the human body had stem cells, but they had no easy way to grow such cells until John Gearhart of Johns Hopkins University and James Thomson of the University of Wisconsin came along. In 1998, these men discovered how to create immortalized stem cell lines from human embryos. They learned how to continually produce stem cells, rather than tediously derive them from minute amounts of tissue from embryos or fetuses.

In effect, Gearhart and Thompson discovered how to make human embryos into tiny biological factories creating stem cells. It is just this "objectification" or "commodification" of human embryos that bothered critics who felt that using human embryos for such purposes demeaned the dignity of human life and led "up" a slippery slope demeaning all human life in all its stages.

Gearhart and Thompson made their discoveries using private funds. Next a larger issue arose: Given that NIH funding was the world's treasure, should it bankroll scientists to study this new area?

ACT Uses Cow Eggs to Grow Human Embryos

In 1998, Advanced Cell Technology (ACT) of Massachusetts announced that it had made differentiated human cells revert to a primordial state by fusing them with cow eggs. Although the cow egg was just the medium for the nucleus of the human cell (the nucleus of the cow egg had been removed), the procedure sounded alarms. Once again, biotechnology seemed out of control. President Clinton and his National Bioethics Advisory Commission (NBAC) condemned any attempts to create children out of such hybrids (although no one wanted to try to create such a being or was suggesting doing so).

NBAC Backs Research on Embryonic Stem Cells

Although it condemned reproductive cloning in 1998, President Clinton's NBAC concluded in 2001 that the government should fund research on stem cells created from human embryos. Congress never accepted this recommendation, in part because cloning had become the Godzilla of bioethics.

Indeed, cloning soon took up more media time and speculation than any issue in the 35-year history of bioethics. With physicist Dick Seed wanting to clone himself, and with Raelians, Pamayiotis Zavos, and Severino Antinori falsely claiming to have a client gestating a cloned human fetus, cloning created one sensational story after another (more on this in the next chapter).

Adult Stem Cells Discovered, 2001

In 2001, scientists discovered stem cells not only in bone marrow but also throughout the human body. Researchers hoped to use them to create stem cells without sacrificing human embryos.

Some scientists challenged the ease of obtaining adult stem cells and denied that they were as valuable in medicine as embryonic stem cells. This dispute had ideological overtones because opponents of embryonic cloning wanted adult stem cells to be just as valuable as cloned embryos.

In the next five years, researchers discovered that many organs and tissues contain precursor cells that act like stem cells. These adult stem cells became specific kinds of cells more quickly than embryonic stem cells, for which scientists do not know how to do the same. One director of an institute for regenerative medicine says, "Brain stem cells can make almost all cell types in the brain, and that may be all we need if we want to treat Parkinson's disease or ALS. Embryonic stem cells might not be necessary in those cases."[5] Similarly, specific adult stem cells can be obtained from the intestine, skin, liver, and bone marrow. About heart disease, the Director of Harvard's Stem Cell Institute says, "If you could find a progenitor cell in the adult heart that has the ability to replicate, it's likely easier to start with that than begin with an embryonic stem cell, which has too many options."[6]

But most adult organs contain few stem cells, not nearly enough to use medically, and adult stem cells are even harder to grow than embryonic stem cells. More fundamentally, "Unlocking the secrets of self-renewal will most likely involve studying embryonic stem cells," says Harvard's Director. So medicine needs both kinds of stem cells to make the most progress.

President Bush's First Press Conference, 2001

On August 11, 2001, President George W. Bush, in the first press conference on bioethics by an American president, announced his policy on federally funded research on human embryos. He rejected using such funds to create embryos for research, but allowed them for research on 60 stem cell lines created from spare embryos. Carried live on television in prime time, his press conference signaled that bioethics had arrived in American politics.

A year after that press conference, the number of stem cell lines appeared to be small, about 15. Scientists then questioned whether President Bush's policy would get them the biological material they needed. Three years later, scientists regarded the 15 stem cell lines as inadequate.[7] Lack of good sources fueled a push in 2006 in the U.S. Senate to fund research on embryonic stem cells.

Cloning and the Law

Senator Sam Brownback (R, Kansas) introduced his Human Cloning Prohibition Act of 2001, which stated: "It shall be unlawful for any person or entity, public or private, in or affecting interstate commerce, knowingly (1) to perform or attempt to perform human cloning; (2) to participate in an attempt to perform human cloning; or (3) to ship or receive for any purpose an embryo produced by human cloning." Also, "It shall be unlawful for any person or entity, public or private, knowingly to import for any purpose an embryo produced by human cloning, or any product derived from such embryo."

Although most Congressmen accepted banning reproductive cloning, Brownback and his supporters, such as Richard Doerflinger of the U.S. Conference of Catholic Bishops, wanted bans on embryonic cloning, too, which medical researchers rejected. So the Brownback bill stalemated.

A similar proposal to ban all forms of cloning worldwide, backed by the administration of George W. Bush, stalemated in the United Nations. Asian countries such as Korea, Malaysia, and China, hoping to excel in biotechnology, aligned with European countries to resist the measure.

With Congress stalemated, action about cloning fell to the states. Californians in 2002 passed Proposition 71, giving $3 billion for stem cell research from human embryos. State legislatures across the land then battled to fund or to criminalize embryonic cloning. Wisconsin, New Jersey, Connecticut, Illinois, Washington, Ohio, and Maryland funded similar research, whereas Massachusetts, Missouri, Arkansas, Indiana, Iowa, Michigan, North and South Dakota voted to criminalize all cloning.[8]

In each of these states, politicians felt the heat surrounding cloning. Journalist Wesley Smith stung politicians in New Jersey and Maryland for supporting "stealth cloning," whereas Massachusetts governor Mitt Romney threatened to veto legislation allowing embryonic cloning, as a prelude to his bid to run for president.

In 2005–2006, Congress tried to fund a bill like California's Proposition 71, but conservative ministers Pat Robertson, James Dobson, and Jerry Falwell, the U.S. Conference of Catholic Bishops, columnists Cal Thomas and Wesley Smith, and House Majority Leader Tom Delay organized resistance to it. Before being forced to resign as a Congressman after being indicted for a felony, Delay said the bill would "kill some to save others."[9]

Leon Kass and the President's Council on Bioethics, 2001–2005

Nowhere did the politicization of bioethics burn hotter than the ideological turn to the right for the national commissions in bioethics typically appointed by American presidents. In 2001, President George W. Bush appointed Leon Kass, the most hostile critic of biotechnology and assisted reproduction of the last decades, to be Chair of his President's Council on Bioethics. Moreover, he allowed Kass to appoint other hostile members, such as Francis Fukuyama, Gilbert Meilander (board member of *First Things*), and Mary Ann Glendon, a member of the anti-gay "Alliance for Marriage."[10]

During the four years under Kass, the council issued reports critical of stem cell research, provoking angry dissent from minority members such as neuroscientist Michael Gazzaniga and the resignation of University of California cell biologist Elizabeth Blackburn.[11]

Other Countries Fund or Ban Cloned Embryos for Stem Cells

In 2005, Dolly's cloning scientist Ian Wilmut was given permission to clone human embryos for stem cells to study motor neuron disease, a wasting illness.[12] Malaysia invested $26 million in its BioValley to house 100 new biotech companies to work on stem cells and raise Malaysia to a world power in biotechnology.[13] China invested in cloning technology, hoping to gain where the West had stumbled.[14]

Hwang Woo Suk Clones Embryos for Stem Cells, 2004

In 2004, seemingly out of nowhere, South Korean researcher Hwang Woo Suk announced that he had not only successfully cloned viable human embryos but had also derived viable stem cells from these embryos.[15] The South Korean team created 213 embryos and grew 30 of these to blastocysts. American researchers at Advanced Cell Technology had previously not been able to grow embryos to blastocysts, which contain an inner mass of stem cells. Hwang's achievement stunned American researchers.

Animal Cloning

In the eight years after Dolly's birth in 1996, scientists cloned animals important for food and research: two calves (1998), the lambs Molly and Polly to create Factor IX (1998), three generations of mice (1998), five pigs, (2002), a goat (2002), a rat (2003), many champion dairy cows and bulls (1998–2004), a horse named "Prometea" (2003), a mule named "Idaho Gem" (2003), and a deer named "Dewey" (2003).

They also cloned animals of endangered species such as the banteng (2003), a bovine native to Indonesia, and the African wildcat (2004). Critics feared that such cloning would lessen preservation of natural habitat for such species.

Scientists also cloned a cat named "Carbon Copy" or "CC" (2001). CC had a striped gray coat over a white base, unlike her ancestor, an orange calico. Critics claimed that this showed that cloning didn't work, while CC's originator, Mark Westhusin, replied that of course CC's coat color differed, because random genetic reprogramming controls coat coloring and patterns.

In March 2005, the South Korean team of Hwang Woo Suk announced it had cloned an Afghan hound that it named "Snuppy." Because of their complex reproductive system, dogs had previously eluded cloning by scientists, but Hwang's team did so (and this achievement remains undisputed).

The Fraud of Hwang Woo Suk, 2005

Hwang Woo Suk again stunned American researchers when he announced in May 2005 the easy cloning of 11 stem cell lines from human embryos. His account emphasized the Buddhist relaxed attention and skills of his team.[16] Importantly, he said these stem cell lines were genetic matches of cells of donors, opening doors to study cells of victims of particular diseases such as Alzheimer's or Lou Gehrig's disease.

The story received almost as much publicity as Dolly's birth. Carefully planned, it was announced at a meeting in Seattle of the American Association of Science. With his handsome face and Western suit, Dr. Hwang seemed to symbolize all that was progressive and therapeutic in medical science. And his successes seemed to be snowballing, showing American politicians the price of their hostility to funding research with cloned embryos.

Of course, controversy continued. Richard Doerflinger of the U.S. Conference of Catholic Bishops called the success a "clear and present danger" to the dignity of human life. Champions of victims of Parkinson's disease, such as the actor Michael J. Fox, hailed it as a major breakthrough.

But one of the biggest medical breakthroughs of the decade was faked, one of the most blatant frauds in the history of science.

Because federally funded American researchers could not perform similar research and because no major medical institution supplied researchers with eggs or human embryos, the Korean's research could not be easily verified.

Questions soon arose about the photos of embryos published in *Nature* and *Science* of Hwang's research, which did not seem to be of different embryos but of the same ones. Pittsburgh scientist Gerald Schatten, listed as a co-author on Hwang's paper, suddenly withdrew his name. Anonymous postings on the Internet from graduate students in Hwang's lab complained that Hwang had faked his results.

In 2005, Hwang's university and the South Korean government thoroughly investigated Hwang's work on cloned embryos. Assistants testified that Hwang had forced them to fabricate results and to alter pictures of embryos.

The investigation concluded that Hwang had not in fact produced any stem cell lines from human embryos, had not discovered easy techniques for doing so, and had not produced matching stem cell lines to cells of donors. Hwang went on trial in South Korea for misusing millions of dollars of funds specially given to him for his work and for violating Korean laws in bioethics. In this year, Hwang admitted to his fraud, but like Enron's Ken Lay and HealthSouth's Richard Scrushy, claimed that underlings had deceived him.

Like the Raelians, Hwang was a fake. Both stories received saturation coverage by the media and both damaged legitimate medical progress.

The Senate Vote and Presidential Veto, July 2006

On July 18, 2006, the U.S. Senate voted to expand federal funding of embryonic stem cell research, passing a bill that had passed the House the year before. The next day President Bush, as he had promised to do, vetoed the bill, the first of his administration. President Bush, at a news conference at the White House explaining his veto, said the bill would be "crossing a moral line and would support the taking of innocent human life." He was surrounded by dozens of Snowflake children, born from embryo-adoption programs, and by their parents. "These boys and girls are not spare parts," the President affirmed.[17]

Representative Nancy Pelosi of California, the House minority leader, retorted that Bush's veto was "saying 'no' to hope." And Senator Orrin Hatch agreed, saying the veto "sets back embryonic stem cell research another year or so."

ETHICAL ISSUE: SHOULD EMBRYOS BE USED IN MEDICAL RESEARCH? FOR AND AGAINST

People for years have argued for and against research with human embryos. The remainder of this chapter explores such arguments.

Valuable from Conception

For Thomas Aquinas in the 13th century, ensoulment occurred at 40 and 90 days for male and female fetuses, respectively, and therefore nothing of value resided in the womb before those points. In 1869, Pius IX announced that abortion at any stage resulted in excommunication.[18] Since then, Catholic teaching has emphasized the value of human life "from the moment of conception." So it was no surprise that in 1982, Pope John Paul II said to a group of scientists,

> I condemn, in the most explicit and formal way, experimental manipulations of the human embryo, since the human being, from conception to death, cannot be exploited for any purpose whatsoever.[19]

Potential for Personhood

Many scientists say that before 14 days, the human embryo has no human form and cannot experience pain. Why then give it value? One reply is that, despite the facts that some zygotes become pathological tissue and some zygotes twin, the embryo is, as Jesuit priest Richard McCormick says, "powerfully on its way" to development as a person. Even though it may later twin or not implant, conservative believers see it as a member of the human family.

Why is that? As McCormick writes about the human embryo:

> . . . it remains [as having] potential for personhood and as such deserves profound respect. This is *a fortiori* weighty for the believer who sees the human person as a member of God's family and the temple of the spirit. Interference with such a potential future cannot be a light undertaking.[20]

Slippery Slope

In addition to asserting the intrinsic value of the embryo, McCormick worries about what happens when human embryos are regarded as mere commodities for research. (In the following passage, "preembryo" refers to the embryo before implantation on the uterine wall.)

> If we concluded that preembryos need not be treated as persons, would we little by little extend this to embryos? Would we gradually trivialize the reasons justifying preembryo manipulation? . . . Furthermore, there is uncertainty about the effect of preembryo manipulation on personal and societal attitudes toward nascent human life in general. Will there be further erosion of our respect? I say "further" because of the widespread acceptance and practice of abortion.

Here we first have a conceptual slippery slope argument, asserting that if trivial reasons justify experimenting on embryos before 14 days, then similar reasons may justify experimenting on first-trimester fetuses, and so on. McCormick also has an empirical slippery slope argument here, predicting that acceptance of the deaths of embryos will generalize to acceptance of deaths of fetuses.

Reductio ad Absurdum

Many commentators think that treating the embryo as valuable because it is a potential person can be refuted by a *reductio ad absurdum:* a line of reasoning that shows that implications of an idea are absurd and thus cast doubt on the idea itself. In this instance, if a woman starts procreating in her teens and continues throughout her fertile years, she can produce a dozen or more children. If each potential person is valuable, then she ought to conceive as many children as possible. Given the consequences of overpopulation, this conclusion hardly makes sense.

If embryos are persons, the following involve killing persons: creating embryos for in vitro fertilization and freezing them for later use, pre-implantation genetic diagnosis, or emergency contraception. Similarly, intrauterine devices (IUDs), which prevent implantation of embryos, also must kill persons.

If these implications are false, then the premise that generated these claims is false, and that premise was that human embryos are persons.

Of course, it might be possible, thinking of Judith Jarvis Thomson, to accept the premise that embryos are persons, but to deny a further premise that persons can never be killed. Also, when no particular woman has a duty to gestate them, there is clearly a philosophical difficulty in claiming a right to life for frozen embryos.

Just Tissue

For some people, a human embryo is not a person but only human tissue. A human embryo has no more moral status than a pint of human blood or a severed appendix.

For them, what gives the human embryos value is a decision by a woman to let it use her body for nine months in gestation. If she makes this decision, the embryo can be gestated, born, and become a baby with moral value. But embryos themselves have no more intrinsic value than any other human tissue.

The Interest View

New York (Albany) philosopher Bonnie Steinbock argues that "having moral status (that is, being the kind of being who must be considered from the moral point of view) is limited to beings who have interests." Generally speaking, a necessary condition of having an interest is being able to desire something. One of the most basic desires is to avoid pain. We don't think vegetables feel pain, so we don't think they have desires. We do think cats and dogs feel pain, so we think they have an interest in avoiding pain.

The law makes a great deal of interests, conflicts among them, and how to resolve conflicts of interest. As such, the concept of interest covers a lot of intellectual territory.

As for embryos, it is commonly accepted that before the emergence of the primitive streak at 14 days, there is no possibility of any neural development such that any being could be "there" to feel pain. The human embryo at this stage is more like a blackberry than a tadpole.

As such, Professor Steinbock argues, the embryo has no desires about what happens to it, so it has no interests and no moral status. So it does not matter whether an embryo fails to implant in the uterine wall, whether it is dislodged by an intrauterine device (IUD), or whether it is used in research. It only begins to matter when neurons form to create *sentience*, the ability to feel pain.

Steinbock distinguishes between moral status and moral value. Beings can have moral value, even if they lack moral status. For her, to say that something has moral value is to say that there are moral reasons for protecting or being concerned about the thing. So wilderness and works of art can have moral value, even if they lack moral status.[21]

For Steinbock, embryos have moral value but no moral status, so there are reasons for protecting how they are used, for respecting them, and for not devaluing them as mere tissue.

Exploiting Women

In his fraudulent research, Hwang Woo Suk used 242 human eggs extracted from 16 women who allegedly volunteered. Even when his research was thought legitimate, critics worried whether these women had been coerced and whether a new stem cell industry would require thousands of young women to work as egg donors.[22]

Lupron (leuprolide acetate) is injected into egg donors to put their ovaries on hold before other drugs are given to stimulate extra release of eggs. Critics say the long-term effects of Lupron have not been well-studied and some women on it have reported adverse effects.[23]

Others criticize the sale of eggs by young women for medical research, even to make stem cells to cure disease. Others worry that harvesting human eggs devalues natural motherhood and makes women into machine-like egg sources, not nurturers and teachers.

To remove danger of exploiting women for eggs to produce embryos, two British researchers proposed creating research embryos from leftover eggs obtained for in vitro fertilization. Women attempting IVF are usually given drugs to induce superovulation and:

> For every 10 eggs collected in a cycle, three or four do not fertilize and are routinely discarded. In our unit alone, this adds up to 2000 eggs per year and, in the UK as a whole, perhaps 50–100,000. If these were matured in vitro and/or injected with sperm from a fertile donor using ICSI, a large number of viable embryos would result.[24]

These researchers think that critics who claim embryonic cloning requires thousands of young women to become egg donors are incorrect: the eggs already exist and now are being wasted. All we need to do is change our attitude and harvest them to make human embryos.

Do Embryos Have Dignity?

The Vatican argues that cloned human embryos "enjoy the same dignity proper to every human being."[25] John Haas, President of the Pope John Center for the Study of Ethics in Health Care, testified about cloning before Congress and made the Catholic position explicit:

> A federal ban against the attempted cloning of human beings would certainly be consonant with Catholic moral teachings. But it must be an honest ban. Human life must be protected from its very beginnings, as soon as there is interior, spontaneous growth.[26]

Haas appeals not to the sanctity of human life but to its dignity, even in its most nascent forms. For this reason, "opposition to cloning [must] include engendering human life for any research or experimental purposes." Similarly for Leon Kass, cloning human embryos for research threatens human dignity because it transforms "procreation into a form of manufacture."[27]

This position on dignity figured highly in the attempt by a coalition of countries in the United Nations, led by the United States and Costa Rica, to ban all forms of cloning. "Every human being has intrinsic dignity and worth from conception to natural death," said Birhanemeskel Abebe, an Ethiopian delegate to the U.N. designated as point man in the attempt to get a U.N.-sponsored worldwide ban on all forms of cloning.[28]

When it comes to treating human embryos with dignity, the concept nearly collapses. As UCLA bioethicist Greg Stock argues, "To claim that legislation that so elevates the status of a pinprick of cells that it blocks research to cure real disease afflicting real people and destroying real lives—to call that respect for human life and dignity is absurd. It's wrong."[29]

Given the frequent charge that embryonic cloning cheapens life, it is amazing that the parents of many embryos refuse to pay anything at all for their continued existence. *The Lancet* revealed that over two-thirds of human embryos stored at two fertility clinics in England had to be destroyed because the couples whose gametes were used to create the embryos would not even respond to a letter asking about their wishes.[30]

Given that such couples are the most affected by the destruction of the embryos and could give them to other couples for use in conception, it seems clear that such couples do not put much value in the dignity of these embryos. At least, they do not when it comes to actually paying money to keep them alive or to writing a letter consenting to keep them alive in public clinics.

The fact that 400,000 embryos are now frozen, deteriorating over time, and becoming nonviable has also created a new kind of adoption. The *Snowflakes* program to date has arranged adoptions of nearly 1,000 embryos, of which about 20 became babies.[31] (The program charges up to $20,000 for this service, as it considers itself arranging an adoption.)

England has allowed its scientists to create human embryos for research and to use them in such research for up to 14 days of development.[32] In the years in which that has been legal, no great changes in the fabric of English life seem to have occurred, nor has there been a massive slide down a slippery slope of loss of human dignity.

Potential Value Is Not Value

Although under ideal conditions embryos have the potential to become persons, such potential itself is not moral value. As Michael Gazzaniga argued about embryos on the President's Council on Bioethics, the goods in a lumber store have the potential to build a dozen houses, but if the store burns down, we do not say that a dozen houses were destroyed, nor do insurance companies reimburse for that larger amount.[33]

Let us put this point a different way. Fertilization after superovulation results in the creation of more than one embryo. Not all are usually implanted, so what is the ethical status of the remaining embryos when they are frozen for future use? About 2,000 spare embryos exist in North America, frozen in liquid nitrogen. If all these embryos were destroyed tomorrow, it is not like a mass murder of 2,000 people occurred. Indeed, would the reader care whether it were 2,000 or 20,000 embryos? What difference would it make to anyone?

Finally, Roman Catholic physician M.V. Viola wrote in 1968:

> A significant number of fertilized ova (some estimate one in three) never implant in the uterus under normal conditions. If in fact these are lost souls, the Church should be consistent and make efforts to administer baptism to them.[34]

But no one is going to baptize embryos that fail to implant because, among other reasons, no one really believes them to be persons.

Potential Value Is Symbolic

Perhaps it is true that potential value is merely symbolic, but that raises just the problem at hand, namely, our growing insensitivity to death and the destruction of human lives. Exactly the same argument could be made about death from a mass killing in a country on the other side of the globe. One might ask similarly, "Indeed, does it make any difference to the reader whether 2,000 or 20,000 people exist now or were destroyed? What difference to anyone the reader knows would it make, either way?"

But is this the moral ideal we want to hold up to our children? Isn't the opposite better, where we strive to make each human life valuable? Even if we usually miss that ideal, is not positing it better than succumbing to the view that no one matters except those within my circle of concern?

Potentiality and Cloning

The strongest argument of opponents of embryo research is the potential of the human embryo, given the right conditions, to become a person. But they have forgotten one thing: what cloning shows is that any cell of the body can become a person. The nucleus of a differentiated cell can be put into an enucleated human egg, a spark applied, and a new embryo can be formed that is a near-copy of the genetic ancestor.

The revolutionary aspect of cloning is that it makes not just embryos special but *any human cell.* The concept of the dignity of the embryo begins to collapse into the concept of the dignity of the cell.

Embryos Must Be Treated with Respect

Bioethicist David Ozar once argued that although an embryo may not be a person, neither is it just a pebble or tissue.[35] Embryos are not simply the property of an owner. They deserve respect in view of their potential as persons.

What does respecting an embryo mean? Well, for one thing, embryos should not be eaten, or be encased in plastic as earrings, or be bred into mixed-species hybrids. Gene Outka claims that respecting embryos also means that human embryos could not substituted for the eyes of rabbits in testing cosmetics.[36]

Another way to put this point is to emphasize that a large amount of bodily products, such as bone, cartilage, blood, and tissue can be legally sold from cadavers. Some firms specialize in such sales and broker them to research institutions and medical schools. Respecting embryos would include banning them from being bought and sold this way.

Respect Is Compatible with Research on Embryos

It is possible to be a good scientist and treat human embryos with respect in medical research. One might make an analogy with animal experimentation. To test new forms of heart surgery or new kinds of lenses for human eyes, we harm animals. But in using animals for our benefit this way, we should minimize their pain and psychological terror, and not make fun of them in any way.

In the same way, researchers who have the privilege of using human embryos should be taught, required, and legally enjoined to treat them with the greatest respect. That respect prevents a slippery slope to devaluing other kinds of human life.

To make another analogy: physicians and medical students should treat the newly dead with respect, and not practice intubation or spinal taps or surgery on them without the family's permission, for to do so is to offer no respect to the life just expired or to those who loved the patient. In the same way, one could argue that human embryos should be treated carefully in view of the persons whom— under different circumstances—they could have become.

What's So Special about an Embryo?

Princeton bioethicist Peter Singer asks us to imagine a sperm and an egg on two sides of an IVF slide.[37] Case 1: Just before the joining of sperm and egg, the couple changes their minds, so sperm and egg are washed down the drain. Case 2: Same as case 1, but the couple changes their minds one minute after the sperm and egg have been joined. Again, the material is washed down the drain. Case 3: Same as case 1, but the technicians discover that the drain is blocked; the sperm and egg may thus have united in the drain, and if not retrieved immediately, the resulting embryo will die of exposure. Singer argues that these three cases do not differ morally, that none of these embryos has a right to life, and that the technician does no wrong in the last case by failing to retrieve the embryo.

The Semantics of the Embryo

Conception takes place when a sperm fertilizes an egg, usually in the fallopian tube. In human embryology, a successful union of sperm and egg is called a zygote, a preembryo, or an embryo. After conception, this entity immediately begins dividing: It first divides into two cells, which then divide to form four cells, which then divide to form eight cells, and so on.

During the 1980s, pro-choice theologians and bioethicists referred to this organism as a preembryo, reserving "embryo" for when it attached to the uterine wall. This was a semantic attempt to divest the embryo of any moral value. In the same way, "therapeutic cloning" is an attempt to put a pro-research twist on this kind of cloning, emphasizing benevolent intentions.

In the 1990s and continuing today, antiabortion speakers took the opposite tactic, speaking of the "embryo/fetus" or "embryo/baby," deliberately running together the ends of a spectrum of gestation. Other phrases used were "embryo/ child," "unborn baby," or "the unborn."

This is conceptually deceptive. The effects of this deception were seen by members of the Human Embryo Research Panel, when they received postcards opposing embryonic research with pictures of human embryos as tiny, fully formed babies inside test tubes.[38]

The Indeterminacy Argument

Although Richard McCormick does not assert that human embryos are persons, he thinks we should treat them as if they were. Why? Because we are unsure exactly where personhood begins in embryonic and fetal development. To use his analogy, if the hunter is not sure whether what is in the bushes is a deer or a human, he should not shoot into the bushes.

It is the same at the other end of life: if we are unsure whether a patient will emerge from a coma, shouldn't we wait as long as possible before declaring that person dead?

A subtler objection emphasizes the indeterminancy of the boundaries of sentience. When under sedation for surgery, well-publicized stories have taught us that patients can hear and perceive. Other patients have been declared dead and then awakened, recalling jokes made in their presence and procedures done on them (an important argument for not allowing medical students to train on the newly dead!).

Similarly, we are not sure exactly when the embryo develops sentience. Perhaps the most rudimentary form is like phototropism, where a plant bends towards light. Even so, when any doubt exists, we should be cautious and, under a general principle of respect, to not subject human embryos to any unnecessary medical research.

What Is an Embryo?

As said, some opponents of embryo research depict the embryo as a tiny baby, one small enough to fit inside a test-tube. In medieval philosophy, the seat of the soul was conceptualized as being occupied by a *homunculus*, a tiny, embodied person with arms and legs and a face. Aristotle thought that sperm injected this tiny human body into a woman's womb, where it simply got bigger during gestation.

Some opponents of embryo research conceive of the embryo as just this way, as a homunculus, rather than more correctly as a blackberry-shaped group of cells. If so, they agree with Steinbock's view that embryos only count morally when they can perceive pain because they think of the human embryo like Aristotle, as a tiny baby from conception who can feel pain. For them, of course, it's wrong to subject such a baby to painful research. But such a view falsely pictures embryos as babies.

More substantially, just when does an entity become an embryo? If no medical research or contraception is to be allowed after the entity becomes an embryo, then the point of demarcation is important. Traditionally, some groups have claimed such status from the moment of conception, but biologically, just when is that moment?

As it turns out, there are several points in a process of conception, any of which might be identified as *the* moment of conception: when sperm penetrates the zona pellucida, when syngamy occurs, when a diploid cell nucleus is formed, when we pass the point of a possible parthenote.[39] Which of these counts as the official moment of conception of an embryo matters, because before that moment, research might be allowed on preconceptive material (such as a human egg stimulated to cellular division by a small electric current).

The Opportunity Cost of Missed Research

We are accustomed to hearing a lot of hype about new medical advances. These exaggerations lead people to falsely believe that medical advance is relentless and proceeding on many fronts. This is more public relations than fact.

In any decade, few really major breakthroughs occur in medical research. The creation of immortalized stem cell lines from human embryonic was one such breakthrough. Not allowing this line of research to be federally funded is a major tragedy.

It is not enough to let private companies or other countries fund the research. American's National Institutes of Health (NIH) are the crown jewel of the world's scientific treasure, and it is a tragedy if such resources could not pursue this new area. Moreover, by allowing federally funded studies, we ensure the highest level of peer-reviewed, objective research—the kind most beneficial in the long run.

Banning use of embryos in federally funded projects, NIH deprives millions of people of new medicines that otherwise might not be discovered for another hundred years. Remember J. Marcia Sims and the hundred years it took to accept AIH.

Not "Just" Tissue, *MY* Tissue!

One of the well-known problems of transplants of foreign organs, blood, and tissue into a patient's body is rejection of the foreign material when recognized by the immune system. After decades of use, drugs that suppress the immune system to allow acceptance of foreign tissue may cause cancer. It would be much better for future use to grow bone, blood, organs, or particular masses of cells from one's own body.

Creating embryos from one's own cells could be used to grow tissue for one's future medical needs. By using a donor eggs, embryos could be created by embryonic cloning that were nearly identical, genetic copies of one's genome.

Libertarians argue that what an individual does with his or her body should be up to him or her. A federal ban on storing "self-made" medicine from one's own embryos allows Big Government to take away this personal liberty. By denying citizens such new medicines made from their own embryonic tissue, it takes away years from their lives.

"It's Not a Person!"

Can someone say, "The Emperor has no clothes on!"? Everyone knows that seven-day-old human embryos are not persons. Why should anyone allow others to pretend otherwise, much less accept this premise in such an important matter as closing down the most important new area of medical research to be discovered in a decade?

Some day we will come to our senses. If a medical building housing embryos catches on fire, and inside were trapped workers, students, and children, would anyone want firefighters to spend as much time rescuing embryos as actual persons? If there are a hundred frozen embryos down the hall to the left and one trapped secretary down the hall to the right, can anyone justify telling the one firefighter to go for the embryos?

What is the opportunity cost of this obsession with embryos? AIDS has orphaned thousands of children in Africa. Does justice focus on frozen embryos of white Americans and ignore these African children?

Deconstructing the Embryo Debate

As Dartmouth bioethicist Ronald Green observes, embryo research became a litmus test of the power of the religious right over American medical research.[40] One may question why this is so, and why the religious right did not choose to focus on starvation or housing or medical coverage for the poor, but the fact remains that one focus has been on cloning and embryonic research (another has been on gay/lesbian marriage).

The involvement of such groups in bioethics raises interesting questions about separation of church and state in North America. This is especially complicated in public debate when such groups do not reveal their religious premises.

Martin Luther King once came to Birmingham, Alabama, in the 1960s to try to peacefully desegregate the city, but city leaders found no way to accommodate him. Then the Black Panthers in California took up guns, and blacks in Watts and Washington, D.C., rioted. When Dr. King later returned, Birmingham's leaders were then glad to talk to the peace-loving King.

We can think of the politics of the embryos the same way. A powerful minority pushes an extreme view to shift the middle ground towards its position, and it has been remarkably successful in doing so about embryonic research in public policy.

Contrasts illuminate here. From 1975 to 1990, conservatives opposed withdrawing respirators or feeding tubes from dying patients and any other form of assisted dying. Why not continue that fight, rather than focus on embryos and cloning? The answers are that interfering with a family as one of its members dies offends many people. Plus, the mortality rate for humans is 100 percent: every person, every family, must deal with dying. No one wants outsiders dictating that Dad must suffer because they say it's immoral to give him extra morphine. So the religious right failed to control dying in America. Oregon's legalization of physician-assisted dying by prescription was just one more blow.

In contrast, opposition to cloned embryos is much easier. No family needs to be confronted and the enemy is a far-away, impersonal medical researcher, who is easy to demonize as a "baby-killer."

Bioethics is now a headliner in politics, and research on embryos is one of the main acts. President George W. Bush vetoed the Stem Cell Research Enhancement Act of 2006, but Americans by then had been educated about embryonic cloning for nearly a decade. By the time of the veto, 72 percent of them then supported embryonic research to study stem cells, a percentage up from the year before.[41]

FURTHER READING AND RESOURCES

Ronald M. Green, *The Human Embryos Research Debates: Bioethics in the Vortex of Controversy*, Oxford University Press, New York, 2001.

S. Holland et al., *The Human Embryonic Stem Cell Debate*, Bradford/MIT Press, Cambridge, Mass, 2001.

In 1991, the *Kennedy Institute of Ethics Journal* had exchanges between Jesuit Richard McCormick and secular law professor John Robertson on the moral status of embryos in research. See Volume 1. In 2001 and 2002, Volumes 11 and 12 had several articles on the same topic.

CHAPTER 7

Reproductive Cloning: Should We Clone Humans?

On July 3, 1996, the Roslin Institute near Edinburgh, Scotland, brought to birth a lamb named "Dolly" originated by cloning, a feat previously thought impossible. The institute waited seven months, until authorities granted it patents on its cloning processes, to announce this feat on February 24, 1997.

Alarmists then predicted that humans would soon be cloned. Such predictions resonated against 50 years of scary tales about human cloning in science fiction. No wonder 97 percent of people polled had a "yuk" reaction to human cloning.

Since then, cloning has become a big issue in bioethics. President George W. Bush's first prime-time television address to the nation in 2001 indirectly concerned reproductive cloning, which he declared to be wrong, echoing the sentiments of most Americans.

In 2003, a sect called the Raelians claimed they had cloned human babies. However, they produced no babies, no scientists, and no evidence for their claim. Nevertheless, and perhaps because there was no other news for one week around Christmas, their claim received saturation coverage by the world's media.

On March 4, just a few days after the announcement of Dolly, President Clinton asked his bioethics commission to decide whether human cloning should be a federal offense. This National Bioethics Advisory Commission (NBAC) recommended making the creation of a human by cloning a federal crime. In so recommending, it went well beyond the previous ban on federal funding of research on embryos and proposed a new federal intrusion into the reproductive life of Americans.

In 1998, rough-hewn Chicago physicist and former fertility researcher Richard Seed (whose name was no Hollywood caricature) caused a sensation by merely announcing that he wanted to clone his genes to produce a child. His announcement revved up anticloning speeches and caused several state legislatures to ban cloning.

The Science of Cloning

In the 1990s, Danish scientist Steed Willadsen, working at Grenada Genetics in Texas, had originated a cloned lamb embryo by enucleating an egg (i.e., by removing its nucleus) and fusing what was left with the nucleus of a cell from the

141

genetic ancestor of the sheep they wanted to re-create. In his first three attempts, in other unpublished work, Willadsen had not only produced a live lamb, he had done far better, cloning cells from embryos that had 120 cells, in contrast to the usual eight-celled embryo.[1]

When Ian Wilmut of the Roslin Institute in Scotland heard of Willadsen's work, it drew him into similar work for the next decade. The rest of the world went in a different direction, pursuing basic research in the new field of molecular biology rather than what was thought to be outdated embryology.[2] Wilmut later created the lamb Dolly from differentiated, specialized cells of her adult ancestor.

"Cloning" is an ambiguous term, even in science, as it may refer to molecular cloning, cellular cloning, embryo twinning, and somatic cell nuclear transfer (SCNT). The latter is what occurred in Dolly and what most people care about. It takes the nucleus of an adult cell and implants it in an egg cell where the nucleus has been removed.

A variant of this process called fusion (which was actually done to produce Dolly) puts the donor cells next to an enucleated egg and fuses the two with a tiny electric current. Because the pulse that produces fusion also activates egg development, a blastocyst—an embryo of about 100 cells—starts to develop. In fusion, mitochondria from both the donor and the egg recipient mix, whereas in strict transfer of a nucleus, mitochondria are only present in the enucleated egg.[3]

At a 1997 conference on mammalian cloning, Wilmut stressed that present techniques were inefficient: he started with 277 sheep eggs and got only one live lamb. Nevertheless, his statement has been widely misunderstood, partly because he has emphasized how many eggs he started with and not how many fetuses resulted in live births. The actual statistics were: 277 eggs fused in oviducts with sperm, 247 recovered from oviducts, 29 of which were transferred at the stage of morula or blastocysts, which created 13 pregnancies in lambs, three of which came to birth, and one of which was healthy and lived, Dolly.[4]

Myths about Cloning

Cloning Does Not Reproduce an Existing Person   Reproductive cloning recreates the genes of the ancestor, not the ancestor himself. Cloning recreates the genetic base of a person, but a person's identity partly stems from nongenetic sources, such as environmental input into the body (e.g., kind of food and drugs ingested), subjective experiences (peak experiences, character formation), and personal decisions based on free will. None of these nongenetic traits would be recreated by cloning.

Many of the portrayals of reproductive cloning in movies convey falsehoods. A child with the genes of an ancestor would not have any memories of the ancestor, as the character Ripley had in the movie *Alien Resurrection*.

This also means that you can't reproduce yourself. Narcissistic people who think cloning a baby with their genes will do so are mistaken. Cloning reproduces about 99.8 percent of the ancestor's genes (the other 0.2 percent come from mitochondrial genes in the host-egg), but even 0.2 percent difference can be significant. Identical twins have small differences in random inactivation of the X chromosome in embryonic development and this results in different personalities and traits as adults.

Of course, the main difference is that a resulting child would not have the memories of the adult ancestor. Nor would the child necessarily have the personality, outlook, or drive of the ancestor. These qualities depend in part on early childhood experiences, chosen acts that mold character, schools the child attends, and the people who mentor the adolescent.

If the 69-year-old Richard Seed had originated a child by cloning in 1998, hoping to re-create himself, he would have been disappointed. Since it would take 20 years for the child to grow to adulthood, Seed would likely have been dead by that time. Even if he did live to see the child as an adult, he would likely have been disappointed to see that the child created by cloning, having grown up in a different environment, in a different time, would be a different person from him.

Cloned Humans Would Not Be Drones but Persons A child created by reproductive cloning would need to be gestated by a human female for nine months, and his birth would be like that of any other child. He would have no distinguishing marks on him to indicate his origins. He would feel, sense, think, and hurt like any other human child.

Today, we do not believe that a child's origins affect his status as a person—it does not matter whether your parents were married, of different races, gay or lesbian, or whether you were conceived in a test tube. Children created by cloning would be persons with all the rights of other persons.

Some widely quoted authors such as Leon Kass have questioned this, implying that prejudiced people might treat cloned children as less-than-human. If this were so, it might not be in the best interest of a child to be originated this way.

But notice that the same logic implies that it might not be best to be created as a child of an interracial couple because "other people" might be prejudiced against such marriages and their children. The effect of such reasoning is to strengthen prejudice, not to weaken it, and to give it too much weight in what, after all, is supposed to be *moral* reasoning. The way to combat prejudice is to expose it and to replace it with knowledge and reasoning, not to give in to it.

For this reason, we must be careful when we speak of children originated by cloning. To call them "clones" is to be prejudicial because it connotes bad things about such children and people who created them. Similarly, to imply that children created by cloning would be raised in batches connotes all kinds of bad, silly things, such as seeing them as zombies, as sources of organs for genetic ancestors, and in general, as less than human.

Cloning Would Have No Effect on the Gene Pool One sometimes hears the objection that cloning will decrease the diversity of the human gene pool. Diversity in such a pool is good for the human race because unknown diseases may appear in the future, against which idiosyncratic genes may offer the best defense to the minority of humans who have them. In this way, it is hypothesized that African-Americans with genes for sickle-cell disease escaped early death from malaria in Africa and whites with genes causing cystic fibrosis escaped lethal airborne diseases caused by viruses (cystic fibrosis creates excess mucus in the lungs and gastrointestinal tract, eventually killing patients but perhaps protecting young people from infection of viruses long enough to reproduce.

Behind this objection is the idea that characteristics of children originated by cloning would not be individually chosen by parents but stamped out, machine-line, in vast, uniform quantities. A variant of the objection is that prospective parents are so easily influenced by a few cultural stereotypes that millions would choose geno-types of famous movie stars, in the same way that names such as "Heather" and "Jennifer" became suddenly popular 20 years ago among white parents.

Even if all the above were true, originating children by cloning would not affect the human gene pool. A few facts explain why. Originating a child by cloning requires in vitro fertilization, which is unsuccessful 75–80 percent of the time and which in over 35 states must be paid for by the prospective parents at nearly $8,000 per attempt. Of the people who use IVF, only a small percentage would consider cloning. So the numbers of children originated by cloning will be tiny.

A little math here goes a long way. Around 2000, the planet held over 6 billion people and by 2010, that number will probably be at 6.5 billion. Even if a million peo-ple were originated by cloning, their genes would have little influence on the 6.5 bil-lion, especially because each person will have free will, grow up, probably fall in love with a person not originated by cloning, and create children sexually with mixed genes. There is no reason to think that people originated by cloning will need cloning to reproduce or prefer cloning over sexual reproduction (which is more fun!).

For this reason, it would be difficult to elevate the quality of the human gene pool by either cloning or by any kind of eugenic-parental selection of traits. In the same way, worries about the deterioration of the human gene pool are also mis-founded, as the next generation will mix its genes with other genes, resulting in new combinations.

The above reasoning illustrates the *law of regression to the mean* in population genetics. If you have a big population reproducing, for example, 6 billion people, then over time, abnormal values will normalize. The crushing weight of the num-bers stabilizes the mean.

When you understand this, you see that the human gene pool is stable. Even a billion superior humans originated by cloning would reproduce with the other five billion normal humans, and within two or three generations, the superior genes would be diluted. But creating a billion humans by cloning is impossible, as it would require five billion successful attempts through IVF at creating babies.

At bottom, worries about effects of cloning on the human gene pool all mis-takenly assume mass production of humans from a cookie-cutter mold. But this assumption is no more true for cloning than it was 30 years ago about test tube babies.

Lack of Informed Consent of Children Created by Cloning   One sometimes hears that attempting to originate a child by cloning would be an unethical exper-iment on the resulting child because such a child could not give informed consent to the experiment. But this objection rests on a misconception.

The misconception is not that it would not be an experiment to create a child this way, for that would be true. The misconception is first, the idea that any child can consent to any experiment before its birth, and second, that to be ethical, such an experiment would require such consent.

Both of these conditions are false. If the second were true, virtually every improvement in the neonatal nursery or pediatric surgery would be unethical. And thousands of experiments have been done on babies without their consent to improve their health and to fix congenital defects. Medical progress depends on them.

It might be countered that such experiments are designed to improve the health of the baby, whereas cloning is not, being merely designed to gratify the ego of narcissistic parents. But that counter begs the usual questions about the bad motives of parents involved in cloning.

Commodification   Originating babies by cloning is often held to be making babies into "things" or commodities, not Kantian ends-in-themselves. Critics assume that people create such babies only for specific qualities, and that creation for such reasons might be imitated by thousands of others (*Newsweek* cover story: "Thousands of parents clone Michael Jordan").

As we saw in the previous chapter, such objections forget that prospective parents make similar choices now in pursuing adoption of babies of a certain race, gender, ethnicity, or health status. As we saw, substantial amounts of money change hands to facilitate adoptions. And yet no one considers the babies adopted to be "commodities" or the parents to be bad for paying large fees for adoption.

The objection also makes the usual mistake of assuming bad motives in parents who utilize a new method of conception. This history of reproductive ethics, going back to artificial insemination and amniocentesis, shows that opponents will greet each new option with this objection.

Brave New World   Conservative Francis Fukuyama believes that originating humans by cloning will destroy the human essence. He and others cite Aldous Huxley's futuristic novel *Brave New World* as an argument against going in this direction.

But such citation is misguided. *Brave New World* is about the dangers of mass conditioning society through behavioral techniques. Only the beginning example is about assembly-line reproduction of prechosen genotypes (admittedly, this is a powerful scene). Ironically, the main message of *Brave New World* is the danger of the state taking away choice from parents about ways of creating children. Yet opponents of cloning cite this novel to do exactly that!

Because people have been so *conditioned* to reject anything associated with "cloning," such citations have added irony.

Scientists Are Not Frankensteins   Dr. Frankenstein, in Mary Shelley's novel of the same name, is the archetype from which scary pictures of scientists are drawn. Arrogant, unfeeling for his creation, working in an isolated lab, seemingly spouse-less and child-less, this mad scientist is meant to be inhuman and scary.

Miss Shelley wrote her book to scare people, to make money, and to become famous. She was not a sociologist who did a careful survey of the qualities of working scientists, nor was she a scientist herself, nor had she ever worked with scientists.

Most scientists are normal, with kids and spouses, who share our fears about runaway technology and dehumanizing medical tools. So let us not impute bad motives to scientists without evidence.

Remember that the scientists who get the most attention from the media—Richard Seed, Panos Zavos, and Raelian Brigitte Boisselier—are not in laboratories working, but constantly working the telephones to make appearances on television and radio. These people seek publicity, not to help infertile couples. They should not be confused with scientists working diligently and ethically in their offices and labs.

ARGUMENTS FOR AND AGAINST HUMAN CLONING

Moral arguments against human reproductive cloning divide into two categories, one that cloning is *intrinsically wrong*, the second that, while not intrinsically wrong, it is *indirectly wrong* because of undesirable things associated with it. This chapter starts with arguments of the first kind.

As said, these arguments are *moral* ones, not *legal* ones. A different kind of argument about reproductive cloning has occurred in the United States, where legislators have made attempts at reproductive cloning a federal crime. The Human Cloning Prohibition Act passed the House of Representatives in 2001 but did not pass the U.S. Senate in 2002.

The legal argument against this bill is that the Bill of Rights or U.S. Constitution does not give Congress the right to make laws about how Americans originate children, choose not to originate children (contraception), or choose to stop children from growing inside them (abortion). While states may do so as a way of regulating medical practice and of protecting children, this is not a power reserved for the federal government.

By 2006, 13 states passed laws making attempts at reproductive cloning a crime, including Arkansas, California, Connecticut, Indiana, Iowa, Maryland, Massachusetts, Michigan, New Jersey, North Dakota, Rhode Island, South Dakota, and Virginia.[5]

DIRECT ARGUMENTS AGAINST HUMAN CLONING

Against the Will of God

Many clergy believe that originating children by cloning is not God's will. God ordained in Genesis that humans should reproduce as did Adam and Eve, man and woman begetting children, and that is God's plan for humanity. To deviate from the plan is wrong. Just as gay men and lesbians were not meant in this plan to have children, so children were not meant to be created asexually.

Notice that this argument is an inference about God's will. Nowhere in any scripture does it say that medical science should not use reproductive cloning to produce children. Notice too that most advances in the history of medicine have been greeted by the same argument that a change is against God's will.

The Right to a Unique Genetic Identity

With Dolly's birth, the possibility emerged of cloning a human baby. Various people began to assert that what was wrong with cloning a human baby from a genetic ancestor's cells was that it would violate the right of each person to a "unique genetic identity." Some theologians at the Vatican made this claim (although they had never made it before Dolly's birth).

An initial problem about this argument concern twins. Since so-called "identical" twins share 99.9 percent of their genes, is their right to a unique identity violated by being a twin? Certain techniques of assisted reproduction, such as implanting many embryos, drastically increase the likelihood of such twins. Are they wrong?

A bigger problem with this objection is the assumption that one's genes are one's identity. This reductionist line of thinking in modern genetics lies behind similar objections that a child created by cloning would not have a soul because it shared the same genes as the ancestor. Both objections assume that genes make the person, the self, the identity, and yet we know that is incorrect because environment also contributes to personhood (and possibly, so does free choice).

Unnatural and Perverse

Many people also wonder about the motives behind cloning. They ask, why would anyone want to originate a child by cloning? Why not use the fun method of sex? If a couple is unable to have a child through sex, why not adopt?

Sexual reproduction is natural. Cloning, or asexual reproduction, is unnatural. What is good for plants or animals should not be used for humans.

Something is wrong with parents who want to clone a child. They are either narcissistic or so desperate—after all other methods of having children have failed—that they will subject their future child to a perverted experiment in which his personhood will be at risk when he later learns that he is "just a clone."

In reply, it should be noted that this objection begs a lot of questions. First it assumes that what is primitive or natural is always best. That is certainly not true for a man and woman who are naturally infertile. Second, it assumes that the new way of making babies is perverse and therefore wrong, a charge that created many other new ways of making babies in the past. Finally, it assumes bad motives on the part of would-be parents.

The Right to an Open Future

Critics claim that parents choose a certain genotype, say, athlete Michael Jordan's or actor Brad Pitt's, for a reason and with certain expectations. After their investment in in vitro fertilization, they would expect the resulting child to have qualities similar to Jordan or Pitt. They would expect the child to become rich and famous through being a professional basketball player or a movie star, respectively.

The future should be open to every child. It is wrong for tennis mothers to impose their wills on their children in their hell-bent determination to make them into tennis stars; it is wrong for East Asian parents to push their children into medical careers from an early age; and it is wrong for soccer dads and Little League coaches to push their children into athleticism.

Why is this so? The heart of the objection about a closed future lies in explaining this answer. At bottom is the premise that parents should not have children to fulfill their own needs, desires, or fantasies, but for the good of the child. In this sense, parenting should be Kantian, not egotistic.

It is certainly not in every child's best interest to have a preconceived career foisted on him or her by parents regardless of that child's abilities and, perhaps more important, their own free decisions. More than one child has felt the agony of being pushed into a Procrustean bed where he or she does not fit, while desperately trying to gain the love and respect of their parents, who only define success as fulfilling unrealistic expectations.

If parents create children expecting specific traits (basketball skills, acting talent), the objection continues, then children can be damaged psychologically when they cannot, or choose not to, fulfill such expectations.

This argument lies behind the widely heard objection about "designer babies," i.e., that it is wrong for parents to try to create children with blue eyes and blonde hair and with a strong interest in music and tennis. Instead, parents should accept whatever God gives them as a gift.

The most dangerous idea of all is that parents should be free to reject, or not love, babies who lack the qualities they want. Already a dangerous tendency has started among some parents to not aggressively treat impaired babies suffering from genetic diseases at birth, followed by equally dangerous practices of death-by-abortion after sonogram after it's been determined that it's a female fetus. If we add to this the possibility of using preimplantation diagnosis during in vitro fertilization to not implant any embryo with cystic fibrosis or Down's syndrome, we are already halfway to the bad place of parents rejecting children in the nursery when they emerge with the wrong genes.

The whole point of this reductio is to challenge the premise that parents should be able to accept or reject babies based on qualities they have or lack. That is to be denied. Since it is to be denied, any practice that would further this is also to be denied, such as the practice of trying to create children with certain specific qualities.

INDIRECT ARGUMENTS AGAINST HUMAN CLONING

Abnormalities

At present, a high rate of abnormalities plagues efforts to create primates by somatic cell nuclear transfer. Any such conception of a human baby by cloning would be an experiment on a child, and no such experiment is justified without a compensating benefit for the child. Such a benefit does not yet exist. As such, attempts to create a child by cloning the cells of a human ancestor and gestating it to birth are wrong.

Indeed, because a child is likely to be born with some genetic defect, conceiving a child from cloning might be a form of child abuse. If the motives of the parent were bad, then deliberately creating a child who was likely to be genetically defective would be like deliberately choosing to implant an embryo with cystic fibrosis rather than a healthy one.

Notice that this objection depends on the existing state of scientific knowledge. If scientists learn to originate baboons and chimpanzees by cloning without defects and learn how to originate all other mammals safely by cloning, then the chances of a defective cloned baby would drop drastically and the force of this objection would correspondingly diminish.

Notice that when we discuss abnormalities, we need a baseline for comparison. Over 50 percent of embryos created sexually, half of which are chromosomally abnormal, do not implant successfully in the human uterus and are lost. About 2 percent of live-born babies have some genetic defect. Millions of babies are born after the mother smoked or drank during their gestation, yet we do not criminalize such smoking and drinking during pregnancy. (Perhaps we should, but why should we focus on the sensationalistic, remote cases of cloning and ignore obvious harm to babies around us?)

Deep Inequality

Some people, through no merit of their own, start out life much better than others. Some children get two parents, four grandparents, lots of gifts at holidays and birthdays, special pre school and after-school tutoring, and the best private schools and universities. It seems unfair that some get so much but others, so little.

Over the last centuries, civilized societies have mitigated some of the more extreme effects of this *environmental inequality:* estate taxes have reduced how much can be inherited from parents, income taxes redistribute money from high earners to those on disability and public assistance, and expanding economies have created new opportunities for hard work and talent to get ahead.

Even so, the gap between rich and poor is astonishing, having widened over the last decade. Given that gap, reproductive cloning could start a new kind of *biological inequality,* much deeper than our existing, environmental inequality. Because reproductive cloning would normally involve a conscious choice to clone the genome of one person rather than another, it is likely that families would choose genomes with good qualities. If cloning could be done successfully, such families could create strong, clever, talented, energetic dynasties that outstripped normal humans. It would be a biological case of "the rich get richer, the poor get poorer." Princeton biologist Lee Silver calls the results the "GenRich" and the "Normals."[6]

This is something new in human evolution. Sexual reproduction randomly exchanges genetic material, and because of regression to the mean, makes sure that the great genetic norm of human nature never rises or falls too much. But in a single swoop, particular families single-mindedly devoted to raising their genetic stature could biologically out-distance normal humans over a few generations.

As such, reproductive cloning poses a grave new danger to social justice. Moreover, because this danger is "written into biology," it would be much harder to undo. People without superior genes would find it much harder to compete against such superior people, even when the competition was completely fair.

But is this the way we want the advanced countries of the world to go? Toward a deeply stratified society that divides into Superiors, whose genotypes were chosen by committed families bent on superiority, and Normals, whose genotypes were randomly assigned by the spin of the genetic roulette ball in sexual reproduction?

DIRECT ARGUMENTS FOR HUMAN CLONING

Good of the Child

Almost all ordinary discussions of cloning beg two important questions: they assume bad motives on the part of parents or scientists involved in creating a child by cloning, and they assume the child would be harmed by knowing he was created this way.

We can see just how much is begged when we counter these assumptions. First, a child created through cloning would know that he was wanted by his parents. After all, creation of such a child would require in vitro fertilization, which at best is successful only 25 percent of the time. Thus, prospective parents probably would have to try several times to create the baby this way, and pay for their efforts.

In contrast, all that many people know about the wishes of their parents is that their parents had sex and did not abort. They have no clear evidence that their birth was planned. This fact especially applies to children created before *Griswold* v. *Connecticut* in 1965 made it legal for physicians to prescribe contraceptives.

To give this argument some play, assume both that technical difficulties are overcome about reproductive cloning and that children produced this way are safe. Besides knowing he or she was wanted, is there anything about being originated this way that could be in the interests of a child?

Well, for one thing, few parents would knowingly recreate the genotype of an adult with a congenital disease. In so far as possible, parents would choose children who would be healthy.

This in itself will be good for the child. Placing aside for the moment worries about eugenics, it is hard to ignore the good of a life where one is not constantly challenged by physical or mental disabilities.

Next, consider that certain traits might be genetically based. We already know that looks and physique are, because we see resemblances in a family. Suppose, too, that intelligence, wit, temperament, sociability, verbal ability, mathematical ability, and analytical ability are partly genetically based. To give the argument more rope, suppose that parents could choose children with some of these traits. Would doing so be good for the child?

It is hard to see why not. Although it may not be politically correct to say it, all other things being equal, it is better to live life as a beautiful, smart, healthy person than the reverse, and it is hard to see why such a life is not in the interests of the person created.

Of course, opponents will say that such a person has been created as a purchased "commodity" and is subject to the unrealistic expectations of the parent. We will consider the objection about expectations below, but for now, notice that this general line of objections applies to any service that parents buy for present children with the same goals in mind, such as sending children to elite private schools. Yet no one considers the latter to be bad for the children.

Finally, we should notice that there is a dilemma that proponents of reproductive cloning encounter in which either way, they lose. If cloning is unsafe, then it hurts the child, and therefore it's wrong to do. If cloning is safe, then it improves the child and is eugenic, and therefore wrong to do. Obviously, trapped in this false dilemma, proponents of cloning can never win.

At bottom, what may scare opponents of reproductive cloning the most is the possibility that it will work, be safe, and be in the best interests of the children created. Then some children will have more, biologically, than others, and some families may create biological dynasties. Be that as it may, these are not objections about the intrinsic evil of cloning, but indirect ones, focusing on harm to equality (and which we consider below).

Only Way to Have One's Own Baby

One of the main reasons to produce a child is to have a child with one's own genes. Whether it's to have one's family line continue or to have "a bit of me going into the future," no one questions the soundness of this parental motive.

Now in some rare cases, asexual reproduction will be the only method by which a parent can have a genetic connection to a resulting child. Men who are azoospermatic (producing no sperm) or women whose eggs are too old to conceive often still want a child who is genetically related. Reproductive cloning would allow each parent to have a child (assuming two children) with a strong (99.9 percent) genetic connection to the respective parent.

Although men with low sperm counts could reproduce sexually through intracyptoplasmic sperm injection (ICSI) into a donated egg, there is no option for a man who lacks sperm and a woman who lacks good eggs and who also want a genetic connection to a child. For either parent, the only route is the asexual one of using a cell from a nucleus of a differential cell, and using the genes inside it via cloning to create a human embryo.

The combination of two forces strengthens this argument in subtle ways. First, as they pursue careers, many women delay age of their first pregnancy, and when they marry so late that they cannot conceive, they are disappointed. At age 42, less than 10 percent of women carry healthy eggs; over 90 percent at this age will fail to bear a child with their own egg. Whatever child they adopt or create with donor eggs will have no genetic connection to them.

Second, intellectuals, bureaucrats, and politicians often underestimate the force of the urge to be genetically connected to a child. When government and private insurance refused to pay for in vitro fertilization in the late 1970s, everyone thought that few parents would pay cash for the experimental procedures, much less that struggling college professors with little money would forsake cars and a house in attempts to have a genetically related baby. But they did, and a $3 billion industry was born.

Hence, the millions of couples with women in their 40s who are trying to conceive a child, and who strongly desire a genetic connection to a child or two, will be the prime movers in the quest to originate children by cloning. Hence, this argument will appeal to more people, and for different reasons, than might have been thought at first.

Stronger Genetic Connection

A child created by cloning would have *all* the parent's genes, not just half, right? So he or she would have not the usual 50 percent genetic connection to a parent, but nearly 100 percent. But if half a genetic connection is good, why is double not also good?

See this as an onus of proof argument. Since people and courts assume in public policy that a biological connection makes for a bond between parent and child, why would a stronger bond not be just as good? Whatever it is that makes genetic bonds good for children, is a stronger bond not also good? If not, why? If it's just the novelty of a stronger bond, that is not an argument against the bond, just a new item for empirical investigation.

Do our law and courts see the genetic connection this way? Indeed they do. In a dozen cases around the country, a baby who was adopted and who spent several years with an adopted family was returned to a parent with whom he shared a genetic connection after one of many disputes arose. The point here is not to judge the merits of the final resolution of custody of the child, but to emphasize how much weight the law puts on binding a parent to a child through shared genes.

In another context, countless talk shows feature unmarried women who have had sexual relations with more than one man, each of whom could be the father of the child. On these shows and often in life, the men say, "If it's mine, I'll support the child." And the law agrees, assigning paternity and requirements of child-support if a DNA test identifies a particular man as the father. All of these cases point to the power we assume of the genetic connection to the child.

But those are sexual connections, where only half a parent's genes are bequeathed to a child. Imagine a total, 100 percent genetic connection. Would that not bind males to sons in an incredibly strong way? Couldn't that be a good thing for some sons, to have a father so tightly bound to him? Or for a girl, to have a mother so tightly bound?

INDIRECT ARGUMENTS FOR HUMAN CLONING

Closed Future?

Opponents argue that children created by cloning will have a closed future because parents will expect, say, tennis stars or professional basketball players. Explaining why that is false gives some important insights into who people created by cloning will be.

First, any adult created by cloning will have free will. Too often in discussions about nature versus nurture, or genetics, people talk as if college students and adults are not responsible for their sexual choices, health behavior, grades, choice of mates, and choice of careers. No parent or script can negate free will or take it away.

Perhaps one reason so many people forget about free will when it comes to reproductive cloning is that, in the back of their minds, the myth from science fiction of clones-as-zombie still operates. When a person created by cloning is thought of as a drone or zombie, it is easy to forget about free will. Indeed, the word "clones" (as in "an army of escaping clones") seems to denote beings with little free will.

Second, many parents have expectations of children, even before birth. But most parents love their children and realize that they cannot go against a child's unfolding nature or desires. No matter how much a parent might want his child to become a physician, if the child hates science, the parent's wish is not going to come true. Most parents understand the wisdom of not subjecting their children to unrealistic expectations. So, too, would parents of children from cloning.

Opponents would retort that parents using cloning will be a special subset of parents, much more likely to impose their expectations on resulting children. Even if this is so, what should we make of it? Notice that it isn't always bad for parents to have high expectations of children. Too many parents have no expectations of their children. Having expectations per se is not necessarily a bad thing.

The best retort to this objection is that it assumes bad motives on the part of parents. Why should we assume this? Why shouldn't the onus of proof be on those who want to see such parents as bad?

If originating humans by cloning becomes safe, we will be in for some surprises. Suppose a child is created from the genes of a girl who was an all-state champion in the breast stroke and who had ability in math, scoring in the top 1 percent of standardized tests and excelling in AP math classes in high school.

What is often overlooked is the role of supportive parents in such achievements. Now suppose that the child cloned never learns to swim and is never exposed to math, and doesn't develop these abilities while she is young enough to. In that case, we will learn, perhaps painfully, that parents of children cloned for certain abilities cannot just sit back and wait for the abilities to unfold, but will need to be just as involved as the ancestor's parents. If they are not, it will be easy to see where the blame should go.

Liberty

Those wishing to curtail reproductive cloning because it might increase social inequality need to put their cards on the table and not hide behind subterfuge. They rarely say exactly what they want to do and that is to decrease the liberty of the average person to have children and to create a family.

Now the liberty to create children and a family is not absolute and may be outweighed by a much greater social good. But in the rest of our lives, we prize liberty highly, especially when it comes to creating families and what goes on inside them.

In most areas of our personal lives, we are not willing to curtail our personal liberty to create more social-political-economic equality. For example, we could make private schools illegal and require all children to attend public schools. This would get the best parents involved in PTAs and community boards, which in turn would raise the level of all public schools, thereby helping equality. In the South, where private academies continue as the vestiges of racially segregated schools, and where elite preparatory schools create a class of highly privileged students, equality is not furthered by giving the best students the most resources.

But few people favor mandatory public schools because it would take away freedom from parents about how and where their children are educated. It is for this reason that some people hate busing, because it forces some children to be bused across the city in the name of equality.

The point is not about busing and public education but about how it is easy to pick on reproductive cloning, sacrificing it to equality, because so few people want to exercise this liberty. But the principle is the same: sacrifice liberty for equality. What justifies sacrifice in one area of reproductive life may be extended to another. For example, if only well-off people can afford in vitro fertilization, shouldn't it be banned too?

A Rawlsian Argument for Cloning and Choice

A surprising number of people are against any attempt to improve the genetic qualities of the human race, labeling such attempts eugenic (and hence, wrong). But one argument of the late philosopher John Rawls may counter this sentiment.

Justice, according to Rawls, applies not to acts between individuals but to the basic structure of society. Rawls argues famously in *A Theory of Justice* that the principles of justice that apply to the basic structure would be chosen in a hypothetical social contract where parties choose under a "veil of ignorance" about their position in society when the veil rises. Now consider the following passage from Rawls:

> I have assumed so far that the distribution of natural assets is a fact of nature and that no attempt is made to change it, or even to take it into account. But to some extent this distribution is bound to be affected by the social system. . . . [I]t is also in the interest of each to have greater natural assets. This enables him to pursue a preferred plan of life. In the original position, then, the parties want to insure for their descendants the best genetic endowment (assuming their own to be fixed). The pursuit of reasonable policies in this regard is something that earlier generations owe to later ones, this being a question that arises between generations. Thus over time a society is to take steps to preserve the general level of natural abilities and to prevent the diffusion of serious defects. These measures are to be guided by principles that the parties would be willing to consent to for the sake of their successors. I mention this speculative and difficult matter to indicate once again the manner in which the difference principle is likely to transform problems of social justice. We might conjecture that in the long run, if there is an upper bound on ability, we would eventually reach a society with the greatest equal liberty the members of which enjoy the greatest equal talent.[7]

To the argument that we should not attempt to improve the human race, Rawls replies: if we were in the social contract—taking the long view of millions of people over many generations—and when the veil lifted, we did not know which generation we would inhabit, would we choose not to make the later generations as genetically talented as possible, compatible with the equal liberty of each to procreate in preceding generations?

It cannot be stressed too much that Rawlsian principles forbid state coercion to improve genetic inheritance of future generations. For Rawls the first principle of civilized life is protection of our basic civil liberties. Any attempt to impose a procreative program on us violates such liberties. Equally, when the state says we cannot reproduce in certain ways, it also violates our liberties.

Under the veil of ignorance, it is in the interest of future children to allow our parents to create each of us with as much natural talent as possible, with the best genes, and with the best chance at a long, healthy life. One could even argue, although this is controversial, that under this intragenerational, Rawlsian theory of justice, people are not just *permitted* to improve the genes of future children, but are *obligated* to do so. Why? Because it is wrong to choose lives for future people that makes them much worse off than they otherwise could have lived.

Politicization of Facts about Cloning

Feminists have noted that gender bias reflects how scientists see the facts: women and men approach a context with different interests and backgrounds, and as such, filter data differently in generating facts.

Worldviews certainly affect how people see the facts. Creationists famously dispute the idea that humans evolved over millions of years by evolving from a chimp-like ancestor. Others dispute the age of the earth and the molecular origins of life from a molecular, Godless soup.

There are many other controversial areas of science where facts about certain topics generate a lot of heat, especially anything to do with sex (homosexuality, lesbianism, or transgender issues). Assisted reproduction and parenting are also hot-button topics.

As a general rule, the more emotion swirls around a topic, the more politicized facts about it are. Reproductive cloning is certainly an emotional topic, so we would predict (and find) that even the most respected scientists often run with their passions when writing about cloning.

It is often easy to emphasize that the glass is half-empty when it's also half-full. You can emphasize that Ian Wilmut started with 277 eggs to get one lamb, or you can emphasize that he brought three cloned lambs (one live, named Dolly) to birth from 13 fetuses from 29 implanted embryos. You can emphasize that Dolly has arthritis and imply that it's from her unique origins, or you can test a thousand lambs of similar age created sexually and describe how many also have arthritis.

Links between Embryonic and Reproductive Cloning

Research on human embryos creates fear in some people of slippery slopes. Leon Kass made such fears explicit in an article that appeared just before the announcement of the recommendations of the National Bioethics Advisory Commission. "And yet, as a matter of policy and prudence, any opponent of the manufacture of cloned humans must, I think, in the end oppose also the creating of cloned human embryos."[8]

Because he fears that allowing cloning of human embryos will inevitably lead to implantation of a human embryo originated by cloning, he wants to test physicians and scientists who favor lifting the ban on embryo research by making them endorse "an absolute and effective ban on all attempts to implant into a uterus a cloned human embryo (cloned from an adult) to produce a living child."

To the criticism that the techniques of human asexual reproduction are not that complicated and that someone in the world will eventually originate a living child by cloning, Kass would put the onus of proof on those who would permit the "horror" of such origination: "Perhaps such a ban will prove ineffective; perhaps it will eventually be shown to have been a mistake. But it would at least place the burden of practical proof where it belongs: on the proponents of this horror."

If it is true that embryonic cloning cannot be divorced from reproductive cloning, then other things also follow. For one thing, if reproductive cloning is not bad, then neither is embryonic cloning. If reproductive cloning is not intrinsically bad, but only bad because of abnormal results, then we should study how to prevent abnormalities by funding research in embryonic cloning.

In other words, the argument above says that because reproductive cloning is evil, we shouldn't fund anything that would help us do it. But if that is false and reproductive cloning is just a tool—just another way to make a baby and help start a family—then we should investigate all ways to create such a tool.

Not funding research on cloned embryos, or on ways to prevent abnormalities in reproductive cloning in primates, seems perverse. If abnormalities are the major reason for prohibiting reproductive cloning, then surely research to prevent them is justified. But if the real objection is the assumption of the intrinsic evil of reproductive cloning, then we should dispense with the cover of arguing about abnormalities and get to the real issue.

Conclusions: The Future

Reproductive cloning will not go away, especially because it will be difficult to police every top scientist in every corner of the world. (Remember: the techniques involved do not require cyclotrons or great financial investment and might be done by scientists who leave North America to pursue their vision, say, in Bangalore, India.)

Whatever happens in the future, the world will undoubtedly overreact to the nature of the first human baby created by cloning. If the baby is abnormal, in whatever way, the world will rush to make cloning illegal. If the baby is normal, by all apparent means, then much of the hysteria about reproductive cloning will die down, just as it did in 1978 after the birth of Louise Brown.

If babies created by cloning develop into normal children, then the argument will shift to possible dangers to children from cloning, and using cloning might be considered more like drinking while pregnant: bad, but not completely evil.

There is also another possibility that could change the world: Children created by cloning could be adorable, bright, healthy, and lovable, and hence become children that everyone wants. Critics such as Francis Fukuyama will say that such a possibility would change "who we are" and our human essence,[9] but others would see it as a happy fact, a blessing to such children and their families, and an area which should be off-limits to federal intrusion.

FURTHER READING AND RESOURCES

Gregory Pence, *Who's Afraid of Human Cloning?* Lanham, Md.: Rowman & Littlefield, 1998.

Gregory Pence, *Cloning After Dolly: Who's Still Afraid of Human Cloning?* Lanham, Md.: Rowman & Littlefield, 2004.

Human Cloning Foundation, www.humancloning.org.

Francis Fukuyama, *Our Posthuman Future*, New York: Farrar Straus & Giroux, 2002.

Leon Kass, *Human Cloning and Human Dignity: The Report of the President's Council on Bioethics*, New York: Public Affairs Press, 2002.

CHAPTER 8

Ethical Theories and Bioethics

A HISTORY OF ETHICAL THEORIES

The Greeks and the Virtues

Ancient Greek philosophers during the fifth century BCE and earlier advocated virtue ethics. Applied to medicine, virtue theory emphasizes physicians with good traits of character.

"Ethics" derives from the Greek *ethos*, meaning "disposition" or "trait." *Ethos* constituted part of the Greek phrase *ethike aretai* ("skills of character"). The Greek word *arete* connotes "excellence," "good," and "skill."

Pre-Socratic ethics emphasized *ethike aretai* in performing roles well. Ethics concerned the role one fulfilled. If one wanted to know about ethics, one asked about, say, the traits of a good soldier, physician, mother, or ruler. If one asked, "What is the goal of being a soldier?" others answered: "To defend one's country." And again, "What excellences are needed to defend one's country?" The answer: physical strength, courage, skill in using weapons, organization in fighting in groups, temperance, and cunning.

Greek ethics were *teleological*: they assumed that things developed towards a natural goal. In Greek medicine, if we want to know what makes a good physician, we need to know the goal of medicine. That goal is to heal the sick. What virtues does this goal require? Answer: compassion, knowledge of healing, and skill in human relations.

In a move of ethical genius, Socrates transcended role-defined ethics and asked about the *ethike aretai* of a good person. His questions were answered best by his student, Plato, and even better by Plato's student, Aristotle. In their view, these *ethika aretai* were courage, temperance, wisdom, and justice (in human relations)—the excellences necessary to function well in human society. Today we know these traits as *the cardinal virtues*.

So we should not only ask, "What virtues should a good physician possess?" but also, "What virtues should a good person possess who is a physician?" The narrow question is, "What should a good *physician* do?" The broader question is, "What should a good *person* do?" They will not always get the same answer.

One way to define a good person is as one who follows God's law. Traditional interpretations of God's law condemn abortion and euthanasia. A physician who is a good person in that sense will not do some acts that naturalist physicians would do. For example, in ancient times, Hippocrates adopted not only a patient-centered, but also a sanctity-of-all-life-centered, ethics.

Based on what they could see or palpate, most ancient Greek physicians took a different, naturalistic approach. So they often helped terminal patients to die. Most such Greek physicians adopted a quality-of-life view, believing that it is futile to maintain lives of suffering.

Christian Ethics, Christian Virtues

In the fourth century C.E., Christianity added to the cardinal virtues its theological virtues of faith, hope, and charity, bringing the total to seven. Christianity also added the Seven Deadly Sins (sloth, lust, envy, greed, wrath, gluttony, and the master vice, pride).

Good physicians always exhibit compassion. This virtue comes from Christianity and its monastic tradition where lives are dedicated to helping others. Etymologically, "compassion" means "to suffer with," as Christians believe that Jesus suffered with, and for, humans on the Cross.

Where naturalistic physicians emphasized technical competence, religious physicians emphasized compassion. When physicians reach the limits of technical competence, compassion becomes important. Because those limits are always reached, because all humans die, compassion is always a virtue in physicians. Moreover, patients always want physicians who are both knowledgeable and merciful.

Role-defined ethics and virtue ethics underlie the apprentice system in medical education, where medical students gradually assume more responsibility in assisting older physicians in treating patients. The attending physician teaches the resident, who teaches the intern, who teaches the fourth-year student. Senior physicians teach not only how to perform procedures, but how to be compassionate, wise, courageous, and patient-centered.

What would virtue ethicists say about a particular issue in medical ethics? The general answer is that physicians-in-training should imitate good, senior physicians. Confronted with a 14-year-old patient who refuses to eat after being paralyzed during an auto accident, most experienced physicians are likely to say: "Let's work with him until he's of legal age, then he can decide for himself to die. By that time, he'll probably find a reason to live."

Socratic virtues celebrated an elitist, antidemocratic ethics that scorned commoners. The Greeks believed themselves superior to the peoples they conquered. Aristotle's student, Alexander the Great, attempted to instill Greek values, culture, and language on everyone, and he had no tolerance for the cultures of other peoples. The Greek ethics that Alexander inherited were perfectionistic, aristocratic, and meritocratic. In this sense, the quality-of-life attitude of ancient Greek physicians was elitist and perfectionistic, whereas the sanctity-of-life ethic of Hippocratic physicians was much less so.

In contrast, the three great religions of the West emphasize duties to the poor and sick: the rabbinic ethics of Bar Hillel stress acts that help one's fellow man, Jesus says that as you treat the poor, so you treat Him, and Mohammed made the *zakat*, the tax on property for the poor, one of the pillars of Islam. So for a Jew, Christian, or Muslim, a good physician is first a Jew, Christian, or Muslim, and second a physician.

As such, a Christian physician must care for the poor as part of being a physician. The physician's license, knowledge, and wisdom are not a proprietary right, but a calling. In the movie *Chariots of Fire*, the Presbyterian Olympic runner says, "I run not for me but to glorify the Lord," and for this reason refuses to compete on the Sabbath. Similarly, to use a medical degree only to make money is to abase a gift given in trust.

Applying virtue ethics to medical ethics has several limitations. One is that they have little to say about how to make particular decisions. Another is that more role-defined ethics becomes, the less it meets universal standards. Finally, both religious and nonreligious theories of the virtues tend to emphasize the status quo over change. For example, physicians adopting a traditional role tend to be paternalistic, treating patients as children.

Natural Law

When Rome conquered Greece, Greek culture in turn captured Rome. Rome's Stoic philosophers elevated one aspect of the Greek world view to a higher level. Rules for human beings, they argued, were so embedded in the texture of the world that they were *law* for humans. These laws came to be known as "natural laws." They were apprehended by unaided reason, without Scripture or divine revelation.

The notion of a Law Giver lies behind natural law. In the 11th century, Thomas Aquinas synthesized Aristotelianism with Christian ideas to create his *Thomistic* worldview.

Aquinas there made explicit the connection between God and natural laws: a rational God made the world work rationally and gave humans reason to discover these laws. So studying Thomistic ethics is a rational process of discovery of those rules. Correct *descriptions* of the world would yield correct *prescriptions* about how to act. To act rationally is to act morally, which in turn is to act in accordance with natural law.

These rules commanded humans to resist their feelings. St. Augustine taught in the fourth century CE that sin contaminated human feeling and therefore lust, sloth, avarice and pride infected humans. In stunning contrast to modern times, for Aquinas, ethics was *not* about examining one's feelings but about following the natural rules laid down by God.

So natural law condemned homosexuality. Aquinas believed that God made two sexes for procreation and that it was natural and rational for a man and woman to mate to have children. On the other hand, for two people of the same gender to have sex was contrary to natural law, and hence, immoral.

One problem with natural law theory is that what is considered against natural law may vary over the centuries. Many today do not consider homosexuality to be unnatural, especially because it has been practiced since the beginning of human history and because some great cultures, such as the ancient Greeks, celebrated it as ideal.

As another example of problems of natural law theory, consider sex in marriage. Augustine held that the *only* permissible justification for sexual relations between a man and wife was to produce children. Modern Catholic teaching is different, and regards loving sexual relations between man and wife as natural and good, even when there is no desire to have children. The Catholic Church today holds in vitro fertilization to be immoral precisely *because* no act of loving sex is involved between man and woman. But which is the true interpretation of natural law? Natural law theory bequeathed to medical ethics the famous *doctrine of double effect*. This doctrine held that if an action had two effects, one good and the other evil, the evil effect was morally permitted: (1) if the action was good in itself or not evil, (2) if the good followed as immediately from the cause as did the evil effect, (3) if only the good effect was intended, and (4) if there was as important a reason for performing the action as for allowing the evil effect.

For example, exceptions could be made to the rule banning abortions in cases of an ectopic pregnancy (an embryo growing in a fallopian tube) and a cancerous uterus (where uterus and fetus had to be removed together). In both cases, this doctrine allowed abortions if the direct intention was to save the life of the mother.

This doctrine forbids physicians from assisting in executions, since it forbids an intention to assist in killings. On the other hand, it allows increasing dosages of morphine for terminal patients, so long as the intention is to relieve suffering, not to kill the patient.

The *principle of totality* also derives from natural law. It says that the human body may be changed only to ensure the proper functioning of that body. The underlying idea is that one's body is not something that one owns, but that one holds in trust for God: "The body is the temple of the Lord." So a gangrenous leg may be amputated or a cancerous breast removed, because these diseases threaten the body's overall health.

According to this principle, we are given our bodies as they are for a reason and we should not change our bodies for frivolous reasons. Thus the principle of totality rules out all forms of sterilization to prevent pregnancy—vasectomy, tubal ligation, and hysterectomy—because producing pregnancy is a natural function of the bodies of men and women. The principle also forbids cosmetic surgery solely to change one's appearance, such as breast reduction, breast augmentation, rhinoplasty, and liposuction. The principle also forbids physicians from assisting athletes to increase muscle strength by using anabolic steroids, or by using germ-line enhancement to create more ideal bodies.

This principle is deeply embedded in our feelings. When people in 1996 saw a genetically altered mouse with a human ear growing out of its back, they were disgusted. The mouse's creators had violated the bodily integrity of both humans and mice. Similar feelings arise about other chimeras, even with such things as putting genes from salmon into tomatoes.

In other words, the Principle of Totality says that God, or Evolutionary Wisdom, may present human bodies, and species, as they are, and that humans don't have the wisdom to fool with these bodies. Doing so thwarts Nature's wisdom or God's plan for us.

Social Contract Theories

The Englishman Thomas Hobbes (1588–1679) first gave weight to the social contract theory. Social contract theory is essentially secular, independent of belief in God. It assumed that people are fundamentally self-interested and that moral rules evolved for humans to get along. For Hobbes, humans agreed to rules because otherwise, everyone was worse off. Almost any rules are better than everyone taking up the sword.

Social contract theory does not separate ethics from politics. Hypothetical political bargaining creates those rules we call ethics. Today, economists do similar analyses using Game Theory.

Hobbes believed that the most detestable condition for humans was the *state of nature*, a premoral agglomeration of self-interested individuals for whom life was "solitary, poor, nasty, brutish, and short." By the use of reason, people realize that each is better off in a society of rules backed by ethics and law. They therefore form a social contract to create "society" to better themselves.

Kantian Ethics

Immanuel Kant (1724–1804) lived during the Enlightenment, and believed in the power of reason to solve human problems. Raised by religiously conservative Protestant parents, Kant accepted conservative religious ethics at his university until he studied science, whereupon he doubted some of his former beliefs. While continuing to accept basic Christian values, he ached to justify those values in some rational way. Rather than basing them on beliefs about God or an afterlife, he based these values on "pure reason."

The distinctive elements of Kantian ethics are these:

a. Ethics is not a matter of consequences but of duty. Why an act is done is more important than its results. Specifically, an act must be done from the right motive, and the right motive is the desire to do one's duty. Indeed, there is only one correct motive in Kantian ethics and that is the desire to be a good person, to do what is right, to have a "pure will."

Kant's ethics celebrate duty (and are therefore called *deontological,* from *deontos,* duty) because they emphasize not having the right desires or feelings, but acting from obligation. Only medical acts done from duty, and not from compassion, are praiseworthy. For Kant, the correct motive for treating a patient well is not because a physician feels like doing so, but because it is the right thing to do. When we act morally, Kant says, reason tells feelings what to do. Contrary to popular culture, we should not consult our feelings about what to do but instead reflect upon where our duty lies.

Kant says the only thing valuable in the world is a good will, the trait of character indicating a willingness to choose the right act simply because it's right. But how do we know what is right? What is our duty? Kant gives two formulations.

b. A right act has a maxim that is *universalizable.* An act is right if one can will its maxim or rule to be acted on by all others. "Lie to get out of keeping a promise" cannot be so willed because if everyone acted this way, promise making would mean nothing.

c. A right act always treats other humans as "ends-in-themselves," never as a "mere means." To treat another person as an "end-in-himself" is to treat him as having absolute, infinite moral worth, not relative worth. His welfare cannot be sacrificed to the good of others or to one's own desires. So patients cannot unwittingly be used as guinea pigs in dangerous experiments to advance medical knowledge.

Consider the case of a radiologist who discovers that he missed a small lesion three months previously on the X-ray of a 60-year old patient. The patient now has level IV untreatable cancer. The patient says, "I guess that cancer just grew out of nowhere because it wasn't there three months ago." Should the physician tell the patient the truth? A consequentialist might argue that he should not because it could do no good for the patient.

But for Kant, the answer is clear: the patient must be told the truth. Why? The only universalizable rule is, "Always tell patients the truth." Such a rule is the basis of trust and of treating patients as ends-in-themselves. If the physician were the patient, he would want to know the truth. The resident may *feel* that he shouldn't reveal the truth but his reason will tell him what his real duty is.

d. People are only free when they act rationally. Kant would agree that much of how we act is governed by our emotions, as well as our biology and genes. But controversially, Kant denies that we act morally when we do the right thing because we are accustomed to it, because it feels right, or because our society favors the act. We only act morally when we exercise our understanding about why certain rules are right and then freely choose to bind our actions to those rules. Kant calls the capacity to act this way *autonomy.* For him, it gives humans higher worth and dignity than animals.

It follows for Kant that few people act morally. Kant accepts that fact. It was also true that in early Christianity, few people were thought to be capable of salvation. The purity of Kant's view entails a moral elitism for the few who can successfully follow ethical rules, like the idea that only a minority will be saved for an afterlife.

Kantian ethics has several problems. First, Kant is regarded as the supreme rationalist in ethics because he claimed that anyone who disagreed him was guilty of a contradiction. But the utilitarian lifeboat commander, when he will not let everyone board to save those in the boat, does not contradict himself when he wills the maxim, "All those in control of lifeboats should maximize survivors, even if it means denying access to some in the water."

Kant is generally regarded as failing in his Enlightenment project. His critic and contemporary, Scottish skeptic David Hume, argued against Kant that ethics is little more than inculcated, socially valuable, feelings. This view in ethics is called *emotivism.* Charles Darwin and the father of psychiatry, Sigmund Freud, later agreed with Hume that reason is the tip of the moral iceberg. Because so much of ethical life is emotional, little is changeable by reason.

Regarding the place of reason in ethics, emotivism and Kantian ethics face each other as poles, while other views lie between, such as those of Aristotle and his modern follower, Martha Nussbaum, who argues that feelings can be educated rationally by culture, therapy, and schooling.

Kantian ethics also fails to tell us how to resolve conflicts between competing maxims. Worse, critics such as John Stuart Mill believe that Kantians indirectly appeal to consequences in thinking about what to universalize. Finally, the ideal of treating each person as if he had infinite value is not always practical: it does not tell us how to deliberate about tradeoffs when, by definition, some humans will die in triage situations.

Nevertheless, Kant provides useful insights to medical ethics. He would favor using a lottery to distribute a lifesaving, scarce drug. His emphasis on people as ends-in-themselves explains the outrage that people have felt when learning of research done by Nazi physicians. Finally, Kant's most important legacy to modern medical ethics is his emphasis on the autonomous will of the free, rational individual as the seat of moral value. Autonomy explains why informed consent is necessary to legitimate participation in an experiment. When combined with the emphasis on personal liberty in our democracies, Kant's emphasis on autonomy sets the stage for modern medical ethics.

Utilitarianism and Consequentialism

Utilitarianism originated in late 18th and early 19th century England as a secular replacement for Christian ethics. Its essential idea is that right acts produce the greatest amount of good for the greatest number of beings, which it called "utility."

Like the Taliban today, the Puritans then wanted everyone to obey their religious rules. In contrast, utilitarians thought morality should minimize harms to people and maximize group welfare. For Christians, Jews, or Muslims, morality is inconceivable without God's existence, but not so for utilitarians.

Utilitarianism aimed to humanize outmoded institutions. Developed by reformers Jeremy Bentham (1748–1832) and John Stuart Mill (1806–1873), it focused on changes that could benefit the majority of people.

Utilitarianism did not urge people to turn the other cheek and hope for justice in another life, nor did it exalt those virtues so cherished by England's aristocracy: stylish dress and manners, personal honor, literacy, scientific and artistic accomplishment, and appreciation of the arts. Hence, to aristocrats, being "utilitarian" is to be crass and too practical.

The foundation for reform by Utilitarians came in 1832 in eliminating boroughs controlled by one landlord and in extending the vote to all citizens with property. Utilitarians also campaigned against slavery and the harsh factory conditions made famous by Charles Dickens in novels such as *Hard Times*. They also attacked the penal system, passed the Corn Laws, ended debtor's prison, opposed capital punishment for petty thefts, and advocated the vote for women. They urged public hospitals for the poor, proper sewage disposal, the penny post so that everyone could send and get mail, and created a central board of health, so that municipalities could create facilities for clean water, waste disposal, and sewers.

Utilitarianism's teaching can be summed up in four basic tenets:

1. *Consequentialism*: Consequences count, not motives or intentions.
2. *Maximization:* The number of beings affected by consequences matters; the more beings affected, the more important the result.
3. *A theory of value* (or of "good"): good consequences are defined by pleasure *(hedonic utilitarianism)* or what people prefer *(preference utilitarianism)* or by some other good thing.
4. *A scope-of-morality premise*: Each being's happiness is to count as one and no more, and beings who count are to be made explicit, whether these are only humans or all sentient creatures.

For utilitarians, right acts then produce three things, the greatest amount of good consequences for the greatest number of beings.

Each of these tenets can be controversial. Bentham emphasized that the meaning of (4) was whether a being could suffer, not whether it was human or animal. As such, utilitarianism includes animals in its calculations of the greatest number.

To ethicist Peter Singer, utilitarianism was enlightened in not differentiating between the sufferings of humans and those of animals. Utilitarianism also seems to imply that every being's happiness on the planet matters, not just beings of my society. Singer agrees that morality doesn't stop at the borders of one's country.

Virtue ethicists and Kantians regard a person's motives as sign of his character. John Stuart Mill says that the drowning man doesn't care why the lifeguard is swimming out to sea to rescue him, just that the lifeguard is coming. Utilitarians think motives only count insofar as they tend to produce the greatest good.

In medicine, it makes a difference whether a physician listens because she really cares about patients or because she's found that having satisfied patients is an effective way to maximize income. A utilitarian might argue that if the physician's techniques are good enough, whether she really cares about her patients matters little; in either case, the behavior produces good consequences to real people.

Utilitarianism also contains a theory of value, that is, a theory about what is a harmful consequence and about what is a good one. The simplest theory of value is *hedonic utilitarianism,* which equates a good consequence with pleasure, and harm with pain. *Negative utilitarianism* focuses on relieving the greatest misery for the greatest number, as in famine relief; *positive utilitarianism* focuses on benefiting humanity. Utilitarian theorists debate whether some things are intrinsically valuable, such as pride and honor *(intrinsic value utilitarianism)*, or whether they are good only because they create good feelings in people over the long-run.

A compromise view is called *preference utilitarianism,* and its adherents believe that utility is maximized by furthering the preferences that people have. Preference utilitarianism is compatible with a base of subjective feelings in ethics, whereas intrinsic value utilitarianism is not.

The maximization tenet can get utilitarians into trouble. Wouldn't utilitarianism be willing to violate the traditional sanctity-of-life principle to save many people? Here, utilitarians bite the bullet: they think that the Nazi generals who tried to kill

Hitler in 1944 at Wolf's Lair were justified; they think that on the expedition to the South Pole, commander Robert Scott should have allowed his crew member with the gangrenous leg to die, rather than slowing down the whole party by carrying the injured man, which resulted in the death of all; they think that if an FBI sniper saw a terrorist about to detonate a bomb in a skyscraper full of innocent people, the sniper should shoot the terrorist.

These are the easy cases. The hard ones come in population policy. If more happiness is better than less, why shouldn't we create the maximal number of people on the planet? So long as each new life has more happiness than misery, and so long as everyone else's life has at least the same, shouldn't we produce more? This "total view" of utilitarianism is universally seen as what philosopher Derek Parfit calls "The Repugnant Conclusion," because we think the average happiness is more important. But it is difficult to see why utilitarianism entails maximizing average happiness and not the total good, so it may be stuck with this counterintuitive implication.

More specifically to medical ethics, wouldn't utilitarianism permit the sacrifice of an innocent, healthy person to transfer his organs to four patients who needed them to live? Aren't four people alive better than one? If consequences and numbers define morality, what's wrong with doing so? Yet it's wrong to chop up a patient like this.

One traditional reply among utilitarians is to distinguish between *act* and *rule utilitarianism*. Rule utilitarians believe that normal moral rules, such as "First, do no harm" in medicine, maximize utility over decades. *Act utilitarians* advocate judging each act's utility. Some act utilitarians think rule utilitarianism has a dilemma: if there are exceptions, then you ultimately have act utilitarianism (since you never know in advance whether a particular situation needs to be judged as an exception); if there are no exceptions, then you are close to a Kantian and only a nominal utilitarian. If the rule, "First, do no harm" has no exceptions in medical ethics, it may explain why it is wrong to chop up an innocent person to transplant his organs to four others.

In medicine, utilitarianism rules public health and triage. The goals of public health fit with this theory. Improvements in public health have helped more people live longer (created more "utility") than all the drugs and surgeries ever invented. When English physician John Snow in 1849 advocated clean water to prevent cholera epidemics (which dirty water spread), he acted like a good utilitarian. Unfortunately, it took 40 years and many cholera epidemics for Snow's ideas to prevail.

Triage allocates scarce resources during emergencies when not all will live. Because consequences count, utilitarian physicians should *not* treat each patient equally, but should focus on those who can be benefited. Rigorous application of this principle gives utilitarianism its famous hard edge: physicians should abandon those who will *die* anyway and, just as ruthlessly, abandon those who will *live* anyway. Physicians at the scene should help only those who waver between life and death and for whom intervention can tilt the balance toward life. The goal is to save the maximal number of lives.

This point illustrates an ambiguity in sanctity-of-life ethics. Traditionally, sanctity-of-life ethics, such as Kantian ethics, emphasize the absolute value of each individual, implying that the physician should at least comfort those who are beyond his help. But utilitarian-triage ethics values life in saving the maximal number of people who can live.

Contemporary Times: Four Principles

One modern method of analysis is to analyze a medical case in terms of four principles. These principles are patient autonomy, beneficence, nonmaleficence, and justice.

Autonomy refers to the right to make decisions about one's own life and body without coercion by others. It honors the value that democracies place on allowing individuals to make their own decisions about whom to marry, whether to have children, how many children to have, what kind of career to pursue, and what kind of life they want to live. Insofar as is possible and to the extent that their decisions do not harm others, individuals should be left alone to make fundamental medical decisions that affect their own bodies and lives.

John Stuart Mill was a political theorist as well as an ethical theorist. In his most famous work of politics, *On Liberty* (1859), he defended this ideal of autonomy against the growing powers of government. He there defends "one simple principle," his so-called *harm principle:* ". . . that the only purpose for which power can rightfully be exercised over any member of a civilized community, against his will, is to prevent harm to others. His own good, either physical or moral, is not a sufficient warrant . . . Over himself, over his own body and mind, the individual is sovereign."

Such political individualism parallels valuing personal autonomy in ethics. Since the beginnings of modern medical ethics in the early 1960s, autonomy has meant the patient's right to make his or her own decisions about his or her body, including dying and reproduction.

The ethics of autonomy evolved as a rejection of paternalistic ethics. Both secular and religious versions of virtue ethics tend to be paternalistic, especially when they emphasize the physician's greater wisdom and when they ignore wishes of patients. During the patients' rights movement in the early 1960s in America, feminists scorned paternalistic physicians as sexist octogenarians who imposed their rigid ideas on a more enlightened, freethinking, younger generation.

In the first two decades of bioethics (1962–1982), bioethicists exalted autonomy above other values, emphasizing the rights of competent adults to end their lives, to control their own bodies and reproduction, and to decline to participate in experiments. Since then, bioethicists have realized that other values are important, such as good of the family and the physician's integrity, which must be weighed with autonomy in finding answers in cases.

Beneficence, or helping others, grounds compassion. It grounds the moral difference between therapeutic and nontherapeutic experiments. If physicians intend to help diabetics, beneficence justifies experiments on diabetics, but if they have no such intent, the experiment may be unjustified.

Beneficence can be seen both as a principle and as a virtue for physicians. Physicians receive special powers, income, and prestige from society, and in return are asked to help patients. Medical training requires this trait, as demands on a student increase on a slope between premedical years and residency. Self-sacrifice is part of medicine. Ideally, physicians should want to help others, but if the internal desire is lacking, they should act this way out of duty. The principle of beneficence spells out this duty.

Beneficence may conflict with autonomy (as any of these principles may conflict with each other). Consider the involuntary psychiatric commitment of schizophrenic, homeless people. Is it better to let such people wander the cold streets of a big city, or to incarcerate and medicate them against their will? Should we let them "die with their rights on" or inject them with sedatives and antipsychotic drugs "for their own good"? Maybe we should do nothing at all and not risk making them worse off. After all, who are we to say that it is beneficent to do so? Maybe homeless schizophrenics want to stay as they are.

How beneficence and autonomy are balanced in particular cases is not easy to understand. Indeed, when John Stuart Mill advocated both utilitarianism and personal autonomy, critics wondered whether he contradicted himself.

Nonmaleficence, not harming others, echoes an ancient maxim of professional medical ethics, "First, do no harm." Above all, this maxim implies that physicians not technically competent to do something, shouldn't do it. So medical students should not harm patients by practicing on them without consent: patients are there to be helped, not to help students learn.

Patients should not leave encounters with physicians worse off than they were before. This crucial principle of medical ethics prohibits corruption, incompetence, and dangerous, nontherapeutic experiments. It explains why the 80,000 deaths per year in American hospitals from mistakes horrifies critics.

The principle of nonmaleficence also accords with Mill's harm principle: the state and society should not attempt to shape all citizens for the better. In a fundamental sense, the first obligation we have is to leave each other alone, especially those who don't want our help. That means that physicians should not harm patients by unsolicited intrusions.

The last principle, *justice*, has both a social and a political meaning. Socially, it means treating similar kinds of people similarly (this is the so-called "formal element" of the larger principle). A just physician treats each patient the same, regardless of his insurance coverage.

Politically, the principle refers to distributive justice, and in medicine, to the allocation of scarce medical resources. Because there are many theories of justice, this principle is not self-evident. For example, Rawls's theory of justice demands that medicine serve the worse-off people.

But another view equates justice with simple egalitarianism: medicine is just if it treats each patient equally. Of course, that goal would not be easy to achieve either, and doing so would go a long way toward realizing Rawls's ideal. At the least, it would mean a guarantee of equal access to medical care for every citizen, such that insurance coverage would not be a factor in selection of which patient receives a liver transplant.

Finally, justice can be interpreted in a libertarian sense of treating anyone with the ability to pay the same. In this sense, it means leaving people alone who do not want to be helped.

In the most minimal sense, justice requires physicians to treat patients impartially, without bias on account of gender, race, sexuality, or wealth. Even in such a minimal sense, justice requires a high standard of behavior among physicians.

These four principles were chosen as a distillation of the ethical theories described above. Their use in medical ethics is controversial. Critics say they are often invoked at the start of the talk, then forgotten. More substantially, critics say that champions of the Four Principles do not tell us how to balance them to find the correct answer in a case. Finally, critics of *principlism* claim that champions do not tell us how to resolve conflicts between principles in particular cases.

Feminist Ethics

In the early 1970s, a modern version of feminism shook American medicine to its foundations and buttressed, the patient rights movement its sister movement. Both movements attempted to take patients' decisions about their bodies and lives away from physicians—especially male physicians—and give women and patients control.

Dissatisfied women patients in Boston wrote the landmark book *Our Bodies, Ourselves*. Although they had access to some of the grandest—some would say, most self-satisfied—medical centers in the world, they couldn't get the information they wanted in down-to-earth, patient-friendly language. So they published a how-to manual covering every woman's issue from breast cancer to abortions. Successive editions sold millions of copies and gave rise in publishing to thousands of books in what is now called "alternative medicine" and "self-help."

During the 1980s feminist philosophers questioned whether traditional ethical theories were the ways to think of ethics or merely *male* ways. Kantianism, Greek ethics, social contract theories, and utilitarianism all looked like male theories: too abstract, too intellectual, and too false to the experience of women. What previous theories ignored were values such as trust, cooperation, nurturing, and bonding.

Harvard education professor Carol Gilligan showed that many women analyzed ethical dilemmas differently than men. Subsequent feminist theorists explored topics of caring, trust, and family relationships in moral theories.

This *Ethics of Care* may be considered a branch of virtue ethics in promoting "female" virtues of caring, nurturing, trust, intimate friendship, and love. But even among feminist theorists, this statement is controversial: some feminists believe that these virtues are not inherent in women but exist only because of traditional gender roles.

Feminist ethics certainly emphasizes the problems of women in medicine. For example, in discussing stopping the global spread of AIDS, they emphasize the vulnerability of women and the necessity of empowering women to stop the spread of HIV.

The Ethics of Care may be seen as correcting previous emphasis in ethical theory on abstract, semi-legalistic concepts, such as rights. It also reflects a turning inward in ethics to the family and to those around the family, fighting battles close at hand and letting far-off concerns take care of themselves. Also, this theory takes a minimal approach to morality—a kind of "within-my-circle-of-relationships" approach—in discussing moral issues within the limited contexts of families or patients in a case. Finally, the Ethics of Care can be seen modestly as supplementing traditional theories that emphasize rights, utility, and duty.

The Ethics of Care has problems. It is not a complete ethical theory, for it does not tell us how to treat people we do not know or people we do not care about. This is important because much of medicine is about treating strangers, at least when patients first meet physicians. Nor does this theory tell us how to resolve conflicts among those we care about, such as when a female physician is torn between checking on a patient and being with her daughter at the birth of her grandchild.

Case-Based Reasoning

Many physicians and some medical ethicists do not find any of the theories described above very useful to their practice of medicine. To force the complexities of many medical cases into a preconceived, abstract framework is often to be guilty of oversimplification, and when that happens, the truth is not discovered.

Since 1990, some bioethicists, including the author of this text, advocate teaching bioethics based on paradigms or seminal cases. These paradigmatic cases serve as a basis to generalize to other, similar cases.

For example, both Karen Quinlan in 1975 and Nancy Cruzan in 1990 went into persistent vegetative states. In both cases, the parents decided after many months that their daughter's biography was over and wanted to end the biological life of the remaining body. Karen Quinlan's case focused on removal of a respirator, Nancy Cruzan's on removal of a feeding tube. Both cases resulted in landmark legal decisions.

Advocates of case-based reasoning believe that study of these two famous cases can teach us a lot about ethics in medicine over the last two decades. Paradigms are bedrock cases from which we generalize in ever-expanding circles of similarity. By understanding and analyzing arguments on both sides about killing and letting die, ordinary versus extraordinary treatment, forgoing versus withdrawing treatment, standards of brain death, and models of proxy consent for making decisions about incompetent patients, we increase our understanding of these issues and prepare ground for analyzing future cases.

So we understand best the Terri Schiavo case in 2005 by first understanding the Quinlan and Cruzan cases. Even the Hugh Finn case, where the governor of Virginia politicized a family dispute, sheds insight on the Schiavo case.

Because thousands of patients may end up in comas like those of Karen Quinlan and Nancy Cruzan, studying how decisions were handled in their famous cases can teach us how to handle future cases better. Case-based reasoning parallels the famous case-analysis of the Wharton Business School and the traditional teaching using cases in rounds in medical schools. It resembles an ancient method of theological reasoning called *casuistry*, and some bioethicists with theological training use this word to describe this orientation.

Case-based reasoning does not deny that ethical theories play a role in moral life. When these are relevant to a case, they must be discussed. It is just that when they are relevant, we need not study ethical theory to see their relevance. If a patient has been abused in a nontherapeutic, psychiatric experiment, we do not need to have a complete theory of justice to understand that the patient has been abused. On the other hand, a good theory of justice may help us decide borderline cases about *whether* a patient was abused.

Case-based reasoning does deny that any overarching ethical principle of morality can guide us in making day-to-day ethical decisions in medicine. Each situation or case will present a unique array of people, interests, conflicting principles, incompatible role-duties, strong passions, and concerns about the larger good, about resources, about institutional policies, and about political consequences. Each set of circumstances will require what the Greeks called *phronesis*, or practical judgment, to find the optimal solution for all parties.

From the viewpoint of case-based ethics, the four principles express four interests or values that appear in some cases in bioethics. But the problem is that many cases contain far more than four factors. For example, feminists rightly emphasize that concerns for the family and exploitation of women are missing from many analyses. Certainly no good analysis of AIDS in Africa, or new reproductive technologies, should be done without these other viewpoints.

Indeed, intriguing cases in bioethics often involve *dozens* of conflicting values and *many* parties who have interests or standing in the case, such as the patient himself, his family, his physician, the nonmedical staff, the agency paying for the medical treatment, and society itself. Any theory that tried to reduce all the values and interests involved in the case to one master value inevitably will slight excluded values or interests.

Of course, if grasping one idea could solve all ethical problems, that would be nice. We might have a decision-procedure for discovering right answers. But that is likely a quixotic quest. Any theory that asks, "What makes an act right?" is probably asking the wrong question in assuming that one monistic thing makes all right acts moral. But rather than moral acts sharing one form (e.g., universalizable) or being an expression of one value (such as utility) it is likely that they only could do so only at the most abstract levels of description.

A wrinkle here is that often in medicine conflicts among traditional ethical theories generate intriguing cases. Clashes over distribution of organs for transplant, or studying vertical transmission from mother to child in Africa, express conflicts between Kantian and utilitarian ethical theories. Clashes over the rule of rescue express conflicts between partial and impartial ethical theories.

For example, the rule of rescue (discussed in Chapters 1 and 13) exemplifies the larger clash in medicine between kinds of ethical theories. On one side are partial theories that favor special regard to identified people such as patients in the hospital, members of one's family, or members of one's country. The Ethics of Care illustrates one such partial theory.

On the other side are impartial theories, such as Kantian ethics or utilitarianism, that regard each person as having the same moral worth regardless of his geographical location or other nonmorally relevant criteria. It is precisely the partiality of the rule of rescue toward an identified person that impartial theories despise, for such partiality seems to disvalue the worth of all the anonymous people who do not receive the medical resource.

This clash looms throughout medicine. Admission to the hospital may illustrate the rule of rescue when a powerful physician decides to admit a patient without medical insurance and to care for him. Obviously, the hospital cannot do so for everyone or it will be sought out by other patients without insurance and go bankrupt. Such an admission may give the patient hundreds of thousands of dollars worth of treatment that she would otherwise not get.

But the important point here is that the *theories themselves* are creating the above problems and cases in medical ethics. Only some super- or meta-theory could conceivably solve such clashes, but that is unlikely.

THREE POLITICAL IDEAS IMPORTANT TO BIOETHICS

Libertarianism

Libertarians favor government for defense and for limited public works, perhaps not even including national parks or a public interstate road system (we could have private toll roads). They disfavor government programs such as Medicare, Medicaid, disability insurance, food stamps, and welfare. Libertarians oppose forced taxation by the government, especially when it redistributes property and income from rich to poor. They champion the property rights of the status quo, but tend to be silent about how those enjoying the status quo acquired their property. Libertarian philosophers such as Harvard's Robert Nozick see forced taxation as equivalent to forced labor, that is, to slavery.

Accordingly, libertarians oppose mandatory F.I.C.A. taxes on workers' pay and taxes for the Medicare and for the Hospital Insurance Trust Fund. Even though federal programs such as Medicare have made American physicians rich, libertarian physicians would rather have no government control over their business. In a libertarian society, physicians would be reimbursed only in cash.

Critics say that in such a system, fewer hospitals would be built, elderly patients would frequently forgo procedures for lack of money, and physicians would earn far less money. In such a system, physicians would be controlled by few federal regulations.

Rawlsian Justice

Rawlsians are named for John Rawls, a Harvard colleague of the libertarian Nozick. Rawls believes that the social contract should have moral restraints imposed on it. The most important restraint is what Rawls called "the veil of ignorance," meaning that in the hypothetical social contract, no one would know his or her age, gender, race, health, number of children, income, wealth, or other arbitrary personal information. Rawls' theory is contractarian in that it assumes that people are self-interested and are forced to form a social contract to choose the basic institutions of their society; on the other hand, it is Kantian (as we shall see in the next section) in that is imposes impartiality on the choosers.

Rawls argues that the only rational way to choose under the veil of ignorance is as if one might be the least well-off person in society (because a person doesn't know anything personal under the veil, he doesn't know what place in society he occupies.) This justifies the choice of his famous *difference principle*: choosers should opt for institutions creating equality unless a difference favors the least well-off group. Everyone should be trained in medicine unless training only a few is better for the least well-off. Choosing the difference principle as the arch principle of justice imposes the Golden Rule on the structure of society.

Rawlsian justice entails that every citizen should have equal access to medical care unless unequal access favors the poor. It attempts to reduce the natural inequalities of fate; hence, children and those with genetic disease must get good medical care. Consider these two classes combined: children with genetic disease. Their care takes up huge resources in children's hospitals, but for Rawls, such children deserve good medical care as a *matter of justice*.

In some ways, we stand under a genetic veil of ignorance about our future illnesses and those of our children and grandchildren. The coming decade will identify who is susceptible to genetic disease and who is not. In the future, it may be much more difficult for those with familial lines of genetic disease to purchase private medical insurance. Some people who now attack universal coverage may find themselves at risk.

Libertarians favor private medical insurance plans in which the healthy do not subsidize the unhealthy. Rawlsians see "healthy" and "unhealthy" as arbitrary distinctions, due more to genetics and fate than individual merit. Libertarians would allow for-profit companies to practice experience rating, whereby citizens with preexisting illness may be excluded (and genetic disease is increasingly being defined in this way). Rawlsians favor community rating, whereby risk and premium rates are spread over all members of a large community, such as a state or nation (for example, a federal, single-payer system).

Mill's Classical Liberalism and Morality

The 19th century political philosopher John Stuart Mill wrote *On Liberty* in 1859. This classic contains an admirable distinction between private life and public morality—a distinction based on the concept of harm.

Mill believed that a civilized society must promote certain ideals and discourage certain vices. He also believed that a society can do this while granting individuals a sphere of private belief and action immune from interference by government. Mill saw that the power of the nation-state could be dangerous when used against the individual, and he held that governments and their agents—such as the police—should be forbidden to meddle in private life. Equally, he held, the majority should be forbidden from becoming tyrannical; it should be forbidden to impose its social or religious beliefs on a dissenting minority.

Where is the line to be drawn between private life and public morality? Mill's rough rule of thumb is called his *harm principle*. According to this principle, private life encompasses those actions of an adult (or adults together) that are purely personal and that do not put other people at risk of harm.

In private life, as defined by this principle of harm, there should be no interference by government—even for a person's own good. For example, consider a certain form of sexual activity between two consenting adults: even if other people consider that activity "immoral," for Mill it will not be a "moral question" if no one else is affected.

Personal Life, Morality, Public Policy, and Legality

Building on Mill's work, this book will make a distinction among four areas: (1) personal life, (2) morality, (3) public policy, (4) legality.

Issues of *personal life* are purely private and affect no one else.

When someone else is affected, issues move from the personal to the realm of *morality*.

When society attempts to promote certain positive values while at the same time tolerating individuals' personal disagreement with those value, issues move into the third area, *public policy*. Actions in the area of public policy, like those in the area of morality, do affect other people's interests, but negative actions in public policy are not necessarily condemned as immoral. For example, consider the consumption of alcohol. Although society tries to discourage this activity (as by taxation) and to regulate it (forbidding alcohol at elementary schools), people may drink in their homes without being seen as immoral. For another example, consider adoption. Society would like adults to adopt needy children (and may offer tax incentives to encourage adoption), but no one thinks it immoral for a childless couple not to adopt a baby.

When society promotes certain actions and discourages others actions, issues move into the fourth area, *legality*. In this area, some actions (such as paying taxes) are compulsory and others (theft, murder) are forbidden. Omitting a legally compulsory action or committing a legally forbidden action is punishable by the force of the state. In general, the more harmful an action is considered, the more likely it is to fall into the area of legality.

The effect of these distinctions is to limit the range of morality from two ends: first by carving out a zone of private, personal life, and second, by allowing society to encourage and discourage behaviors without explicit moral judgment. In summary, then:

> *Personal life*. Concerns actions that are purely private and that affect no other person (or persons).
>
> *Morality*. Concerns interpersonal actions—situations where one person's actions affect other people.
>
> *Public policy*. On the one hand, concerns actions that affect other people negatively, but which society tolerates, though it attempts to discourage such actions (as by education). On the other hand, concerns actions that affect other people positively and that society attempts to encourage (as through incentives).
>
> *Legality*. Concerns positive actions that are, by law, compulsory; and negative actions that are, by law, forbidden. Penalties (such as fines and incarceration) are imposed for omitting compulsory actions or performing forbidden actions.

Here are some further examples: smoking is a personal issue; smoking in your child's room is a moral issue; taxing tobacco products heavily is a public policy issue; and forbidding sale of cigarettes to minors is a legal issue. To repeat: according to these distinctions, not every evaluative issue is a moral issue. Issues such as masturbation, littering one's own car, or the personal religious beliefs of one's relatives, are not moral issues at all.

Conclusions

The study of ethical theories enlightens the study of modern medical ethics, but the study of modern medical ethics is not the same as merely applying one ethical theory to a case. The study of these theories does not give us a definitive, absolute answer to each case in medical ethics. Our society has inherited many different ethical theories from the past, the most important of which have been sketched above. Although each theory has its champions who believe that it alone is completely correct, most sophisticated people today believe that the best part of each of these theories needs to guide us in a particular case, such that in analyzing some cases, we will use parts of many different theories together.

FURTHER READING AND RESOURCES

Michael Slote, "Ethics," *Encyclopedia of Bioethics*, 2005.
Alasdair MacIntyre, *A Short History of Ethics*, MacMillan, New York, 1982.

CHAPTER 9

The Ethics of Treating
Impaired Babies

In recent decades, the rate of premature births rose from 9.8 percent in 1985 to 12 percent in 2002.[1] In 2005, it rose to 12.5 percent and reached the historic marker in America of a half million.[2]

Although babies born at 28 weeks have a 90 percent chance of survival, extreme prematurity at 22 to 25 weeks causes many problems. About 80 percent of such babies will have neuromotor or mental disability.[3] Compared with only 2 percent of babies born full term and at age six, 41 percent of babies born extremely premature will be moderately to severely mentally impaired.

Most obstetricians believe that, unless the babies are born dying or irreversibly comatose, the Americans with Disabilities Act (1990) requires them to aggressively treat all newborns. Whether that interpretation is correct will be discussed later, but for now, notice that it gives parents no say in whether their premature or impaired baby is aggressively treated.

Every issue in bioethics has a pedigree, and aggressive treatment of impaired babies has a long one. That pedigree includes the Baby Doe cases, the Baby Doe rules, and the Baby Doe squads during the 1980s. Baby Doe cases arise when parents of impaired neonates forgo treatment to let their baby die. This chapter discusses the Infant Doe case in Indiana, the Baby Jane Doe case in New York in 1983, the Baby Doe rules, and the legal and ethical issues of all these cases. At the end, the chapter returns to treatment of premies.

HISTORY AND CASES PRECEDING THE BABY DOE RULES

In ancient Athens, both Plato (in *The Republic)* and Aristotle (in the *Politics*) advocated killing impaired newborns. In ancient Sparta, a cyclops baby (that is, an infant born with single eye or with the two eyes fused) would be left to die in a country field. Later, in ancient Rome, babies who looked grotesque were also abandoned by exposure. During the next four centuries, exposure remained common: such letting die was legal and not considered infanticide. The Bedouin tribes of Arabia, the Chinese, and much of India have practiced female infanticide for two millennia.[4]

Around the year 300, Roman emperor Constantine converted to Christianity and, because Christianity condemned both abandonment and infanticide, banned infanticide. However, the church had neither funds nor people to care for abandoned babies. Foundling hospitals for abandoned babies did not start until the eighth century in Milan.

During the Middle Ages, wet nurses acted as agents for parents wishing to rid themselves of children (a practice that would continue well into the 19th century). In the 18th century, when the population of Europe exploded, exposure-as-infanticide was used as birth control. During the reign of Napoleon, women abandoned so many babies that Napoleon established his own foundling hospitals, where parents could deposit a baby on a turntable set into the front entrance, spin it to send the baby inside, and depart unseen. In France in 1833, over 100,000 babies—20 to 30 percent of all newborns that year—were abandoned.[5]

Just as respirators and feeding tubes during the 1960s first allowed comatose patients to stay alive, so neonatal intensive care units (NICUs) during the same period allowed premature babies to be kept alive. During the 1970s, small respirators and feeding tubes began to be used on such babies. They saved babies with congenital disabilities who otherwise would have died.

Treating such infants created an ethical dilemma. Even with premies with no genetic disease, about a third will have a significant life-long disability.[6] A similar dilemma arose in the McCaughey septuplet case, where implanting seven embryos resulted in several disabled children. Moreover, treatment in NICUs is expensive. Both the expense of NICU treatment and the low quality of life of some of its survivors began to raise questions in the 1980s about whether such babies should be treated at all. Such questions led to the events described below.

Preceding Cases and Controversies

By 1983, when the Baby Jane Doe case took place, and as a result of several earlier cases, a set of rules known as the *Baby Doe rules* had already been developed. These earlier cases are described below; the following section discusses the rules themselves.

The Johns Hopkins Cases, 1971

Down syndrome is a genetic condition that always causes retardation and a characteristic facial appearance; it is often accompanied by cardiac or intestinal problems. In the early 1970s—at the time of the Johns Hopkins cases—parents of children with Down syndrome were told by physicians that although the eventual IQ of a person with Down syndrome could not be predicted at birth, the usual range was between 25 and 60, with some severely impaired individuals below 25. (Whether or not this information was correct will be discussed later.)

In 1971, when NICUs were new and physicians omitted aggressive treatment from most impaired newborns, three babies with Down syndrome in the NICU at

Johns Hopkins Hospital in Baltimore, Maryland, had life-threatening intestinal defects. Physicians and parents allowed two of them to die.[7]

One of the babies allowed to die had *duodenal atresia,* a blockage between the higher duodenum and the lower stomach that prevents passage of food and water. The mother of this baby—a nurse who had worked with children with Down syndrome—knew that if she did not consent to surgery to open the atresia, her infant would die. She refused to do so, as did her husband, a lawyer. Pediatric surgeons at Hopkins honored their decision and did not go to court to force them to operate.

The mother of the second baby who was allowed to die already had children. According to theologian James Gustafson, she explained her decision to forgo treatment by saying, "It would be unfair to the other children of the household to raise them with a mongoloid."[8] (Because of the facial characteristics associated in Down syndrome, it was at one time called "mongolism.") Gustafson describes this mother's decision as "anguished" but also notes that when she learned her baby had Down syndrome, she "immediately indicated she did not want the child."

The two babies whose parents refused treatment were not killed; they were simply allowed to die—a course that was thought to be more acceptable morally and less likely to incur legal prosecution. One of these babies took 15 days to die; ordinarily, the baby would have died in about four days, but some staff members surreptitiously gave the infant water.

The parents of the third baby eventually accepted treatment, and this baby lived. This baby's parents had originally been given a pessimistic prognosis for Down syndrome by an obstetrician who referred them to Hopkins because Hopkins had been willing to allow the other two babies to die. However—and perhaps significantly—the staff at Hopkins then gave them a more balanced view.

Pediatric Intensivists Go Public, 1970s

In the early 1970s, because of the increasing incidence of cases like the Johns Hopkins babies, several well-known pediatricians went public. R. Duff and A. Campbell at Yale-New Haven Medical Center admitted they had forgone treatment for 43 impaired infants, who died early.[9] They caused a minor sensation, which led to soul-searching by pediatricians at other NICUs, who wondered if they too were doing the right thing.

English physician John Lorber argued that some babies are so severely impaired that they are better off being allowed to die without treatment.[10] Lorber specialized in spina bifida.

Spina bifida literally means "divided spine" and is a hernial protrusion through a defect in the vertebral column. It is the most common serious neural-tube defect, occurring in 1 in 1,000 live births. It may occur in the form of a *meningocele,* a protrusion of part of the meninges; or it may take the form of a *myelomeningocele,* a protrusion not only of part of the meninges but also of the spinal cord (the nervebundle).

A baby with spina bifida is almost always paralyzed below the level of the opening and thus has bowel and bladder problems. The opening makes the baby vulnerable to infections such as meningitis. Quality of life depends on two factors:

first, the level of the meningomyelocele; and second, the degree of associated problems such as hydrocephalus—a swelling of cranial tissue which commonly accompanies spina bifida and that often causes increased intracranial pressure and decreased blood flow to the brain, resulting in mental retardation. However, the probability of mental retardation can be reduced by aggressive surgical treatment involving tubes called *shunts* to decrease this pressure. (Hydrocephalus was present in Baby Jane Doe.)

Lorber developed criteria to predict which spina bifida babies, if left untreated, would die: the higher the meningomyelocele on the spine and the larger the affected area of the spine and its coverings, the greater the probability of attendant problems and of death. These criteria had risks and a dilemma: if left untreated, not all infants with spina bifida die, and for infants who live, nontreatment makes them worse off.

Lorber's criteria seemed to make it possible to identify babies who would die: all those in his lowest category did die. During the 1970s, criteria like Lorber's were apparently used at Oklahoma Children's Hospital, where it was decided not to treat 24 babies with spina bifida who were in the lowest category and who all subsequently died.[11]

The Mueller Case: Conjoined Twins, 1981

In 1981, conjoined twins joined at the trunk and sharing three legs were born in Danville, Illinois, to Pamela and Robert Mueller.[12] Robert Mueller, a physician, was in the delivery room when their family physician, Petra Warren, delivered the babies, who were named Jeff and Scott. The Muellers and Warren decided together not to treat the twins aggressively, so they could die. However, other physicians in Danville were deeply divided over the ethics of the Muellers' decision. An anonymous caller alerted Protective Child Services, which obtained a court order for temporary custody of the children.

The Muellers were initially charged with neglect; at a later hearing, that charge was dismissed, but the Muellers were denied custody. In September 1981, they regained custody after pediatric surgeons testified that successful separation was unlikely and the prognosis for the twins was therefore bleak.

Subsequent events in this case tell a different tale. The twins lived, still joined, for about a year, at which time they weighed 30 pounds.[13] Shortly thereafter, they were separated in a long operation. Scott, the weaker twin, died; but Jeff, the stronger twin, survived, and later he entered a regular school.

The Infant Doe Case, 1982

The Infant Doe case in Bloomington, Indiana, took place about one year after the case of the Mueller twins, but only over the course of a few days—from Infant Doe's birth on April 9, 1982, to the baby's death on April 15. Infant Doe had Down syndrome with a tracheoesophageal fistula, and once again physicians split over forgoing treatment.[14]

The prognosis for tracheoesophageal fistula is more serious than for duodenal atresia and depends on the severity of the fistula, or gap. In Infant Doe's case, the gap was fairly small, and an early operation to close it would have had a 90 percent chance of success. However, in discussing the case with the parents, the referring obstetrician, Walter Owens, downplayed this fact and emphasized that some people with Down syndrome are "mere blobs" and that the "lifetime cost" of caring for a Down child would "almost surely be close to $1 million." Infant Doe's parents decided not to allow the operation.

In this case, hospital administrators and pediatricians disagreed with the parents' decision and immediately convened an emergency session with a Monroe County judge, John Baker. Testifying at this hearing, Owens repeated his grim prognosis: even if surgery was successful, "the possibility of a minimally adequate quality of life was nonexistent" because of "the child's severe and irreversible mental retardation."

Infant Doe's father, a public school teacher who had worked closely with Down children, agreed with Dr. Owens and felt that such children never had a "minimally acceptable quality of life." It is noteworthy that this hearing was held late at night in a room at the hospital where it was not recorded, and that Judge Baker did not appoint a guardian ad litem for Infant Doe. Judge Baker ruled the parents had the right to make the decision about treatment versus nontreatment.

The county district attorney appealed to the county circuit court, and after losing there, to the Indiana Supreme Court. Both appeals failed: each time the court ruled for the parents. He then appealed to United States Supreme Court Justice Paul Stevens for an emergency intervention, but Infant Doe soon died.

Seven years later in 1989, the U. S. Civil Rights Commission cited the Infant Doe case as a landmark case of prejudice against disabled infants. Owens wrote about his role in the Infant Doe case, maintaining that he was "proud to have stood up for what I and a large percentage of people feel is right"; he also said he was glad that Infant Doe had died in only a few days and with little suffering, and glad that the parents were able to have another baby—a healthy child who, if the couple had been forced to treat Infant Doe, would not have been born. The Commission concluded that Owens's evaluation was "strikingly out of touch with the contemporary evidence on the capabilities of people with Down syndrome."[15]

THE BABY DOE RULES, 1982–1986

National media extensively reported the Infant Doe case, which prompted President Ronald Reagan to direct the Justice Department and the Department of Health and Human Services (HHS) to mandate treatment in future cases. Reagan, who opposed abortion, had appointed C. Everett Koop as Surgeon General. Koop opposed both abortion and nontreatment of impaired newborns.[16]

Because states define crimes such as homicide and gross negligence and not the federal government, Reagan's Justice Department needed to find an indirect route to make nontreatment illegal. It creatively hit upon a way to do so, but revealed contradictions in the views of conservatives about the role of government in personal life.

The executive branch can set social policy by reinterpreting prior Congressional legislation. In the 1960s, President Lyndon Johnson used orders to fight laws against racial discrimination. Institutions violating them risk losing all federal funds. Through similar executive orders, the Justice Department and HHS developed the *Baby Doe rules*, which required physicians to treat all impaired newborns.

The first step was taken in 1982 when lawyers defined nontreatment as violating Section 504 of the Rehabilitation Act of 1973, which forbade discrimination solely on the basis of handicap. This interpretation by the Justice Department created a new conceptual synthesis: imperiled newborns were now handicapped citizens who could suffer discrimination against their federal civil rights. Congress had originally meant this Act to apply to adults and children with handicaps, not babies.

HHS then required large posters to be displayed on the outer glass walls of every NICU:

DISCRIMINATORY FAILURE TO FEED AND CARE FOR HANDICAPPED INFANTS IN THIS FACILITY IS PROHIBITED BY FEDERAL LAW

HHS also posted a toll-free 800 telephone number on the poster so anyone around an NICU could report abuses—including concerned nurses, disgruntled parents, ambulance-chasing lawyers, and anonymous cranks. "Baby Doe squads," composed of lawyers, government administrators, and physicians, investigated complaints.

The contradictions in conservatism about the Baby Doe rules lay along two fronts. First, some conservatives claim that politicians and judges should not interpret the Constitution and previous law, especially for their own evaluative agenda. When they attack such interpretation, conservatives cite abortion and *Roe* v. *Wade*. Clearly, the Baby Doe rules reinterpreted previous law. Second, once upon a time, some political conservatives believed that federal government should not intrude in a family's life, leaving such decisions to parents. Clearly, the Baby Doe rules intruded on such decisions.

In 1983, the American Academy of Pediatrics successfully sued in a federal district court to block implementation of the Baby Doe rules. While appeals of this decision continued in 1983, the famous Baby Jane Doe case began.

Before we turn to the case of Baby Jane Doe, it will be interesting to briefly consider the Baby Doe hotline and the Baby Doe squads. As long as they existed, the Baby Doe squads were ready on an hour's notice to rush to airports, fly across the country, and suddenly arrive—as a squad arrived one day at Vanderbilt University—like outside accountants doing a surprise bank audit. Records were seized, charts were taken from attending physicians, and all-night investigations took place. The attitude of the squads was that time was of the essence because an innocent baby's life was at stake. Besides Vanderbilt, the University of Rochester also suffered (in the words used privately by some pediatricians) a "blitzkrieg by the Baby Doe Gestapo." Eventually, because of the objections by pediatricians and the national press, the squads were called off.

What was the ultimate effect of the hotline and the squads? One study discovered that Baby Doe squads did in fact *force* more treatment for six infants, who were given operations they otherwise might not have had, but in no case did the squads *prove* a violation of the Baby Doe regulations.[17]

THE BABY JANE DOE CASE, 1983–1984

On October 11, 1983, Baby Jane Doe was born at St. Charles Hospital of Long Island, New York. Because she had several major defects, she was transferred for care by neonatal specialists to an NICU at University Hospital of the State University of New York campus at Stony Brook (SUNY).

Her parents—who were known only as Linda and Dan—were lower-middle-class people working hard to improve their lives; Linda was 23 and Dan was 30. They had been married four months when Linda became pregnant, and Dan had built two extra rooms onto what has been described as their "modest suburban home" in the "flatlands of eastern Long Island."

Baby Jane weighed six pounds and was 20 inches long. According to testimony, she was born with spina bifida, hydrocephalus, a damaged kidney, and *microcephaly* (small head, implying a minimal brain or lack of most of the brain). Her defects must have been traumatic for her parents. For one thing, her spine was open with the meningocele protruding prominently.

At Stony Brook, surgeon Arjen Keuskamp recommended immediate surgery to minimize retardation by draining the hydrocephalus. When Baby Jane was examined by George Newman, a pediatric neurologist, he told Dan that Baby Jane would either die soon without surgery or could undergo surgery and be paralyzed, retarded, and vulnerable to continual infections of her bladder and bowels. According to Newman's later court testimony:

> The decision made by the parents is that it would be unkind to have surgery performed on this child. . . . On the basis of the combination of malformations that are present in this child, *she is not likely to ever achieve any meaningful interaction with her environment, nor ever achieve any interpersonal relationships*, the very qualities which we consider human.[18] (italics added)

Keuskamp withdrew from the case and did not testify in court. About midnight on October 11, 14 hours after Baby Jane was born, Newman probably told Dan something like his testimony in court.

After a good deal of soul-searching, Dan and Linda decided not to allow the surgeon to drain the hydrocephalus. They acted on their understanding of the distinction between extraordinary and ordinary treatment, disallowing surgery but allowing "comfort care:" food, fluids, and antibiotics.

Based on what they had been told, they naively assumed that Baby Jane would soon die, but four days later, she was still alive. A social worker wrote at this time that Dan was in "despair" because Baby Jane had not yet died; she also noted that Linda was determined to give Baby Jane "as much love as possible" while the infant still lived. "We love her very much," Linda said, "and that's why we made the decision we did."[19]

Newsday reporter Kathleen Kerr broke the Baby Jane Doe story nationally on October 18, 1983. Kerr, who had numerous firsts on the story, was also the first and only reporter to interview the parents. She described the interview:

> Each time he began a sentence, Mr. A. let out a deep sigh, as though seeking strength to answer. Mrs. A. continually touched her husband's arm and rubbed it soothingly. Mr. A. shed his tears openly. . . . Mr. A. said, "We feel the conservative method of treatment is going to do her as much good as if surgery were to be performed. It's not a case of our not caring. We very much want this baby." . . .
>
> "We're not being neglectful, and we're not relying on our religion [Catholicism] to give us the answer to what we're doing here."[20]

Baby Jane Doe continued to survive, and—as occurs naturally in some cases of spina bifida—her open spinal wound closed.

Baby Jane's Case in the Courts

On October 18, 1983 (the same day that Kerr broke the story), Lawrence Washburn, a municipal-bonds lawyer who lived in Vermont and who promoted right-to-life organizations, filed suit in a state court to force treatment for Baby Jane. Over the following weeks, the case of Baby Jane Doe proceeded through the courts with enormous speed; everyone seemed mindful of the earlier Infant Doe case, in which the child had died while appeals were still continuing.

An emergency lower-court hearing was held on October 20, with Judge Melvyn Tannenbaum presiding. Because Washburn did not have legal standing to sue, Tannenbaum appointed another attorney, William Weber, as Baby Jane's guardian *ad litem* ("for this action or proceeding"). Weber, was temporarily empowered to make decisions regarding Baby Jane's medical care.

At first, Weber supported the parents, but then there was an interesting development. Having talked to Newman, when he read two items in Baby Jane's medical chart, Weber abruptly changed his mind. Why? First, Weber had read that Newman had written that after surgery, Jane would be able to walk with braces.[21] Second, her chart said that the initial measurement of her skull was 31 centimeters (cm), which is within normal limits. A measurement of 31 cm would indicate that Baby Jane had a brain, perhaps even a normal one.

Yet Newman had testified that the baby had microcephaly and would never be able to recognize her parents. Weber concluded that what Newman had written on the chart conflicted both with what he had told the parents and with his testimony in court. In regard to the microcephaly, Weber decided that this was, "a lie." So on October 20, Weber authorized surgery.

The case ended up in the appellate division of New York courts. The justices there decided that the law left decisions up to parents when a choice was available between two *medically reasonable options*. Interestingly, previous rulings of courts had required a "medically reasonable option" to be an option that was not only supported by evidence, but also in the interest of the child. The new judgment contradicted these precedents.

It is interesting to compare this decision in 1983 to the 2006 decision by the U.S. Supreme Court blocking Attorney General Ashcroft from enforcing a traditional definition of "legitimate medical purpose" (see Chapter 3). The 1983 interpretation clearly wants to let parents make important medical decisions in the nursery; the 2006 decision clearly wants to let physicians and Oregonians decide whether helping terminal patients die is a legitimate purpose of medicine.

The court hearings in this case were front-page news across America. Perhaps everyone else in the country was too influenced by the immense publicity surrounding the case. The courts seemed to have completely forgotten about the traditional doctrine of *parens patria*, according to which the state protects helpless people against those who might neglect them.

After these court proceedings concluded, the parents said:

> I just want [all this] to end. Just to have a baby like this and deal with it is so much to go through right now. Just let us be with our daughter and leave us alone. . . .
> If there's hell, we've been through it.

By this point, however, the federal government had begun to act.

In October, the Justice Department informed Stony Brook Hospital that federal investigators were coming to see Baby Jane's medical records. The parents were outraged by this intrusion: "They're not doctors, they're not the parents, and they have no business in our lives right now."[22]

Stony Brook's lawyer then announced that the hospital would not let the government examine the records. HHS turned the case over to the Justice Department, which filed suit against the hospital in federal court, charging possible discrimination against the handicapped. Attorney General Edwin Meese and Surgeon General Everett Koop personally acted in the case.

Soon federal judge Leonard Wexler ruled that the Justice Department could not have the medical records and that the parents had not decided against surgery for "discriminatory" reasons. (It is not clear if Judge Wexler had examined Baby Jane's hospital chart.)

Dan and Linda were pleased, but exhausted: "I'm drained physically, mentally, and emotionally," Dan said; "I believed that you couldn't look at what we were doing and say we were wrong."

In 1984, the case reached the federal Court of Appeals for the Second Circuit, which denied the government access to Baby Jane's records. This decision, which would presumably apply in similar cases, had the practical effect of making the Baby Doe rules useless: because the government could not obtain medical records from NICUs or hospitals, it could not enforce the Baby Doe rules. The Justice Department appealed to the United States Supreme Court, but two years later in 1986 in *Bowen* v. *American Hospital Association et al.*, the Supreme Court declared that no records needed to be released and, in effect, ended the saga of the Baby Doe Rules, their national hotline, and their possible investigators.

During the court battles over Baby Jane, Linda and Dan changed their minds and permitted surgery to drain her hydrocephalus—a decision that became known only months later.[23] After contracting pneumonia, the baby had been given strong antibiotics (without these antibiotics, she might have died). Baby Jane continued to live and was taken home on April 7, 1984, at age 5 1/2 months. At the time she went home, one physician predicted that she would "probably always be bedridden."[24]

Five years later, Jane lived at home with her parents. According to Kathleen Kerr, whose stories about the case won a Pulitzer Prize for local reporting and who visited with the family over those years, Jane was:

> . . . doing better than anyone expected—talking, attending school for the handi-capped, and learning to mix with her peers. She still can't walk and gets around in a wheelchair but her progress has defied the dire predictions.[25]

Some disturbing questions were raised by the reporting of Baby Jane's case in the print and visual media, particularly when we consider that Jane not only survived but was able to live at home and even attend school. Recall that Dr. Newman had testified that Jane would never achieve any meaningful interaction with her environment, never achieve any interpersonal relationships. Why did Newman's opinion prevail? That is an interesting question.

During the fall of 1983, the momentum of the media in support of the parents—and with it the momentum of medicine and medical ethics—became so strong that dissenters were perceived as bigots. People read reports of the Baby Jane Doe case with their minds made up. Ed Bradley on *60 Minutes* did a hatchet job on Koop and the case.

The nadir was reached in November when Lesley Stahl on *Face the Nation*, grilled C. Everett Koop and implied that she was interviewing a fundamentalist, parent-baiting Big Brother. From today's perspective, Koop's answers are impressive: He said that there were discrepancies in the medical chart and that he wanted to see the records to learn what was best for the child.

One pediatric neurosurgeon who had treated over 1,000 patients with spina bifida said that children whose heads measured 31 cm (as Baby Jane's did) are among "the very brightest" of such children, presumably implying that Baby Jane's IQ could be normal or better.[26] The public was not informed that although hydro-cephalus generally accompanies spina bifida, if shunted immediately, it may not cause retardation.

All the major media simply accepted George Newman's negative prognosis, and almost all dismissed William Weber, the child's court-appointed guardian, as a fanatic. The media's stance may have unduly influenced not only the general public but even many physicians and medical ethicists, who took Newman's depressing prognosis as fact.

In retrospect, another astonishing aspect of the story escaped the public's notice. When Stony Brook Hospital resisted Koop's attempt to see Baby Jane's medical chart, the hospital's motives might have been not to protect the privacy of the family but to protect itself from a suit. Given that what Newman wrote in the chart contradicted what the parents heard him say, one can see that the hospital had a problem.

Beyond a doubt, pediatricians disagreed about which treatment was best for Baby Jane, about the "medically reasonable options" in this case. Unfortunately, the public never read about the two real sides of this medical controversy. As a result, the public came to believe that the case involved only moral questions about parental decisions and low quality of life, when in fact it raised questions about making decisions based on incomplete, biased information and about a hospital protecting itself from suit.

It is astonishing that a story for which the journalist won a Pulitzer Prize was seriously inaccurate and incomplete. It is also astonishing that neither the *New York Times* nor the *Wall Street Journal* checked the story's facts independently. The media during this time so much favored the parents that perhaps it was politically impossible for any reporter to present another side.

Perhaps, too, that just shows how hard the story was to understand and how difficult it is for nonphysicians to get the real story. Physicians usually will not talk to reporters about a controversial case and will not criticize their colleagues to reporters. So the public only finds out in court what is really going on.

In 1994, another reporter interviewed Jane Doe and her family:

> Now a 10 year-old . . . Jane Doe is not only a self-aware little girl, who experiences and returns the love of her parents; she also attends a school for developmentally disabled children—once again proving that medicine is an art, not a science, and clinical decision making is best left in the clinic, to those who will have to live with the decision being made.[27]

In 1998, Paul Gianelli, who represented the parents in their legal battles, told reporters that Jane was 15-years-old and still living with her parents, who guard her privacy and theirs. "It was a very sad case and yet satisfying," said Gianelli, who ultimately won in court for the parents.[28]

ETHICAL ISSUES

Selfishness

Theologian James Gustafson said Baby Jane Doe's parents selfishly did not want Baby Jane to live.[29] Living one's life for others, he said, is the primary ethical requirement of Judaism and Christianity. C. Everett Koop argued similarly: "Why not let the family find that deeper meaning of life by providing the love and the attention necessary to take care of an infant that has been given to them?"[30]

In contrast, the late John Fletcher, a former Episcopalian priest who later became a secular medical ethicist, said that he could "stand by the parents" in such cases and "would not want to come down real hard on them" for letting a baby die by forgoing treatment.[31] Others asked whether, if living for others was a religious value, nonreligious people should be forced to adhere to it.

Reluctance to raise a profoundly disabled child is not necessarily selfish but may be simply realistic. For a couple who both work, raising a severely disabled child usually means that one parent must give up a job and hence that the couple will lose income. Moreover, caring for such a person is generally a life-long job: people with Down syndrome in 2002 had an average lifespan of 49, and some live into their 70s (and all Down adults who live this long develop Alzheimer's disease). So some children with Down syndrome will outlive their parents. Is it really always selfish for parents to decide that they are not called to spend their own lives caring for such a person, especially if at birth they can choose a different life?

Disability advocates argue that disadvantaged children cannot be allowed to die merely because they don't fit into their parents' preconceived plans. Part of the responsibility of having sex, and accepting childbirth, is to accept whatever comes along. We can't let parents adopt the attitude of, "I'll only be a parent if my child is healthy and normal." They also stress that family values mean that everyone in a family pulls together to help the least well-off member, whether that person is Baby Doe or Granny Doe. They reject the conceptualization of this case as one about the autonomy of parents to make decisions and to prevent the intrusion of Uncle Sam in the nursery. Instead, they argue, the case should be seen as one of communitarian ethics, where "it takes a village" to see the potential of a child with Down syndrome.

On the other hand, if we do not consider the family's good in some way, are we not in effect saying that the random birth of an impaired child must be fatalistically accepted by every family, no matter what hardships it entails? As an institution, the family today seems shaky enough; how much more stress can most families be expected to manage?

Fred Bruning, a writer for *Newsday*, urged everyone to leave the parents in this case alone:

> Travelers familiar with Beirut claim it is a city lost to hope because consensus is impossible. Perhaps it can be said that parents of severely damaged children inhabit a Beirut of the spirit, a place where innocence has no armor, where there is no distinction between suffering and survival. The rest of us are strangers, and we ought to let the parents consult the doctors, reach their decisions, tend to their babies, grapple with their lives. We ought to respect their heartache and their wishes. We ought to leave them in peace.[32]

Abortion versus Infanticide

Today, some pregnant women undergo amniocentesis or sonograms, and if the results indicate a fetus with a chromosomal abnormality, some terminate the pregnancy and try for a healthy baby. Such abortions can take place legally late in the second trimester, when the fetus is large and perhaps at a stage of development where some premature babies are saved. This practice raises a significant ethical issue.

When amniocentesis indicates spina bifida, the fetus will almost always be aborted. But if spina bifida justifies abortion, why doesn't it also justify letting a newborn with spina bifida die? Similarly, if an abortion is permissible because the fetus has Down syndrome, why shouldn't Down syndrome justify allowing a baby to die?

Birth, after all, does not change the medical condition: in this sense, it can be argued that the significance of birth is merely symbolic or emotional. Note that this logic is neutral between opposed moral conclusions about nontreatment. That is, if there is no good reason why a neonate with, say, spina bifida should be allowed to die, then presumably there is no good reason why a fetus with spina bifida should be aborted.

If parents want to forgo treatment in these cases, then should they be required to justify the decision, or should they simply be left alone? When a woman decides to abort even a healthy fetus, she is not required to give good reasons. Why are we so much more concerned when an impaired newborn is involved?

Conceptually, the problem is to find a consistent position that includes accepting abortion but opposing letting parents decide to forgo treatment in Baby Doe cases. If one accepts choice with regard to abortion because of a Down fetus, why not with regard to letting a Down newborn die? Or perhaps one should oppose both?

Killing versus Letting Die with Newborns

In a famous article, the late James Rachels asked whether it would not be more compassionate to simply kill impaired and imperiled newborns than to let them die slowly by forgoing treatment.[33] Rachels argued this way: In both forgoing and infanticide, the motive—the death of the baby—is the same, and so is the result: in both, the baby dies. If the motive is the same in both decisions, and if both decisions lead to death, how can the two decisions differ morally? This might seem to be a matter of simple logic: whatever makes one decision good (or bad) should also make the other decision good (or bad). If so, the kind of action itself, as to its active or passive nature, should make no difference.

Some bioethicists disagree with Rachels, especially about nontreatment of newborns and infanticide. One reason they do is because people are not perfect, make mistakes, and killing is too quick and too final. Merely allowing an infant to die leaves the door open for a while, in case parents or physicians have a change of heart. Another argument for forgoing treatment is that it shows more respect for the value of life: a quick end cheapens life, but when treatment is forgone, parents and professionals must suffer through the ordeal.

Personhood of Impaired Neonates

Before he became surgeon general, C. Everett Koop wrote that "each newborn infant, perfect or deformed, is a human being with unique preciousness because he or she was created in the image of God."[34] On the other hand, Catholic theologian Richard McCormick argued that an infant can realize some "good" of its own only if it can potentially form human relationships.[35] So Koop assumed that any human newborn is a person, whereas McCormick's criterion would rule out anencephalic babies as persons.

McCormick's *potential-for-relationships standard* is a reasonable attempt to delimit personhood, but it has problems. It can be difficult to predict potential for relationships, which seems to depend on the attitude of parents. And what about orphans?

Associations of parents of babies with spina bifida hold that a person's potential cannot be known until his or her life is lived. So every child deserves a chance to fulfill his potential.

One theory of personhood asserts that the developmental stage of the fetus/baby really does matter morally. After all, a crying baby differs a lot from a two-day old embryo. Several cognitive scientists and bioethicists believe that personhood develops along a gradient, such that the further along this continuum, the more the fetus is a person. This *gradient view of personhood* rejects the all-or-nothing fallacy that an embryo or fetus is not a person one moment and a person the next.

On the gradient view, it's worse to kill fetuses than embryos, and it's worse to kill fetuses just before birth than in the first trimester (which explains why many physicians are reluctant to perform so-called "partial birth" abortions). Similarly, a baby with Down syndrome differs from a fetus with Down syndrome: the former has more moral status and rights. The death of the baby requires more justification than the death of a fetus.

The distinctions of the gradient view are just what drive some opponents to claim that no difference in personhood or moral status exists between human embryos and human babies. Both sides agree about the gradient and its smooth continuum of development; they just disagree about the proper inferences to draw from this fact.

In Baby Doe cases, some bioethicists champion the *cognitive criterion of personhood*. It identifies certain characteristics, including reason, agency, memory, and self-awareness, and assumes that without them, personhood does not exist.

With regard to impaired infants, bioethicist Peter Singer once used the cognitive criterion to argue that children should not be regarded as persons until "a few months" after birth; physician and philosopher Tristam Engelhardt once held that infants are not persons until they form a self-concept, around the age of two (he has since given up this position). Philosopher Michael Tooley holds that they are not persons until they can use language.[36] For Singer, the early Engelhardt, and Tooley, newborns fail to meet the cognitive criterion.

As noted before, many families use the cognitive criterion in letting adult relatives die. However, its application to impaired newborns may be more questionable. Allowing parents to forgo treatment for an imperiled neonate is one thing; claiming that a child is not a person until age two seems to be quite another.

Personal versus Public Cases

Was Baby Jane's case a private, personal family decision or a case of neglect that public policy must not tolerate? One member of a group advocating recognition of the sanctity of life in public policy criticized the parents, maintaining that "private individuals and private groups of individuals don't have the right to make life or death decisions in private in an unaccountable manner."[37] On the other hand, many people argued that Baby Jane's parents should have been left alone to make decisions.

Do problems of personhood effectively prevent us from applying Mill's concept of harm in this context? Can we distinguish between private life and morality here? Mill's harm principle calls for government not to interfere with decisions that put no other person at risk of harm, but his principle may not help us in Baby Doe cases, if we think that impaired babies are persons.

If we decide that every impaired newborn is a person, it follows that no parent could decide to let such a child die, and this would severely limit a family's range of choices. But if we allow a wide range of choices, we allow each family to decide what personhood is. Can we allow that?

For example, the state of Tennessee intervened in 1983, over a father's religious objections, to allow chemotherapy for 12-year-old leukemia patient Pamela Hamilton. Another such case occurred in Boston in 1988, when a young child became ill; the child's parents, who were Christian Scientists, called a practitioner instead of a physician; after apparently improving for a while, the child suddenly died five days later. Boston district attorney Newman Flanagan charged the parents with manslaughter.

Clearly society must strike a balance between allowing parents some choice about medical treatment of their children and protecting vulnerable children from misguided parents. But which parents are wise, which misguided? That is the question in what follows.

Conceptual Issue: Taxonomy in Ethics

Cases of treatment versus nontreatment are often grouped together, and sometimes even lumped together with cases of assisted suicide and physician-assisted dying, as "euthanasia." This is confusing and possibly dangerous. As argued previously, we should differentiate physician-assisted dying, which involves terminally ill competent adults, from assisted suicide, which involves nonterminal competent adults; we should also distinguish these from nontreatment of incompetent adults in PVS; and distinguish the above from allowing impaired newborns to die.

One reason why such distinctions matter has to do with criteria for forgoing treatment. Criteria for nontreatment of *never-competent* patients should presumably be much higher than the criteria for competent or formerly competent patients whose own wishes can be known or inferred. With never competent patients, the decision to forgo treatment must be based on evidence which is beyond a reasonable doubt, and this would also be true for babies who are presently incompetent but who later may be competent.

Degrees of Defect

In practice, criteria for nontreatment of impaired babies tend to be based on long-term prognoses and degrees of defectiveness in newborns.[38] Babies whose problems are less serious should be treated, whereas it would be permissible to let babies who are most serious or gravely ill die.

Cases between these two poles—cases such as spina bifida and Down syndrome—are controversial because prognosis is far from absolute and may be influenced by moral frameworks. Consider John Lorber's predictive criteria for spina bifida. One vocal critic of Lorber's approach is his colleague at the same hospital, pediatric surgeon R. B. Zachary. Zachary argues that the only options for babies with spina bifida are either to kill them or to do everything possible for each one of them. Basically, he is saying that there is no category of babies with spina bifida who can be allowed to die.

Lorber and some other pediatricians say that the mortality rate is high for babies they place in the "worst" category of spina bifida, but Zachary maintains that these physicians do not simply withhold treatment. According to Zachary, they "push the infant towards death" by giving:

...eight times the sedative dose of chloral hydrate recommended in the most recent volume of Nelson's Pediatrics and four times the hypnotic dose, and it is being administered four times every day. No wonder these babies are sleepy and demand no feeding, and with this regimen most of them will die within a few weeks, many within the first week.[39]

Prognoses about the intelligence of impaired people seem to be influenced by social views. Down syndrome is a good example, especially because of the external characteristics associated with it. Let's briefly consider Down syndrome in more detail.

During the last 50 years, a Copernican revolution has occurred in thinking about people with Down syndrome.[40] Many earlier studies of IQ on those who were institutionalized were flawed. A sampling bias failed to take into account the higher IQs of people with Down syndrome who lived with supportive families.

At present, although most people with Down syndrome will have IQs below 70, less than one-third (some studies say only 10 percent) will have IQs lower than 25 (profoundly retarded and untrainable).[41] Most people with Down syndrome who receive good early care, maximum stimulation, and support will have IQs between 50 and 70.

What does this imply about quality of life for a person with Down syndrome? IQ is a measure of intelligence, of course, and academics and physicians often associate intelligence with happiness. However, it is an unwarranted conclusion to infer that people with IQs between about 50 and 70 must be unhappy, unless we simply define unhappiness in those terms.

Given reasonable stimulation, love, and supervision, most people with Down syndrome will, to use a phrase made important in ethics by philosopher Tom Regan in another context, "have a life."[42] Almost every person with Down syndrome will have a narrative history, and lives that will go (to use another famous phrase from Regan), "better or worse for them." Under almost any criteria of quality of life, most people with Down syndrome would not be better off dead.

Note the mention of early care, stimulation, and support; the prognosis for Down syndrome varies with treatment: early stimulation can raise IQ, whereas mere custodial care will lower it. At birth, we cannot predict whether a baby with Down syndrome will be at the low or the high end of the IQ range; consequently, the best interest of these babies is maximal treatment. Whether maximal treatment best benefits their families is another question.

Sanctity of Life versus Quality of Life

It is interesting to realize that although the ethical frameworks loosely described as sanctity of life and quality of life are commonly held to be incompatible, these two standards would agree on the early treatment of most babies with Down syndrome and spina bifida. It would seem that a neonate with spina bifida has a good chance of "a life"—that is, neither genetics nor probable IQ predetermines a life of misery. Often, it cannot be predicted at birth whether a child with spina bifida will be in the high, normal, or low range of IQ; but most such children will *not* be profoundly retarded. If we cannot assume that low IQ precludes any happiness in life, it can be argued that such children should live—that an IQ described as "borderline," "trainable," or even "imbecile" does not make life so bad that nonexistence would be better.

However, sanctity of life and quality of life diverge when a prognosis predicts a life of total pain: in such a case, considerations of quality of life or "the good of the child" support nontreatment. If this outcome could be known in advance, it would be immoral, from a quality of life standpoint, to save the neonate. These cases are the ones that traumatize pediatric neurologists. Because most of these children die, nontreatment is best—but not all of them die, and those who do not die will be worse off.

What about the *family's* quality of life? How does that figure into moral thinking? Into family values? Caring for an impaired child imposes enormous burdens on other children and stressed parents. If the quality of life standard applies to the entire family, rather than just to the baby ("the good of the child"), it implies nontreatment.

This interpretation of quality of life is unusual. When we think of quality of life in, say, cases of PVS or physician-assisted suicide, we are of course thinking of the *patient's* quality of life. Applying this standard to a neonate's family is like arguing that a patient in PVS should be allowed to die, or that a terminally ill patient should be helped to die, not for their own good but for that of the family.

Wrongful Birth versus Wrongful Life Suits

Parents can sue physicians in civil courts for allegedly causing babies to be impaired. Today, few parents simply accept birth defects as God's will; standards of health continue to rise, and couples expect healthy babies. When babies are disabled, parents often blame physicians.

Both wrongful life and wrongful birth suits fall into the general classification of tort law, and in both kinds of actions compensation for a harm or "tort" is sought.

It is important to distinguish between different meanings of harm. Like the concept of good, the concept of harm covers a broad range of meanings. For our purposes here, we can distinguish three broad meanings of harm.

In the first way, both a baseline and a temporal (time) component are necessary, so that a change occurs that makes someone worse off. *Baseline harm* requires an adverse change in someone's condition. With baseline harm, someone who doesn't yet exist cannot be harmed, because he or she has no baseline from which change can occur.

The second way of defining harm compares a present deficiency with what normally would have been. In this *abnormal harm,* someone is injured by being brought into existence with some defect that could have been avoided by taking reasonable precautions. Here, the event or omission that causes the defect is the cause of harm.

Third, harm may be defined as a life of total pain and injury, such that no hope exists. Perhaps this is the lot of many pigs raised in industrial factory-farms, confined their whole lives and squashed together for maximal profits in tiny metal pens with their tails cut off. Let us call this third harm, *total harm.* To some of its critics, reproductive cloning would be so bad for the child as to constitute total harm.

Preventing abnormal harm underlies the belief that parents should do everything possible to have healthy, unimpaired babies; that anything less than the maximal effort is blameworthy; and that it is wrong for a woman to take risks with a future person's intelligence or health. In this sense, deaf parents harm their children when they only implant embryos genetically disposed to be deaf.

Total harm in the law is called *wrongful life*. In such cases, lawyers claim that the lives of some babies are so miserable that their existence is a tort. In contrast, *wrongful birth* assumes abnormal harm, and claim not that the child's life is totally miserable, but that the child has been damaged by being born less than normal, and that a physician's action or omission caused the relevant defect. Courts have almost always rejected wrongful life suits because courts have rejected the implication that killing a baby can benefit it.

An instructive case containing aspects of both wrongful birth and wrongful life was a suit in 1967 involving Jeffrey Gleitman. His mother had contracted German measles during the pregnancy; Jeffrey was born nearly blind and deaf, and she testified that her obstetrician had failed to warn her of this outcome. She was one plaintiff, suing for the expenses of Jeffrey's lifelong care (this was the wrongful birth aspect); in addition, Jeffrey was another plaintiff, and the brief for Jeffrey argued that he was so impaired that he would have been better off not existing (this was the wrongful life aspect).[43]

The Gleitmans lost, evidently because of the wrongful life element of the case. The judge found that if Sandra Gleitman's physician had warned her about probable fetal defects she would have had an abortion, and concluded that Jeffrey "would almost surely choose life with defects against no life at all." Since 1982, courts in New Jersey, Washington state, and North Carolina have agreed that, while life itself can never be an injury, parents may recover damages to pay for care that would not have been required if physicians had not made errors.

Conceptually, the main problem with the wrongful life aspect of the Gleitman case is that, if you accept wrongful life and its idea that some kinds of life are so bad as to be worse than nonexistence, it implies that *it would be a benefit to a child to kill him*. Few judges are willing to accept that implication.

Several well-publicized wrongful birth suits by parents against physicians have transpired. In New Jersey, parents of a baby with Down syndrome sued pro-life obstetrician James Delahunty, whom they say discouraged them from pursuing amniocentesis when a sonogram showed a fetus with a thick neck (a possible sign in utero of this condition).[44] The jury awarded the couple nearly $2 million and found Dr. Delahunty guilty of "failing to recognize, appreciate, and discuss the results of the tests, particularly ultrasound" with his patients. The verdict may have stemmed partially from his combative behavior in the courtroom.

At least 27 states allow parents to sue for wrongful birth, although Michigan and Georgia recently disallowed them. In a case in 1999, as well as another case in 1990, the Georgia Supreme Court ruled that a couple with a child born with Down syndrome could not sue their physician for failure to perform amniocentesis or other prenatal tests.[45]

In France, an uproar occurred when, after 13 years of litigation, a court ruled in 1995 that parents of a child born with German measles and not offered an abortion were entitled to compensation for wrongful birth. In two subsequent cases, damages were also awarded to parents of children with disabilities where parents argued that had they had known prenatally of the disability, they would have aborted. Critics in France assailed these results, saying they had established a "right not to be born," re-started Nazi eugenics, and would increase premiums for malpractice. The French legislature in 2002 banned wrongful birth suits.[46]

New Legislation

In 1984, Congress amended its Child Abuse Prevention and Treatment Act of 1974 (not the Rehabilitation Act), to count nontreatment in Baby Doe cases as *child abuse*. The Child Abuse Amendments (CAA) circumvented the injunction against the Baby Doe rules. They made states, not the federal government, responsible for such cases—getting Uncle Sam out of the neonatal nursery. These amendments were never repealed and are technically still in force today.[47]

The only exceptions to the CAA are: (1) when an impaired child is "chronically and irreversibly comatose," (2) when a child is inevitably dying, and (3) when treatment would be "futile and inhumane." These exceptions are often interpreted narrowly, so as to give parents few choices. As one law professor sums it up, "Since passage of the CAA, ethical and legal controversy over parental authority to withhold treatment from handicapped or disabled newborns . . . has largely ceased."[48]

Problems resulting from such narrow interpretation were illustrated dramatically in the Rudy Linares case, which took place in Chicago in 1989. Dan Linares held an NICU staff at gunpoint while he disconnected the respirator of his 16-month-old son Rudy, who had gone into PVS 9 months earlier, after swallowing a balloon at a birthday party; Rudy soon died, and Dan Linares was charged with first-degree murder.[49] Because there was no doubt that Dan Linares was a caring parent, a grand jury refused to indict him for homicide; he later received a suspended sentence on a minor charge arising from his use of a gun.

In 1990, the *Americans with Disabilities Act (ADA)* was passed and went into effect over the next few years. It protects Americans with a wide range of disabilities from discrimination. Nevertheless, the application of ADA to newborns with congenital defects—and thus to Baby Doe cases—is so far unresolved.

In 1994, a federal court specifically cited ADA in mandating treatment for a 16-month-old anencephalic infant, Baby K, who had been brought to a hospital emergency room in Virginia in respiratory distress.[50] Baby K had been on a respirator since birth. When the case was heard, her physicians wanted to disconnect it and let her die; but for religious reasons, her mother insisted on continued care. At its heart, Baby K's case was about whether physicians may overrule parents' decisions about continuing futile, expensive treatment without incurring charges of discrimination against the handicapped. For over a year, Baby K continued to receive treatment, but died in 1995.

After two decades of legal wrangling about Baby Doe cases, the results are equivocal. On the one hand, some impaired babies who would once have died as a consequence of nontreatment now undoubtedly survive to lead meaningful lives. On the other hand, the right of parents to make choices in cases of disabled newborns has declined dramatically. As a result of the amendment to the Child Abuse Act, most NICU physicians usually overtreat severely impaired newborns.[51]

The ADA does not make it criminal for physicians to withhold treatment from impaired newborns. Rather, it threatens to withhold federal funding from a state for its programs. Even under this threat, no state has ever been found to be out of compliance. Moreover, although thousands of such infants have had life-sustaining treatment withheld or withdrawn, contrary to the guidelines in these regulations, no legal charges have been brought against physicians, hospitals, or states for doing so.

Nevertheless, while the ADA imposed no criminal charges on physicians who failed to comply with it, most obstetricians perceived it as requiring a presumption in favor of treatment. And subjected to a barrage of lawsuits with every disabled baby, obstetricians are not risk-takers these days.

History is repeating itself in bioethics with premature babies, whose numbers have recently soared.[52] The prospects are dire for such babies under 750 grams, yet they do not fall under exceptions to the ADA, so most physicians treat them aggressively. This treatment takes away choice from parents; such lack of choice is being increasingly challenged by parents in court.[53]

The Rise of Disability Advocates

Many pediatricians claim that in the 1950s, it was rare for a baby with Down syndrome to live long.[55] Even after institutionalization, nontreatment intending death was the norm, not the exception. Babies who survived were sent to be warehoused in custodial institutions, where they were never stimulated or educated. They almost always became severely retarded.

Within pediatric neurology, opinion about treatment in Baby Doe cases changed dramatically over the past decades. In the 1960s and early 1970s, the consensus was that many such cases should not be treated; today, all but the most hopeless cases are treated.[54]

For example, Lorber's criteria concerning spina bifida initially swung the pendulum toward nontreatment in many NICUs; but during the 1980s, right-to-life organizations and disability advocates swung the pendulum back toward treatment. Also, breakthroughs were made in urology, neonatology, neurosurgery, and CAT scan diagnosis, and these not only increased the accuracy of prognoses but also improved quality of life for such children. These changes have led to a new understanding:

> Mild to moderate degrees of microcephaly are compatible with normal or even exceptional intellect. This is particularly true in cases of untreated meningomyelocele in which loss of cerebrospinal fluid through the unrepaired hole in the back may decrease the total mass of the head .... Essentially all children with severe meningomyelocele have hydrocephalus .... Children with hydrocephalus who are treated reasonably early and who do not develop meningitis have a better chance than 50 percent of being intellectually normal.[56]

The Spina Bifida Association has stated:

> Since we have found it virtually impossible to predict at birth which infants with meningomyelocele will become competitive, ambulatory, and intellectually able, we have not relied on arbitrary guidelines to determine which children should or should not be treated. On the contrary, we believe that all such children should be treated, and we feel that our data show this philosophy to be correct.[57]

The outcome in the Baby Jane Doe case, chosen for discussion because of its fame but otherwise typical of spina bifida, makes this statement seem reasonable. Moreover, the unexpected outcome of the Mueller case and the newer prognoses for Down syndrome suggest that similar reasoning may be appropriate regarding other defects.

Conceptual Dilemma: Supporting Both Choice and Respect

The parents of spina bifida child Leilani Duff-Fraker, born in 2004, love their daughter, but if their obstetrician had ordered the right tests, they would have aborted her and tried again for a healthy child.[58] Is that inconsistent? Can you love a child who you might have deliberately stopped developing as a fetus?

In some aspects, this question is analogous to the Ayala case, where parents deliberately conceived a child to be a source of bone marrow for her older sister with leukemia. The Ayala parents claimed that they would and could love Marissa, and not just see her as a resource for her sister. Jodi Picoult's *My Sister's Keeper*, a work of fiction, tells a different story.

Public policy reveals a similar dilemma writ large. Is it consistent to do prenatal testing for genetic diseases while at the same time telling adults with the same diseases that they are respected? Is it consistent to test babies at birth for genetic conditions such as PKU and at the same time tell adults with PKU that they are valued? Do funds for prevention of disabilities compete with funds for services for disabled adults?[59]

On another front, is history repeating itself with the half million premature babies born in America each year? Given that the ADA has taken away almost all choices about treatment from physicians and parents, must all extremely premature babies be aggressively treated? Notice that if some are "let die" and do not die as planned, we repeat the scenario of the Baby Jane Doe case.

Finding a consistent, defensible policy on these questions is not easy. Each day, bioethicists and physicians struggle to find it.

FURTHER READING AND RESOURCES

Fred Frohock, *Special Care: Medical Decisions at the Beginning of Life*, University of Chicago Press, Chicago, Ill., 1986.

Loretta Kopelman, "Are the 21-Year Old Baby Doe Rules Misunderstood or Mistaken?" *Pediatrics*, 115, no. 3, March 2005, pp. 797–802.

John Freeman, "On Learning Humility: A Thirty-Year Journey," *Hastings Center Report*, May–June, 204, pp. 13–16.

John Robertson, "Extreme Prematurity and Parental Rights After Baby Doe," *Hastings Center Report*, July/August 2004, pp. 32–39.

Peggy and Robert Stimson, *The Long Dying of Baby Andrew*, Little, Brown, Boston, Mass., 1983.

U.S. Commission on Civil Rights, *Medical Discrimination Against Children with Disabilities*, September 1989.

CHAPTER 10

Medical Research on Animals

This chapter discusses the ethics of using primates and nonhuman animals in medical research. It gives a historical overview of opposition to using animals in such research and takes up philosophical concepts underlying the recent animal-rights movement. Its central cases are the research of Thomas Gennarelli, who injured primates to mimic the effects of such injuries in humans, and the research on primates to study learned helplessness to help stroke victims. Publicity about these cases changed the way American researchers use animals.

ANIMAL LIBERATION FRONT AND GENNARELLI'S RESEARCH ON PRIMATES

On Memorial Day in 1984 when everyone was gone, members of the Animal Liberation Front (ALF) quietly entered a building of the University of Pennsylvania Medical School in Philadelphia. They broke into a laboratory where they found—and stole—32 audiovisual tapes covering years of experiments on primates.

In stealing the tapes, these ALF members broke the law, but there is disagreement over how much other damage, if any, they did. One university official claimed that they had done $2 million worth of damage; but although *American Medical News* reported this figure prominently, no evidence was offered for the exact dollar amount. Subsequent newspaper reports omitted that claim, and it is not mentioned in the final report to the National Institutes of Health (NIH).

The stolen tapes had been made over 15 years by the neurologist Thomas Gennarelli, who was trying to produce exact brain damage in primates—adult monkeys and baboons. For this purpose, a device had been developed to make a reproducible model of brain injury: a live monkey or baboon, wearing a helmet, would be strapped down, and the animal's head would be subjected to terrific force at a 45-degree angle. Gennarelli had initially used monkeys in these experiments, but the studies with monkeys failed to simulate human head injuries, and as of 1980 he used baboons. All together, Gennarelli's laboratory studied this topic for over 15 years: 1970 to 1985.

There were about 60 to 80 hours of tape in all; ALF edited them to produce a 25-minute segment that showed only abuses. This edited version, called "Unnecessary Fuss" (a quotation from a defender of the project who therein described the protests), was distributed widely to television stations. It was wrenching and emotionally persuasive; as a reporter for the *New York Times* said:

> One sequence showed a monkey strapped to a table pulling against its bonds. The animal's head was encased in a steel cylinder to a pneumatic machine called an accelerator. Suddenly, a piston drove the cylinder upward, thrusting the animal's head sharply through an arc of about 60 degrees.
>
> . . . In another sequence, as an animal lay in a coma, a researcher's recorded voice was heard saying, "You'd better have some axonal damage, monkey," and calling him "sucker."[1]

As shown on the edited tape, the researchers made derogatory and taunting remarks about the animals; these comments sounded adolescent or macho and damaged the credibility of the researchers. They used profanity, performed unsterile surgery, and had sloppy care of animals.

Researchers claimed that the baboons were sedated and felt no pain; but, as the quotation above describes, several segments showed baboons twisting and struggling to free themselves just before the pneumatic hammer smashed their heads. Thomas Langfitt, the principal investigator of the overall head-injury program and chairman of the university hospital's neurosurgery department, maintained that even though the animals moved before the tests, they had been anesthetized; when watching the videotape, his claim is hard to believe.

Perhaps most repugnant to many nonscientists were several segments showing the researchers making fun of injured baboons, holding the animals up by broken arms or laughing at conscious, brain-injured baboons. The effect of these tapes, filed by the researchers themselves, undermined their cause more than an ALF documentary could have.

Several key members of Congress had previously opposed a bill to strengthen regulation of animal experiments. In 1984, People for Ethical Treatment of Animals (PETA) showed the edited tape in two briefings on Capitol Hill; that same evening, the tape appeared on ABC's news show, *20/20*. Viewing the tape were Senator Weicker and Congressman William Natcher, the chairs of the Senate and House committees responsible for the NIH budget.[2] The two chairmen and 16 other members of Congress decided the public would not like what it was going to see on television that night, and they sent letters to the NIH demanding suspension of Gennarelli's studies.

As predicted, the public did not like what it saw on the tapes, which forced Margaret Heckler, Secretary of Health and Human Services (HHS), to review them. Officials in Pennsylvania denied that Gennarelli had abused animals "gratuitously" in his laboratory.

In April 1985, PETA turned the stolen tapes over to the NIH for review. A branch of HHS, the Office for Protection from Research Risks (OPRR), appointed a committee to evaluate Gennarelli's research. This committee, which consisted of a neurosurgeon, a veterinary anesthesiologist, and a veterinary pathologist, all of whom used animals in research, assumed nothing to be intrinsically wrong with injuring baboons to study head injuries in humans: "The research, as proposed, is likely to yield fruitful results for the good of society."[3]

The committee found Gennarelli guilty of nine of ten charges: lack of anesthesia, inadequate supervision, poor training, inferior veterinary care, unnecessary multiple injuries to the same animals, humor, smoking, statements in poor taste around animals, and improper clothing. It concluded: "Taken collectively, these conclusions constitute material failure to comply with the Public Health Service Animal Welfare Policy." Gennarelli's lab had violated most rules designed to protect animals, and the university had no mechanism to ensure that it followed such rules.

HHS Secretary Margaret Heckler suspended Gennarelli's research, the first time a lab had been closed because of abuse of animals. To Carolyn Compton—a physician, pediatric researcher, and spokeswoman for scientists using animals—this was a "tragedy."[4] To ALF, it was a momentous victory.

One member of the original team defended the break-in as follows:

> We may seem like radicals to you, but we are like the Abolitionists, who were regarded as radicals, too. And we hope that 100 years from now, people will look back on the way animals are treated now with the same horror as we do when we look back on the slave trade.[5]

Six weeks after its Memorial Day raid, ALF struck the University of Pennsylvania's veterinary school, "liberating" three cats, two dogs, and eight pigeons. The dean of this school said the raid "would set back research efforts, including a study to determine the cause of sudden infant death syndrome."[6] Another dean said the stolen cats were being used in studies of breathing during sleep, a missing dog had a steel plate inserted to study osteoarthritis, another was being studied for ear-canal infections, and the pigeons were part of a study of broken bones intended to benefit all birds.[7] He aid that the work on dogs would benefit other dogs, adding that it had to be done and that more dogs would end up having to be used as subjects.

In 1984, ALF struck in California, taking two rabbits injected with oral herpes and numerous dogs with cancer, along with 100 other animals, from City of Hope National Medical Center in Duarte. In the lab, ALF painted: "ALF IS WATCHING AND THERE'S NO PLACE TO HIDE!" Ingrid Newkirk of PETA called City of Hope a "concentration camp" where animals were "being used for painful experiments."[8]

The associate director of City of Hope said the theft of these animals had disrupted $500,000 worth of research on emphysema, cancer, and herpes. ALF had targeted a study testing tobacco carcinogens in dogs. The associate director refused to comment on whether the abducted animals had been treated cruelly but did say that 36 cancerous dogs, 12 cats, 12 rabbits, 28 mice, and 18 rats had been stolen and added, "We're concerned that very important research work may not now be completed."[9]

In 1985, in the largest animal raid to date, ALF hit the biology and psychology laboratories of the University of California, Riverside, taking 467 animals, including a stump-tailed macaque whose eyes had been sewn shut to study a device to help the blind navigate. PETA said these animals had been used in painful, unnecessary experiments, some involving starvation; NIH investigated the charges but found no evidence of abuse. The University claimed $683,000 in damages.

In 1987, arson gutted the $2.5 million veterinary research animal lab at the University of California, Davis; ALF claimed responsibility. In California in 1988, ALF destroyed a new building for animal research at the medical school in San Diego and burned down a veal-packing plant in Oakland. Masked ALF spokespersons took credit for these attacks in televised interviews, vowing to continue them "until the killing of the innocent animals stops."

Also in 1988 in Connecticut, Stephanie Truit planted a bomb outside a company that made surgical staples and used animals to train surgeons in handling them. She was arrested for attempted murder.[10]

Several experiments reviewed by NIH in the 1980s fared poorly. The City of Hope Medical Center in Duarte, California, was fined $25,000, lost $1 million in grants, and lost its Animal Care Assurance, a semi-legal document in which an institution promises to abide by federal regulations. After ALF released pictures of poor lab conditions and inspectors made an unannounced visit, Columbia University lost all its grants involving vertebrates.

To prevent further abuses, Congress mandated in 1986 *Institutional Animal Care and Use Committees* (IACUCs) for all institutions receiving federal funds for research on animals. These committees try to reduce the number of animals involved in experiments, the amount of pain inflicted on research animals, and the kind of species used from higher to lower.

Although IACUCs are composed mostly of researchers themselves, they do force experimenters to justify their projects to fellow scientists—some of whom can be critical. Since the existence of IACUCs is directly attributable to the exposure of Gennarelli's experiments, his work can be called the Tuskegee Study of animal research.

PETA AND EDWARD TAUB'S RESEARCH ON MONKEYS

In 1981, Alex Pacheco volunteered in the primate lab of psychologist Edward Taub in Silver Spring, Maryland. Pacheco told Taub that he wanted to become a research scientist, but he really intended to videotape Taub's research on animals for PETA.[11] Taub was studying "somato-sensory deafferentation" in monkeys by surgically cutting all the nerves in one limb and then trying to stimulate regrowth. He hypothesized that *learned helplessness* caused some of the damage in stroke, and this was his animal model mimicking stroke. Each year, strokes disable a half-million Americans, who often lose use of a limb.

Pacheco entered the lab late one night and photographed Taub's experiments. The tactics used by PETA in the Taub case were sensational. To obtain evidence for the trial, Alex Pacheco invited activists such as Donald Barnes, John McArdle and Michael W. Fox to search Taub's lab at night; when warrants were served on Taub shortly thereafter, several television stations recorded the event while PETA leaders distributed press releases outside. During the trial, PETA seemed to orchestrate each element for maximal emotional impact in the media—with the predictable result that the media portrayed Taub as another Josef Mengele and PETA as the animals' Robin Hood.

Taub was convicted of failing to provide proper veterinary care, a charge based on the fact that he did not bandage the animals' wounds. Professor Taub testified that it was better to leave the wounds unbandaged because years of experience had convinced him that the monkeys would only tear the bandages off, making their wounds worse.

Veterinarians disagreed about this; but eventually the American Psychological Association's Ethics Committee, the National Institutes of Health, and an ad hoc committee of the American Physiological Society exonerated Taub of any failure to provide adequate veterinary care. After its own investigation of the charges, the psychology department at the University of Alabama at Birmingham hired him as a full professor.

The 1991 Story of the Year for ethics in *Discover* magazine concluded that four of Taub's monkeys showed:

> dramatic new evidence of the adult brain's capacity to "rewire" itself, something previously thought to be impossible. And ironically, it was PETA's success at keeping the monkeys away from research for a decade that made the discovery possible.[12]

The 15 surviving monkeys had been transferred in 1986 to the federally funded Tulane Regional Primate Center in Covington, Louisiana. In 1990, in an experiment which PETA opposed, a brain researcher—Timothy Pons—tested Taub's hypothesis by examining the brain of a dying monkey before euthanization. Pons was "flabbergasted" to discover that "the entire patch of the cortex corresponding to the arm—about half an inch wide—had been rewired to receive input from the face." Pons concluded, "The results offer hope that the brain can be coaxed into rewiring itself after injury." Data from other monkeys in the study supported this finding.

Neural rewiring is the Holy Grail in rehabilitative medicine, something offering hope to victims of stroke and spinal cord injury. Whether Taub has achieved such rewiring is still uncertain.

In 2000, Taub achieved a breakthrough, which CNN and ABC News reported extensively.[13] Taub reported that all stroke patients using his *Constraint-Induced Movement Therapy*, or CI therapy, had significantly improved in function. For an affected arm, 30 percent of patients gained close to normal use.[14]

Taub's treatment built directly on two of the most criticized experiments on animals in psychology: Martin Seligman's experiments on dogs demonstrating learned helplessness and 20 years of his own work on monkeys.

So can the brain reorganize after a stroke? Some people think that CI therapy jump-starts self-repair of surviving, healthy cells in the brain or spinal cord. CI therapy tries to "wake up cells that have been stunned," says Taub.[15] "CI therapy appears to produce a rewiring in the brain that leads to improved motor function of the affected limb."[16]

"Right after a stroke, a limb is paralyzed," he says. "Whenever the person tries to move an arm, it simply doesn't work." But often the cells that represent the arm are still alive. The patient assumes the arm is permanently dead, expects failure from trying to use it, and does not. "We call it learned non-use," Taub said. The more the patient relies on the good arm, the less likely recovery becomes in the bad arm.

Timing is critical. Immediately after a stroke, if movement is induced in the bad limb, damage increases to the brain. But in the second or third week, therapy can begin.

Requiring scarce rehabilitation therapists trained in the new techniques, the therapy goes six to seven hours every weekday for 10 consecutive weeks. Patients move around with good limbs tightly-bandaged. Because of lack of therapists and space, and with little publicity, most patients seeking the new treatment cannot be accommodated.

To begin to meet the demand, in 2001 UAB opened the Taub Clinic for CI therapy. Although neither private insurance nor Medicare pays for the costs, which run $6,000 to $13,000, over 5,000 stroke patients are on the waiting list. Demand for therapy has also created ethical problems similar to that of Seattle's God Committee, which struggled to allocate scarce, life-saving hemodialysis machines in 1962 among many candidates.

The National Institutes of Health funded in 2004 the first multicenter national trial to prove the benefits of CI.[17] In 2006, a placebo-controlled study proved that benefits of CI therapy for victims of stroke lasted two years after therapy.[18] In a separate result, Taub proved the benefits of CI therapy last five years after a stroke. Twenty-one survivors underwent the standard CI therapy, while 21 other survivors merely had a general fitness program. Two weeks after CI therapy, patients in the treatment group had a "large to very large" improvement in use of the affected arm, whereas those in the control group had no change.

BACKGROUND: MILESTONES IN ANIMAL RESEARCH

In 1992, the Farm and Animal Research Facilities Protection Act made it a federal crime to break into a research facility or the premises of a company that breeds research animals. Violators face prison sentences of up to one year for illegal entry and fines up to $5,000. A vice-president at UAB Medical Center, which had originated the bill, said that this legislation would protect scientists against "activists who use terrorist techniques to interfere with potentially life-saving research."[19]

In 1993, animal rights activists won a significant victory for dogs and primates used in laboratory research. Judge Charles Richey ordered the Agriculture Department to enforce and advance the Improved Standards for Laboratory Animals Act of 1985, the act creating the IACUCs. Judge Richey concluded that the Agriculture Department had violated the act by giving all power to interpret it to local IACUCs: he implied that members of such committees, including veterinarians, were employed by the institutions they were supposed to regulate and had conflicts of interest.

Psychological experiments that have drawn severe criticism and scorn from activists include Harlow's study of baby monkeys deprived of their mothers, and Seligman's original research on learned helplessness in dogs and monkeys that subjected them to electric shocks. According to activists, not only are experiments like these extremely painful, but the results have been trivial. Psychologists regard Harlow's and Seligman's work as landmarks.

Richey also criticized the government for taking nine years to implement some of its own rules, and he implied that some of the rules were intended more to increase profitability than to ensure the welfare of research animals.

Judge Richey recently rejected the claim that "a rat is a pig is a dog is a boy" and dismissed claims that American researchers had to keep detailed records for their 21 million rats and mice. He said researchers could treat rats and mice differently than dogs and primates.

Animal activists see IACUCs as window dressing and claim the committees do little good. They say that the Department of Agriculture, which must inspect labs, has a too-cozy relationship with animal-abusing agribusiness. They lament that veterinarians on IACUCs are caught in the middle, charged with protecting animals but salaried by researchers.

During the 1980s, faced with what they perceived as devastating losses in public confidence, scientists decided they could no longer ignore animal rights activists. They established the Foundation for Biomedical Research, which lobbies for 350 universities, drug companies, manufacturers of medical devices, and commercial animal-supply companies. It has a paid staff member in most states and maintains lobbyists in Washington, D.C., to counter the numerous lobbyists of PETA.

During the 1990s, positions of animal activists and animal researchers hardened, with activists seeking to abolish all research using animals and researchers branding activists as sentimental "bunny huggers." Researchers adopted a siege mentality, using electronic surveillance and branding anyone who talked to outsiders as a traitor.

This movement to extremes made it difficult for reformers, such as F. Barbara Orlans of the Kennedy Institute of Ethics at Georgetown University, whose life-long goal is implementing the "Three R's" of *replacement* of animals by in vitro methods; *reduction* of their numbers through statistical analysis; and *refinement* of experiments to cause the least suffering.[20] The European Union is far ahead of America in implementing this plan, although Congress directed NIH to do so in 1993.

In the past 20 years, a number of celebrities campaigned against use of animals in medical research, including Loretta Switt, Lindsay Wagner, Clint Eastwood, and Johnny Carson. Former game show host Bob Barker fought the University of Southern California Medical School's primate research program. Filmmakers took up animal rights in movies such as *Star Trek IV* and *Project X*.

BACKGROUND: ANIMALS IN RESEARCH

How many animals do American researchers use each year? No federal law requires such data to be kept, so estimates vary. The Office of Technology Assessment estimated 14 million, *Newsweek* estimated 17 million, and activist Andrew Rowan, former dean of Tufts Veterinary School, estimated 71 million.[21]

Regardless of the exact figure, scientific research uses immense numbers of animals. America has nearly 130 medical schools. These, as well as a dozen pharmaceutical and private research foundations, use millions of animals each year, mostly rats and mice, but also dogs, pigs, cats, rabbits, and primates. In 1983 alone, Charles River Breeding Laboratories (the General Motors of animal breeding), produced 10 million animals for research.

Basic research uses many animals—far more than most people realize. For every practical success in human medicine, such as cyclosporin or knee replacements, dozens of failures occur in studies with human subjects and hundreds of failures occur in animal studies. To arrive at each success, the sad truth is that researchers maim and kill millions of animals each year.

According to Rowan, 40 percent of experimental animals are used in basic and applied research, 26 percent in drug development, 20 percent in safety testing, 8 percent in science and medical courses, and 6 percent in other scientific programs.

Animal rights activists made two tests controversial: the LD-50 tests and Draize tests. LD stands for *lethal dosage,* and LD-50 tests determine what amount of a substance will kill 50 of 100 animals. Done routinely across species for substances ranging from soap to chemotherapies, these tests have been criticized as crude, blunt measures (one wit said they tell mice how much of something to take for mass suicide). Because of such criticisms, use of LD-50s declined 96 percent since the early 1970s, most replaced by LD-10s.[22]

The Draize test estimates how much of a product will irritate the human eye; a concentration of the product is dripped into a rabbit's eye, which is particularly sensitive. Activists have sought alternative tests using cell cultures and computer models.

ETHICAL ISSUES

Concept: What Kinds of Beings Feel Pain?

Since prehistoric times humans have used animals for many purposes, but experimentation on animals did not arise as a specific issue until the beginning of modern science. Rene Descartes in the 17th century set the premises for the modern debate.

Not only a mathematician and philosopher, Descartes was also a physiologist and studied the circulation of blood by dissecting live animals without anesthesia (which was not invented until the early 1900s). To understand why he considered that permissible, it is necessary to understand his basic philosophical approach, which is known as *Cartesianism* and has deeply influenced western science and philosophy.

Descartes is known for his famous argument "Cogito ergo sum": "I think, therefore I am." According to him, what distinguishes human beings from other animals is *res cogitans,* or "thinking stuff," a substantial mind or soul. For Descartes, this mental substance held together transient mental states such as perceptions, feelings, thoughts, and dreams and served as a ground for free will, reason, and moral values. Nonhuman animals, Descartes believed, lack *res cogitans,* mind or soul, and are therefore ultimately only *res extensa,* or "extended, physical stuff." Thus in Cartesian philosophy, animals were merely fleshy machines; their eyes reflected no soul and no pain lay behind their external pain behavior.

Descartes's idea that animals lack a soul was not unique as this was also Christian doctrine. Descartes accepted Christian teaching that humans have souls created by God whereas animals do not. But Descartes assumed further that *soul* is identical to *mind,* so if animals have no soul, neither do they have a mind; and if animals have no mind, they are not conscious and if they are not conscious, they cannot feel pain.

For Descartes, in order to feel pain, a mind is needed, and—to repeat—only human beings have minds. In Descartes' view, no middle ground exists between a human being, who has a soul and a capacity to experience pain, and an animal that has no soul and no capacity to experience pain.

Cartesianism represents an attempt to deal with the tension between science and religion by demarcating proper areas for each: the province of science is the study of matter, mathematics, animals, and the human body; that of religion and the humanities is mind, art, and ethics. Obviously, however, it has not come to represent a consensus, or even a widely accepted solution—even for Christians, who are still struggling with the concept of how mind and soul are related, how they relate to morality, and whether animals count in the grand scheme of things (clergy are often asked whether pets go to heaven).

Among Descartes' followers during his own century was an infamous group of early physiologists and *vivisectionists* (researchers operating on live animals without anesthesia) at the Jansenist seminary of Port Royal. Here is how 18th-century writer Nicholas Fontaine describes them:

> They administered beatings to dogs with perfect indifference, and made fun of those who pitied the creatures as if they felt pain. They said the animals were clocks; that the cries they emitted when struck were only the noise of a little spring that had been touched, but that the whole body was without feeling. They nailed poor animals up on boards by their four paws to vivisect them and see the circulation of the blood which was a great subject of conversation.[23]

To some extent, the Cartesian concept of animals has persisted into modern times. Some behavioral psychologists argued against assuming rats were conscious and drew a distinction between "pain behavior" and the experience of pain. Rats and chickens, they said, exhibited "pain behavior," but whether they had mental states and thus had an experience of pain like humans was another matter.

The 20th-century Christian writer C. S. Lewis tried to find a middle ground between the above Cartesian extremes. Lewis rejected the view that animals feel nothing and argued that animals indeed do feel. But in what sense? Lewis distinguished between *sentience* (the ability to feel pain) and *consciousness* (awareness of feeling pain). All mammals are sentient, he argued, but only human beings are also self-conscious.[24]

According to Lewis, animals feel pain, but not as humans do. A rat receiving three electric shocks feels the pain of each shock—the rat is sentient—but it does not think, "I have had three shocks." The thought, "I have had three shocks," requires what Lewis calls "consciousness or soul" (he runs these together). Lewis agreed with the 18th-century philosopher David Hume, who argued that self-identity requires a permanent self or mental substance which unites all of a person's thoughts as "his" or "hers" (Hume famously thought that, even for humans, this deep self was a myth).[25] For Lewis, a baboon would have a "succession of percep-tions," but not the human experience of pain as "my pain."

Lewis, then, identified consciousness with self-consciousness or soul (for which he also used the term "deep self"). Some critics have disagreed with this idea, particularly since Lewis assumed that memory depends on self-consciousness. These critics observe that if self-consciousness were needed for memory, animals would never remember anything, and studies of learning in animals would be senseless; but everyone knows that animals remember—a dog who has been kicked by a mailman remembers when he returns.

Today, philosophy of mind and animal ethics agonize over answers to the fol-lowing kinds of questions: how much pain do animals feel? To what extent is their pain like our pain? On the ladder of evolution from, say, an amoeba to a baboon, at what point does an organism become sentient? At what point can an organism react to pain? At what point can pain be anticipated? How much "mental" pain can be experienced by fish, cats, dogs, or pigs? When can an animal remember pain as "my" pain? How can we know an animal is experiencing pain as "mine"? Is there a difference between being sentient and being conscious? If so, how can we know this? If we cannot know, why should we use two different words? Is there a difference between being conscious and having a mind? Is there a differ-ence between being aware of the capacity to feel pain and being aware of a "self" as the subject of awareness?

These are not simple questions; they raise some of the deepest problems in philosophy of mind and lie behind many controversies about animal research.

Clearly, with regard to questions like these, philosophy of mind blends into ethics. As discussed previously, two standards of personhood are the cognitive cri-teria and the gradient theory. On either one of these standards, some nonhuman ani-mals may count as persons if they have enough of the relevant cognitive abilities.

What cognitive capacities qualify an animal for membership in the moral com-munity? In other words, what qualities does an animal need to count in the moral calculus? (Sentience? Consciousness? A soul?) How can we verify such capacities in a species, especially if those capacities have important ethical implications? As we consider various answers to such questions, do we have, as a species, a conflict of interest? Do we have any bias toward accepting some answers and rejecting oth-ers? We explore answers to these questions in some of the sections below.

Even if animals are not aware of pain, or do not remember pain the same way as humans, that does not mean they suffer less in medical experiments. When humans consent to be subjects of medical experimentations, the purpose and risks of the study are explained to them. So they have some understanding of the exper-iment. This does not occur with animals who have no idea why they are being subjected to these procedures. Having less ability to understand may cause ani-mals to suffer more in research.

The Philosopher's Offense I — Peter Singer on Speciesism

Before 1975, groups promoting animal welfare focused on humane treatment of research animals. In that year, the Australian philosopher Peter Singer published

Animal Liberation, where he argued that animals must morally count for some-thing.[26] To say animals do not count because they are inferior by nature, Singer held, is like saying slaves or women do not count because they are inferior by nature. Just as racism and sexism are evil, Singer said, so is *speciesism.*

According to him, the argument that supports equal rights for minorities and women—without begging any questions—also supports animal rights. If our moral concern for children, women, and minorities stems from their sensitivity to pain, family ties, and ability to reason, why wouldn't these factors also be a basis for concern for animals?

Note that we treat humans with *equal* human rights despite the obvious fact that they are *unequal* in their ability to suffer, in their intelligence, strength, and character. Inequality of ability does not dictate inequality of treatment. Such argu-ments put speciesists on the defensive: if the principle of equality applies to all people, despite their obvious differences in ability and intelligence, why should not it also apply to animals?

Singer also argued that a medical experiment using animal subjects must be speciesist unless humans would be willing to substitute irreversibly comatose human subjects. This is an interesting approach. Most people who accept the idea of using, say, a chimpanzee in medical research would cringe at the idea of using an anencephalic baby (an infant born lacking most of the brain). But if the chim-panzee is active, gregarious, sensitive, and responsive, whereas the anencephalic baby is hopelessly mute, comatose, and unresponsive, why should the chimp be the victim? If the answer is simply that the baby is human and the chimp nonhu-man, that answer is mistaken because it assumes what it must prove, in other words, it's speciesist.

Let us put the point differently. Suppose an institution exists with hundreds of profoundly retarded human children and adults who have been abandoned by their families to the State. They are so profoundly retarded as to have virtually no recognizably human interactions with each other or the staff. Even so, most peo-ple would be horrified to learn that a drug company was using them as subjects to test promising drugs for toxicity in humans.

Now move to a large center for primates, such as one near San Antonio, Texas, that holds hundreds of chimpanzees and baboons. Only these primates are *more* social, *more* interactive, and *more* intelligent than the humans described above. Yet these are precisely the beings drug companies use to test new drugs for toxicity. Why do we tolerate such testing on them and not on the retarded humans?

In addition to his argument about speciesism, Singer also used *utilitarian rea-soning.* According to utilitarian ethical theory, right acts produce the greatest good for the greatest number; for instance, research on presently sick patients is right if it helps a greater number of future sick patients.

Singer maintains that stipulating that the "greatest number" must refer only to humans begs the key question. Once animals count for something, however small, in utilitarian reasoning, then radical conclusions follow. Experiments that inflict horrible pain on many animals cannot be justified on the ground that they save a few human lives because the number of animals suffering outweighs the small good to humans.

Ironically, researchers themselves employ utilitarian reasoning to justify their research. In other words, they use secular, results-oriented, quantitative reasoning to defend their research. They say, "Yes, some patients now suffer in finding new cures for cancer and in testing potential cancer-fighting drugs, some of which may be toxic, but the greatest good for cancer patients in the future justifies such experiments."

The founder of utilitarianism, Jeremy Bentham, argued in the 19th century that animals' suffering should count in the moral calculus. He held that the important question was not whether animals could reason, but whether they could *suffer*. If any being can suffer, then its pain should count morally in the actions of people.

Consistent application of utilitarianism obligates individuals to make great sacrifices to help victims of famine, improve the lives of future generations, and relieve the suffering of animals. That is because utilitarianism takes seriously the number of beings affected in calculating which actions are right.

Some people will reject utilitarianism's implications, preferring a within-a-mile-of-me kind of morality. On the other hand, utilitarianism does seem to explain why bioethics should be global, why reduction of spread of HIV may be the most important issue in medicine today, and why global warming may obligate us to drive fuel-efficient vehicles.

For many people, the most shocking implication of Singer's interpretation of utilitarianism is that the current system of factory farming is evil. Billions of animals suffer and die each year so humans can enjoy their flesh. Arguably, vegetarian eating is healthier for humans today than a meat-centered diet, yet giving up meat is where many people balk at following Singer or utilitarian.

On the other hand, if animals count morally and should not be used as mere resources in medical experiments, then they should not also be used as resources for our food. Singer's *Animal Liberation* and many other books explain how veal calves, pigs, and chickens are raised in small, confining cages in industrial-type farms.

The Philosopher's Offense II — Tom Regan and Animal Rights

Underlying the controversy over Gennarelli's experimentation on primates is a more basic issue: whether scientific research on animals is *ever* justified. Tom Regan, an American philosopher and animal rights activist, thinks not:

> I argue that the whole system of animal experimentation [and] the whole system of commercial and sport trapping and hunting are morally bankrupt institutions. The only way you change these things fundamentally is by eliminating them—in much the same way as with slavery and child labor.[27]

Regan argues that human beings have rights because they *have a life*. That is, humans have lives that can go better or worse for them, and this is true for each human being independent of whether or not others value him or her. In other words, people have inherent, not instrumental, value. Where Singer applied utilitarianism to animals, Regan applied a Kant-type ethics to animals, asserting the rights-based idea that each animal's life should be treated as an "end in itself."

So Regan condemns research using animals because it treats them as a means to the good of helping humans. For Regan, animals have rights not to suffer at the hands of humans, rights to be respected in their own habitat, and rights to enjoy a natural life-span. So eating them is also immoral. In other words, each animal's life has *inherent value.*

Of course, once the premise is accepted that each animal's life has inherent value, it follows that medical research to benefit humans is unjustified. For if a life has "inherent value," no competing value trumps it.

Regan maintains that like humans, many species of animals have lives that can go better or worse for them, and he draws this crucial inference: "They too have a distinctive kind of value in their own right, if we do; therefore, they too have a right not to be treated in ways that fail to respect this value."[28] Regan reasons that if humans count in the moral calculus because they possess a quality, and if animals possess the same quality, then it is inconsistent not to count animals equally. Anyone who wants to argue that there is some difference here must prove why.

Regan's critics say that his argument runs several unjustified inferences together. First, they ask, if any being (human or nonhuman) has a life that can go better or worse, does that fact give every life a distinctive value? Second, and more important, just because an animal "has a life," that doesn't mean it is equal in value to that of humans.

Note, however, that Regan includes a qualification: he says that animals (like humans) have lives which can go better or worse *for them.* By qualifying his claim this way, no comparison is possible between human and animal lives. If fish in an aquarium "have a life" that can go better or worse *for them,* from that standpoint, we do not have a right to destroy them.

Charles McArdle, a scientist, also agrees. Suppose that either a dog or a man can remain in a lifeboat: Regan implies that because "animals aren't there to be used as our resources," it is morally wrong to kill the dog to save the man, and McArdle concurs—"I would seriously have to question whether I would allow an animal to die just to protect me."[29] On the other hand, the pediatric researcher Carolyn Compton disagrees: "I love animals, but there's no question in my mind that if I were able to sacrifice an animal life to save a human being, I would do it."[30]

The philosopher Carl Cohen asserts, "Rights arise, and can be intelligently defended, only among beings who do, or can, make moral claims against one another."[31] Because animals cannot make claims, he says, they have no rights.

But this seems a little too quick and question-begging. When a dog pesters his owner to be taken for a walk, isn't the dog making a claim on the owner? If so, Cohen must say that the dog has a right to the walk. Perhaps, then, our pets have rights?

He rejects the analogy between racism, sexism, and speciesism: although racism and sexism are indeed bad, speciesism is not. "I am a speciesist," he declares, and he adds, "Speciesism is not merely plausible; it is essential for right conduct, because those who will not make the morally relevant distinctions among species are almost certain, in consequence, to misapprehend their true obligations." That is, they will take the dog from the burning building and not the child.

Evaluating Scientific Merit

Critics of animal research may compromise by claiming they don't want to stop all research, but only trivial or repetitive research. They are willing to continue using animals in worthwhile research.

Stopping research typically takes the form of cutting off funding, and one suggestion has been that only worthwhile research should be funded. This sounds reasonable, but deciding what is worthwhile is difficult.[32] In practice, this decision is the job of NIH committees of peer reviewers that consider applications for grants. These reviewers are experts, and if they knew in advance exactly which projects were worthwhile, they would fund only those—but of course they don't know in advance. Sometimes an apparently insignificant project can yield important results, and sometimes an apparently important project can yield little of value.

Also, when critics cite specific examples (Harlow's research on maternal deprivation in monkeys, say, or Seligman's research on learned helplessness in dogs), researchers often defend the importance of these studies. Indeed, Taub's research was once cited as a paradigm of worthless research, but that changed dramatically with his unexpected breakthrough with stroke patients.

Scientific research might be compared to an iceberg. The results or findings that will be applicable to humans are the tip of the iceberg, visible above the water. This small tip is supported by the much larger part of the iceberg, the part that is invisible under the water; that large invisible portion consists of basic research which goes on quietly in labs and is rarely discussed in national media.

For example, in 2006 a paralyzed man had a tiny chip implanted in his brain in a system called BrainGate. With it, his thoughts were able to move a computer's cursor on a screen and then the computer could do things for him.[33] The device had been developed in primates, some of them at Stanford University.

At bottom, researchers have faith that the costs of basic studies—in terms of money, effort, time, and the suffering of animals—will one day be outweighed by benefits. At bottom, animal activists are skeptics who doubt or deny that the benefits to humans outweigh the costs to animals.

Evaluating the Philadelphia Study

Gennarelli can be described as working at the bottom of a pyramid of basic research on head injury. To him, it may have seemed obvious that the first step in such research would be to produce one head injury precisely and reliably, so it could be replicated and studied by others. Scientists point out, for example, that knowing how to produce different kinds of burns in animals is the first step in studying the physiology of burns and the metabolism of healing.

On the other side, animal activists held that Gennarelli had merely bashed primates' heads for a decade without getting anywhere. They argued that even if he had succeeded in devising a reproducible model of head injuries, such a model would offer little help in treating such injuries (an argument that scientists have denied).

A committee of his peers reviewed Gennarelli's grant and said that his research would contribute information about the drug mannitol in reducing brain swelling after trauma, and about management of metabolic balance in comatose patients.

Later, the university's investigator, Thomas Langfitt, claimed that Gennarelli's research had provided the first evidence that regeneration of damaged nerve cells may be possible.

On the other hand, critics said these conclusions papered over a lack of findings. Nedim Buyukmichi, an activist and veterinarian, argued that Gennarelli's studies were too inconsistent to result in a reproducible model of head injuries and too limited in scope to adequately mimic injuries sustained by human victims of accidents: "After 15 years and $11 million to $13 million, essentially nothing has come out of this research that hasn't already been known from studies of human head trauma."[34] Other critics were unimpressed by the purported findings about regeneration of nerve cells, comparing that claim to the ubiquitous trumpeting of possible cures for cancer.

Gennarelli's treatment of animals is another issue. In turn, this issue has two aspects. First, there is the question of how badly or insensitively the animals were treated. Some of Gennarelli's defenders have said that the apparently insensitive comments and behavior of researchers on the tapes were comparable to the type of cynical humor typical among medical residents; also, as noted above, the university's investigator, Langfitt, said that the animals had been anesthetized.

These arguments have been attacked, and in light of what the tapes show, neither convinces. Activists argue that the researchers were pursing lucrative grants and professional prestige and were blinded to their subjects' plight by conflicts of interest.

The second question is this: If the animals were indeed mistreated and the researchers were insensitive, does that necessarily affect the scientific value of the research? In other words, could researchers conduct an excellent project even though they mistreated their subjects? For animal activists, Gennarelli's treatment of his animal subjects proved that his project was immoral and thus unjustifiable. Were they right? Can the scientific value or merit of a study be assessed independently of the researchers' behavior?

Protecting Humans and Children: Animals in Research

Consider what would happen if legislators banned using all animals in medical research. Consider first drugs.

By federal law, drugs must first be tested on animals to detect toxicity and to check for promising results. Scientists use mice to test many kinds of anticancer compounds, such as extract of grapes. Scientists also give mice cancer in order to test anticancer drugs.

If no mice were available, such tests would need to be done on humans or not at all. It is inconceivable that humans would be given cancer to have subjects to test anticancer drugs, so we would need to fatalistically accept the reality of cancer and that it will never be eradicated. We would also cease to have proof that any compounds prevent or ameliorate cancer, as we would have no evidence from animals.

In Phase I of testing drugs on humans, scientists strive to see how much of the drug can be given without producing toxic effects. Phase I is only done after extensive testing of the drug in animals. Without such testing, many more toxic reactions will occur in humans than before.

The same argument could be made for how scientists test new heart pumps, artificial pumps, cures for burns, antibiotics, and new kinds of surgery. If they did not test these first on animals, making their mistakes and gaining skill, many more humans would be injured or harmed than at present.

Finally, Taub's research is a telling example. Chosen originally as an example of research considered infamous and suspect, Taub had to endure countless criticisms and hurdles to gain his breakthrough. Stroke victims will benefit now, perhaps even more so in the future, if his research can be refined and generalized. But none of it was possible without research on animals.

In sum, assuming we want medical research to continue, using animals in research is indispensable to reducing harm to humans from medical research. It is true that most people do not understand how many animals scientists use in research or how much such animals suffer. But the judgment is that such suffering is justified to benefit humans and, to a much lesser extent, veterinary medicine.

Once a year in medical school, students pause in a ceremony to remember those who dedicated their bodies to be cadavers for students to learn on in gross anatomy. Scientists and physicians need the same kind of ceremony to commemorate what animals have given us.

We should also keep medical research on animals in perspective: in the United States each year, 22 million dogs and cats are abandoned, killed, or lost each year by owners who fail to make adequate provisions for their care.[35] Many of these owners simply replace the lost animal with a new pet, as if it such replacement were no big deal. At the same time, medical research uses only about 180,000 dogs and 50,000 cats. For every dog used in medical experiments, perhaps 100 dogs kept as pets will die early because of neglect or abandonment by their owners.

Capacities, Moral Standing, and the Gradient

Over the last three decades, reformers have focused on varying *capacities* in human and nonhuman animals. This idea motivates Barbara Orlans's (previously discussed) movement for the "3 R's" of reduction, replacement, and refinement.

Raymond Frey and others argued that the greater capacity of humans to exercise autonomy and plan gives them more value than pigs, chimpanzees, and horses, and these in turn possess more value than chickens, mice, and oysters. The corollary is that the lesser the capacity to suffer like humans, the easier it is to justify use of the animal in medical research.

Interestingly, the capacities argument cuts both ways: it entails that some medical research should be allowed on brain-dead patients, i.e., on cadavers, and on brainless neonates such as anencephalic babies.

The proper use of animals in medical research also raises a deeply philosophical issue that strikes at the heart of ethical theory. It concerns the question of *moral standing*.

Moral standing refers simply to who counts when trade-offs are made or calculations occur. For example, in some versions of utilitarianism, the death of human fetuses counts little, but the pain of farm animals counts a lot.

How do we delineate the boundaries of moral theory? This is another way of asking about the outer limits of proper moral concern.

Perhaps the question is not as difficult as it might appear, once we note something else. Many discussions about animal suffering, animal rights, or animal consciousness only offer us two options: animals suffer like us or they do not; animals have rights like us or they do not; animals are conscious like us or they are not.

This may be the classic false dilemma, the either-or fallacy of only offering two all-or-nothing options in a complex world. In discussing abortion and end-of-life care, we explored the *gradient theory of personhood*. Now here we might extend that theory to nonhuman animals.

As evolution teaches, humans evolved through primates from even lesser animals. As such, we share nervous systems, receptors for pain, and fight-or-flight reactions with our predecessors. Moreover, it is precisely because of sharing so much with primates and mammals that the latter make such good subjects for medical research: they predict well how drugs and surgeries will work in humans.

If we think of proper concern for animals and humans as a continuum, then we will ask different questions and get different answers. We will not ask, whether animals have rights. But ask instead, if a chimpanzee is a lot like a human baby, shouldn't we care a lot about both? Maybe some kinds of research (such as a chimp in a metal canister, breathing through a tube), should be banned on chimps, out of respect for the similarity.

Continuing about concern, a gradient also explains, and perhaps somewhat justifies, why we are and should be more concerned about those around us much more strongly than those in distant lands. Even the best of us only has so much moral concern, which is like a battery that only has so much power and which periodically must be recharged. And all of us start life as nonbatteries and end life that way, such that we go from being the ones concerned to being the objects of the concern of others.

So we have only a limited amount of concern to spread around, and we should do so judiciously. We want first to take care of our family and friends, our neighbors, colleagues, and people in our neighborhood, professional community, or university. And in that circle of concern, many people will include animals, especially their pets.

Of far less concern will be the suffering of people in poor African countries and the suffering of unseen animals. It is not that the average person wants anyone to suffer in Africa or an animal to suffer in being raised for his food, but rather, one person has only so much concern and one person's efforts seem relatively ineffectual to bring about much change.

Other Kinds of Medical Research on Animals

Creation of new kinds of animals for human purposes riles some people. Such creations include cloning of livestock and transgenic animals used as models for research on human diseases, such as the onco-mouse and SCID mouse, useful in research respectively on cancer and the human immune system and xenotransplants.

Opposition stems from two premises. The first is that some kinds of creation are intrinsically wrong. One intuition here is that humans should not play God: God created species just as they are, for the benefit of human beings, and humans should not tamper with this divine plan. Another intuition behind the same premise is secular and often embraced by environmentalists: humans should not tamper with Mother Nature or violate evolution's wisdom, especially by creating hybrid or transgenic animals.

A second premise fueling opposition to creation of new kinds of animals for medical research stems from a public distrust of medical researchers using animals, aka the Frankenstein objection. The public does not see animal scientists as trying to cure human diseases, but sees them as arrogant, cruel, and greedy.

These issues and their objections raise different kinds of questions than previously considered in this chapter. They concern not the ability of animals to suffer and judgments about risk/benefit, but objections to a whole field of research and a hostile view of all scientists. They are therefore beyond the scope of this chapter to discuss.

But we will end by noting how the two objections often work in tandem. One kind of transgenic pig can easily be created by inserting a gene for an enzyme that results in a 60 percent reduction in phosphorus in pig feces. Pig farms smell notoriously bad, and the phosphorus has a lot to do with that smell.[36] Moreover, preventing the phosphorus from contaminating local rivers is a major problem.

So one would think transgenic pigs producing less phosphorus would be welcomed, but such news is greeted by skepticism by environmentalists who retort that farmers will use such technology to grow 60 percent more pigs on the same farm.

FURTHER READING AND RESOURCES

Deborah Blum, *The Monkey Wars*, New York, Oxford University Press, 1994.

Peter Carruthers, *The Animals Issue: Moral Theory in Practice*, New York: Cambridge University Press, 1992.

R. G. Frey, *Rights, Killing, and Suffering*, Basil Blackwell, Oxford, England, 1983.

Tibor Machan, *Putting Humans First*, Lanham, Md.: Rowman & Littlefield, 2004.

F. Barbara Orlans, *In The Name of Science: Issues in Responsible Animal Experimentation*, New York: Oxford University Press, 1993.

Denise Radner and Michael Radner, *Animal Consciousness* Prometheus Books, 1989, Buffalo, N.Y.

James Rachels, *Created from Animals*, New York, Oxford University Press, 1990.

Tom Regan, *The Case for Animal Rights*, University of California Press, Berkeley, 1983.

Richard Ryder, *Victims of Science: The Use of Animals in Research*, London: Davis-Poynter, 1975.

Peter Singer, *Animal Liberation*, New York Review Books, New York, 1975.

Susan Sperling, *Animal Liberators*, University of California Press, Berkeley, 1988.

CHAPTER 11

Research on Human Subjects

This chapter describes the Tuskegee study of untreated syphilis in Alabama between 1929 and 1972. It also discusses medical experimentation by Nazi physicians, secret American medical research, studies in Africa to prevent transmission of HIV from mother to child, the death of Jesse Gelsinger in 2000, and the growing problem of financial conflicts in medical research.

INFAMOUS MEDICAL EXPERIMENTS

In 1822 in a famous case of abuse of an experimental subject, physician William Beaumont, "the father of gastric physiology," treated Alexis St. Martin for a bullet wound in the stomach; St. Martin survived, but the wound healed strangely, leaving a hole. To observe the hole, Beaumont employed St. Martin as a servant, and proved the previously unknown fact that stomach juices digest food. St. Martin soon ran away and Beaumont had him caught to continue to exhibit him. Hospitals today in Texas and Michigan bear his name.

Nazi Medical Research

Besides participating in the Holocaust, physicians during the Nazi regime conducted heinous experiments on human subjects. The physicians reasoned that the people in the concentration camps were going to die anyway, so why not use them to benefit medical science?

Across the globe during the same war, Japanese physicians carried out deadly experiments on Chinese prisoners at unit 731 in Harbin, killing 3,000. To study the natural course of diseases, physicians injected prisoners with anthrax, syphilis, plague, and cholera.[1]

From 1943 to 1945, gay men, convicted criminals, Russian officers, Polish dissidents, Jews, and Gypsies on Ward 46 at Buchenwald in Germany got experimental vaccines against typhus. Physicians injected blood infected with typhus into 40 involuntary subjects, who served as a treatment group. Overall, they infected a thousand prisoners, 158 of whom died. They established no thresholds of infection.[2]

In experiments at Buchenwald, physicians tried to cure gay men with hormone shots, had inmates shot to study gunshot wounds, starved inmates to study the physiology of nutrition, and amputated women's bones and limbs to study regeneration. To study malaria, physicians used anopheles mosquitoes to infect subjects. Physician Ernst Grawitz infected legs of women with staphylococci, gas, and tetanus bacilli. In testing sulfa drugs, he rubbed particles of glass and stone into wounds.

In experiments at Ravensbrück, physician Sigmund Rascher devised his "sky ride wagon" to simulate rapid changes in altitude. Victims were locked inside an enclosed box on wheels with monitoring equipment inside.[3] Rascher also froze a hundred nude Jewish and Russian prisoners in icy waters to study techniques to revive downed pilots in similar waters. In one study, he forced nude Jewish women to revive the subjects sexually. Since such women would be unavailable to revive pilots downed in icy seas, this exercise simply degraded the women.

Josef Mengele

The most infamous Nazi physician, Josef Mengele, known as the Angel of Death, participated in the death of 400,000 victims in concentration camps.

Ambitious, the young Mengele sought fame. To get it, he studied medicine and anthropological genetics in Munich between 1930 and 1936, when eugenics movements swept Germany and America. The Nazi party and its ideology of racial purity were then centered in Munich.

Contrary to some accounts, German medical schools did not resist Nazi eugenics and killing undesirables, but led these movements. To advance, Mengele joined the Brownshirts, a fanatical Nazi movement.

Mengele needed groundbreaking research to reach his goal of appointment as a Professor. In 1943 at the Auschwitz concentration camp, he began experiments to overcome the effects of genetics by modifying environments. He wanted to produce blue eyes, blonde hair, and healthy bodies free of genetic disease. As subjects, he needed identical twins, natural controls for environmental differences.

Mengele greeted incoming trains of boxcars filled with Jews destined for execution. He examined them, looking for twins and other usable subjects, signaling his choices with a flick of his wrist.

Describing Mengele's experiments is painful. He injected blue dye into children's eyes to see if he could create blue eyes. He forced female twins to engage in coitus with male twins to see if twins could be produced. He interchanged blood of identical twins to observe results; he interchanged blood between pairs of twins.

One pair of fraternal twins consisted of a hunchback and a normal child; Mengele surgically grafted the hunchback to the normal child's back, creating the effect of conjoined twins; he accentuated this effect by sewing their wrists back to back. A witness reported that when these conjoined children returned to the barracks: "There was a terrible smell of gangrene. The cuts were dirty and the children cried every night."[4]

Mengele obtained between 150 and 200 twins, most of whom died. As one participant observer related:

> After that, the first twin was brought in, a fourteen-year-old girl. Dr. Mengele ordered me to undress the girl and put her head on the dissecting table. Then he injected the Epival into her right arm intravenously. After the child had fallen asleep, he felt for the left ventricle of the heart and injected 10 cc of chloroform. After one little twitch the child was dead, whereupon Dr. Mengele had her taken to the corpse chamber. In this manner, all fourteen twins were killed during the night.[5]

Mengele also tested endurance by subjecting 75 prisoners to electric shock; 25 of them died immediately. To study sterility, he severely burned Polish nuns by giving them high dosages of radiation.

He once found a hunchback and the hunchback's son; he had both of them killed, their bodies boiled, their flesh stripped, and their skeletons dipped in gasoline for preservation for his anthropological studies of body types. When he came upon seven dwarfs from a Rumanian circus family, he kept them alive to exhibit them to visiting physicians.

Cool, impersonal, and detached, when 300 Jewish children escaped a gas chamber and fled to a nearby field, Mengele had them recaptured, lit a gasoline fire set in a large pit, and had the children thrown in. Some children, on fire and screaming for their lives, clawed their way over dead bodies to the top, where Mengele and his men kicked them back in.

When the Russian army approached Auschwitz in 1945, Mengele escaped to Paraguay. He lived there for 40 years, eluding Israelis who tried to capture him as a war criminal. In later conversations with his grown son Rolf, he expressed no regret for his actions: it was not his fault that Jews had to die at Auschwitz, he said, so why not use them to advance medical knowledge and his own chances for a professorship? Never captured or tried as a war criminal, Mengele died in Brazil in the summer of 1985.[6]

American Military Research during World War II

In 1941, American researchers experimented on orphans at the Ohio Soldiers and Sailors Orphanage, on retarded inmates at New Jersey State Colony for the Feeble-Minded, and on patients at a mental institution in Dixon, Illinois.[7] To develop a vaccine against shigella, they injected deadened forms into subjects. None died, but many got sick.

Some questionable research used military personnel as subjects. Cornelius Rhoads, Director of Memorial Sloan Kettering Cancer Hospital in New York City, became head of the military's secret chemical warfare service. Rhoads

> supervised the long secret and now infamous tests where thousands of American troops were intentionally exposed to mustard and other poisonous gases. Rhoads discovered that the mustard gas killed white blood cells and other cells that divided rapidly. After the war he and others began to experiment with mustard gas as a cancer treatment and also to search for other systemic poisons that kill dividing cells.[8]

In research conducted by the armed forces on poisonous agents, 60,000 subjects did not know what they were undergoing.[9] Between 4,000 to 5,000 subjects inhaled mustard gas in gas chambers.

During the war, Franklin Roosevelt established the Committee on Medical Research, which approached its work with a wartime mentality that carried over into researchers' attitudes after the war: disease was the enemy, researchers were the soldiers, and victory could be won—with enough resources and enough will. During the war, ethical concerns about experiments carried little weight:

> A wartime environment also undercut the protection of human subjects, because of the power of the example of the draft. Every day thousands of men were compelled to risk death, however limited their understanding of the aims of the war or the immediate campaign might be. By extension, researchers doing laboratory work were also engaged in a military activity, and they did not need to seek the permission of their subjects any more than the selective service or field commanders did of draftees.... In a society mobilized for war, these arguments carried great weight. Some people were ordered to face bullets and storm a hill; others were told to take an injection and test a vaccine. In philosophical terms, wartime inevitably promoted utilitarian over absolutistic positions.

When subjects of secret chemical research later applied for treatment at veterans' hospitals, the Veterans Administration (VA) denied that they had been exposed to these agents. This scenario recurred after the war in Vietnam and after Operation Desert Storm.

World War II institutionalized some doubtful attitudes in medical experimentation. When the war ceased, the fight against diseases did not: "The prospect of winning the war against contagious and degenerative illness gave researchers in the 1950s and 1960s a sense of both mission and urgency that kept the spirit of the wartime laboratories alive."[10]

The Nuremberg Code

After World War II at the Nuremberg trials in 1946, German physicians defended themselves against charges of war crimes by saying that they had merely been following orders, that their experiments had been properly related to solving medical problems of war, and that what they had done did not differ from similar research done on captives by American physicians.

The judges at Nuremberg lacked a code of ethics for experimentation on captive populations, so they created 10 principles for ethical experimentation, known as the *Nuremberg Code*. Its most important principle was that people should freely consent to participation in any experiment.

Postwar Criticisms

By the 1970s, faith waned in scientific and medical progress. Rachel Carson's *Silent Spring* described the ravages of pesticides; the Cuban missile crisis brought America close to nuclear war; and drugs such as thalidomide (an antinausea drug during pregnancy), once hailed as miraculous, were found to cause children to be born lacking arms and legs.

In 1966, Harvard medical professor Henry Beecher criticized 22 specific medical experiments published in medical journals that had not obtained consent of subjects, asserting that this was the norm.[11] About the same time, physician Henry Pappworth similarly criticized 500 medical experiments.[12] That year, the United States Public Health Service began to require informed consent of subjects.

THE TUSKEGEE STUDY (OR "THE STUDY")

Nature and History of Syphilis

In the past, victims who suffered from untreated syphilis included Cleopatra, King Herod of Judea, Charlemagne, Henry VIII, Napoleon Bonaparte, Frederick the Great, Pope Sixtus IV, Pope Alexander VI, Pope Julius II, Catherine the Great, Christopher Columbus, Paul Gauguin, Franz Schubert, Albrecht Dürer, Johnann Wolfgang von Goethe, Friedrich Nietzsche, John Keats, and James Joyce.[13]

For hundreds of years, syphilis was attributed to sin and associated with prostitutes, though attempts to check its spread by expelling prostitutes failed because their customers were disregarded. Efforts to eradicate it by quarantine also failed.

Between 1900 and 1948, and especially during the two world wars, American reformers mounted the *Syphilophobia Campaign*. Reformers emphasized that prostitutes spread syphilis, and that syphilis rapidly killed. As an alternative to visiting prostitutes, they advocated clean, active sports, a view known as "Muscular Christianity."

Antisyphilis crusaders split twice over methods to prevent spread of syphilis: once during World War I over giving out condoms, and again during World War II over giving out penicillin. In each conflict, reformers who wanted to reduce the harm of syphilis battled those who wanted to reduce illicit behavior.[14]

This conflict repeated over the next century in battles about venereal diseases, prostitution, alcoholism, drug addiction, gambling, and sex education. *The Harm Reduction Movement (HRM)* focuses on reducing the associated harms of these behaviors, not on moral censure or eliminating the behaviors. Popular in public health, moralists who oppose HRM attack the illicit behavior and view HRM as enabling it, for example, by teaching men how to use condoms.

The armed services during the world wars were pragmatic. Commanders who needed healthy troops overruled moralists and ordered the release of condoms in the first war and penicillin in the second. After the wars, returning troops continued to use condoms and to get penicillin, normalizing these practices among Americans.

Schaudinn discovered in 1906 the spirochete that causes syphilis. It is a chronic, contagious bacterial disease, often venereal and sometimes congenital.

Syphilis has three stages. In the first, *primary syphilis*, spirochetes mass and produce a primary lesion, a chancre (pronounced "SHANK-er"). During this stage, syphilis is highly infectious. After the chancre subsides, the disease spreads silently for a time, but then produces an outbreak of secondary symptoms such as fever, rash, and swollen lymph glands.

In the second state of *latent syphilis*, spirochetes disseminate from the primary lesion throughout the body, producing systemic and widespread lesions, usually in internal organs. Syphilis then spreads silently from one to 30 years. During this stage, symptoms vary so widely that syphilis was once known as the Great Pretender.

In the last stage of *tertiary syphilis*, chronic destructive lesions damage the cardiac and neurological systems. Syphilis then may produce paresis (slight or incomplete paralysis), gummas (gummy or rubbery tumors), altered gait, blindness, or lethal narrowing of the aorta.

Today syphilis is treated with penicillin. Such treatment has been possible only since 1948, when penicillin became available to everyone.

Beginning in the 16th century, to treat syphilis, physicians applied the heavy metal mercury as a paste on the back. During the 19th century, they administered another heavy metal, bismuth, the same way. Neither mercury nor bismuth killed the spirochetes, though they ameliorated symptoms.

In 1909, after the spirochete of syphilis had been identified, two researchers—a German, Paul Erlich, and a Japanese, S. Hata—tried 605 forms of arsenic and discovered a "magic bullet" against it in combination 606 of heavy metals (which included arsenic). Erlich humbly called this Salvarsan (implying salvation from syphilis) and patented it; its generic name is arsphenamine.[15] After finding that it cured syphilis in rabbits, Erlich injected it intramuscularly into men with syphilis.

At first, Salvarsan seemed to work wonders, and during 1910, physicians greeted Erlich with standing ovations. Later, however, syphilis recurred in some patients treated with Salvarsan, and some of them died, both from syphilis and worse, from Salvarsan. Erlich maintained that the drug had not been given correctly, but he also developed another, less toxic form, Neosalvarsan.

Physicians injected Neosalvarsan intramuscularly in 20 to 40 dosages over a year, charging patients a dollar a visit. To get full treatment, patients needed both the time and money for these visits. As most did not, it was no one-shot, magic bullet for syphilis.

Between 1890 and 1910, Norwegian Caesar Boeck studied the natural course of untreated syphilis in 1,978 subjects. He believed that heavy metals removed only the symptoms of syphilis. Because heavy metals killed some syphilitics, he studied whether they might do better untreated.

In 1929, Boeck's successor, J. E. Bruusgaard, selected 473 of Boeck's subjects for further evaluation.[16] Bruusgaard learned that of subjects who had had syphilis for more than 20 years, 73 percent were asymptomatic. This discovery dramatically contradicted the Syphilophobia Campaign, so people resisted the fact that syphilis did not universally kill, much less did not do so rapidly. Even more disturbing to the Syphilophobia Campaign, Bruusgaard confirmed that some latent syphilitics might never develop symptoms at all.

So when the Tuskegee study began in 1932, Boeck's and Bruusgaard's studies had caused physicians to question the received views about the natural course of untreated syphilis, as well as the medical view that all syphilitics should be treated with heavy metals.

The Racial Environment

In the 1930s, American medicine was racist. Most physicians condescended to African-American patients and held stereotypes about them, as in this example from a 1914 *Journal of the American Medical Association*:

> The negro springs from a southern race, and as such his sexual appetite is strong; all of his environments stimulate this appetite, and as a general rule his emotional type of religion certainly does not decrease it.[17]

Physicians saw African-Americans as dirty, shiftless, promiscuous, and incapable of personal hygiene. In 1900, a Georgia physician wrote, "Virtue in the negro race is like 'angels' visits'—few and far between. In a practice of 16 years in the South, I have never examined a virgin over 14 years of age."[18] In 1919, a medical professor in Chicago wrote that African-American men were like bulls in *furor sexualis*, unable to resist copulation around females.[19]

Given such racism, white physicians around 1929 saw syphilis as a natural consequence of low character in African-Americans, described by one white physician as a "notoriously syphilis-soaked race."[20] Such physicians also assumed that African-American men would not seek treatment for venereal disease.

Historian Alan Brandt argues that in the early 1900s, almost all white American physicians were racists and most remained so throughout the decades of the Tuskegee study. Brandt writes, "There can be little doubt that the Tuskegee researchers regarded their subjects as less than human."[21]

DEVELOPMENT OF THE TUSKEGEE STUDY

A Study in Nature Begins

Physiologist Claude Bernard in 1865 distinguished *studies in nature* from normal *experiments* by saying that in experiments, some factor is manipulated, whereas studies in nature merely observe what would have happened anyway. In centuries before the Tuskegee study, physicians sough to understand the natural history of diseases and in doing so, they relied on studies in nature.

The great physician William Osler once said, "Know syphilis in all its manifestations and relations, and all other things clinical will be added unto you."[22] Yet as late as 1932, syphilis's natural history had not been documented, and because of Boeck's and Brussgaard's results, physicians doubted the inexorability of its course.

This explains why the United States Public Health Service (USPHS) in 1929 believed that a study in the nature of syphilis was needed. A second factor was that USPHS discovered an opportunity for such a study. Around 1929, several counties in America had extraordinary rates of syphilis and a philanthropical organization—the Julius Rosenwald Foundation in Philadelphia—started a project to eradicate it. With help from USPHS, the foundation intended to treat with Neosalvarsan all syphilitics in six counties with rates of syphilis above 20 percent. In 1930, the Rosenwald foundation surveyed African-American men in Macon County, Alabama, which was 82 percent black, and found the highest rate of syphilis in the nation, 36 percent. The Rosenwald Foundation planned to treat these African-American syphilitics with

Neosalvarsan, and it did treat or partially treat some of these 3,694 syphilitics. Tuskegee is the chief town in Macon County.

Then something unforeseen happened: in 1929 the great Depression began. As it ground on, funds for philanthropy plummeted, and the Rosenwald Foundation pulled out of Tuskegee, hoping that USPHS would continue the treatment program. Funds available for public health also plummeted, and the USPHS saw its budget drop from $1 million to less than $60,000 in 1935.

In 1931, USPHS repeated the Rosenwald foundation's survey of syphilis in Macon County, testing 4,400 African-American residents, and then found a 22 percent rate of syphilis in men, as well as a dangerous 62 percent rate of congenital syphilis. Of great importance for the Tuskegee Study, this survey identified 399 African-American men who had had syphilis of several years' duration but who had never been treated.

It was the identification of these 399 untreated men in 1931 by the USPHS that created the opportunity for a study in nature of syphilis. The Surgeon General himself, Raymond Vonderlehr, suggested that these 399 men should be merely observed rather than treated. In 1936, he wrote in the *Journal of the American Medical Association* that the Tuskegee Study was "an unusual opportunity to study the untreated syphilitic patient from the beginning of the disease to the death of the infected person."[23] His decision was the key one that began the study.

Three points deserve emphasis here. First, the 399 subjects had *latent* syphilis, not infectious syphilis. During this stage, syphilis is largely noninfectious during sexual intercourse. Second, the 399 subjects were not divided into the typical experimental and control groups: they were all simply observed. There was, however, another group of natural controls, 200 age-matched African-American men living in Macon County who never had syphilis. Third, these men were perfect for a study in nature because they were *so vulnerable*; they were poor, illiterate, and tied to the land as tenant farmers. As such, unlike other people with syphilis over the next four decades, *they were unlikely to ever leave Macon County*. Partly because of this vulnerability, Vonderlehr implied, they presented an "unusual opportunity."

Vonderlehr had no sense that it might be wrong to use such vulnerable subjects in a life-long experiment. Perhaps he assumed, like many of his time, that people with syphilis got what they deserved, as some also assumed later about the first victims of AIDS.

The Middle Phase: Poor Design

No one physician oversaw this study. It lacked written protocols, and the subjects in the no-treatment group of 399 syphilitics were often mixed up with the 200 controls without syphilis. Record keeping in the Tuskegee Study was poor, records were often lost, and the names of the syphilitic subjects were often confused with the controls.

Researchers assumed that controls would remain uninfected, but in a county where one in three people had syphilis, many controls eventually contracted syphilis. So they were switched to the no-treatment group of syphilitics.

The study had gaps. Federal doctors visited in 1939 and then not again until 1948; seven years passed between visits in 1963 and 1970. Only Eunice Rivers, an African-American nurse permanently assigned to Macon County, held the shaky study together.

During the course of the research, many of the 399 syphilitic subjects, who were supposed to remain untreated, did get Neosalvarsan or penicillin outside Macon County. James Lucas, a CDC physician, said that "effective and undocumented treatment had been given to the vast majority of patients in the syphilitic group."[24] As a result, researchers could not know whether a subject observed really represented the consequences of untreated syphilis.

Even as a study in nature, the study proved nothing. Before it began, physicians knew that syphilitics had greater morbidity and mortality than nonsyphilitics, and from Bruusgaard's discovery, that not all men in the latent phase died of syphilis. The Tuskegee Study added nothing to that knowledge.

Spinal Taps

When physicians returned, they wanted to know, first, if they had a subject in the study group; and second, if so, how far his syphilis had progressed. To determine progression, they did spinal punctures on 271 of the 399 syphilitic subjects.

In doing spinal taps, they inserted a 10-inch needle between two vertebrae into the cerebrospinal fluid to withdraw a small amount of fluid. Because this is a delicate and uncomfortable process, subjects were warned to stay still, lest the needle swerve and puncture the fluid sac, causing infection and possible paralysis.

Some physicians then and now regard spinal taps as insignificant, justified by the need to prove a diagnosis. On the other hand, professionals who describe a spinal tap this way may be thinking about administering it rather than receiving it.

A spinal tap is not a minor procedure, like taking blood. Some patients experience side effects, such as being unable to stand for a week without a severe headache. One person in a million will become paralyzed or permanently comatose.[25]

Tapping someone involuntarily, without obtaining informed consent, is legally a battery. Researchers who need healthy volunteers for spinal taps offer as much as $1,000 for them. Even then, some people will not undergo a nontherapeutic tap for $5,000 or for any amount. That should tell us something.

Deception

To induce subjects to travel to town and undergo these painful taps, physicians offered a series of freebies: free transportation, free hot lunches, free medicine for any disease other than syphilis, and free burials. In return for these benefits, physicians did spinal taps and later, autopsies, to inspect for damage from syphilis.

But these freebies and the persuasion of Nurse Rivers failed to get all men to come to town for the "round-ups," so researchers resorted to deception. *Infamously, they told the black men that they had "bad blood" and that the spinal taps were treatment for their bad blood.* Researchers sent the subjects the following letter, under the imposing letterhead "Macon County Health Department," with the subheading "Alabama State Board of Health and U.S. Public Health Service Cooperating with Tuskegee Institute":

> Dear Sir:
>
> Some time ago you were given a thorough examination and since that time we hope you have gotten a great deal of treatment for bad blood. You will now be given your last chance to get a second examination. This examination is a very special one and after it is finished you will be given a special treatment if it is believed you are in a condition to stand it.[26]

The "special treatment" mentioned was the spinal tap to culture for neurosyphilis. The subjects were instructed to meet Nurse Rivers for transportation to "Tuskegee Institute Hospital for this free treatment." The letter closed, in capitals:

> REMEMBER THIS IS YOUR LAST CHANCE FOR SPECIAL FREE TREATMENT. BE SURE TO MEET THE NURSE.

To repeat, the researchers never treated the subjects for syphilis. *Although penicillin was developed around 1941–1943 and was widely available by 1948, the subjects in the Tuskegee study never received it, even during the 1960s or up to 1972.* In fact, during World War II, the researchers contacted the local draft board and prevented any eligible subject from being drafted, and hence from being treated for syphilis with penicillin by the armed services.

The First Investigations

In 1966, Peter Buxtun, a USPHS venereal disease investigator in San Francisco learned about the Tuskegee Study and criticized it. By this time, supervision of the study (and Buxtun) had moved to the newly created Centers for Disease Control (CDC) in Atlanta, but CDC stonewalled Buxtun and threatened to fire him.

By 1969, Buxtun's protests led to a meeting of a small group of physicians at CDC to consider stopping the Tuskegee Study or revealing it. At the end, the committee voted to continue the study and to keep it secret.

In 1970, a monograph on syphilis was published by the American Public Health Association. It stated that treatment for late benign syphilis should consist of "6.0 to 9.0 million units of benzathine penicillin G given 3.0 million units at sessions seven days apart."[27] The first author was William J. Brown, head of CDC's Tuskegee section from 1957 to 1971. Brown had been on the CDC committee in 1969 and had argued for continuing the study in which, of course, subjects with late benign syphilis received no penicillin.

The Story Breaks

In 1972, Peter Buxtun told his story to Jean Heller, a medical reporter for the Associated Press. Six months later, on July 26, 1972, her story began to appear on front pages of newspapers nationwide.[28] Her series of stories described a medical study run by the federal government in Tuskegee, Alabama, in which poor, uneducated African-American men had been used as guinea pigs. After noting the terrible effects of tertiary syphilis, the story said that in 1969 a CDC study of 276 of the untreated subjects had proved that at least seven subjects died "as a direct result of syphilis."

Heller's story had an immediate effect. Congressmen were amazed to learn of the study. Senator William Proxmire called it a "moral and ethical nightmare." J. D. Millar, chief of Venereal Disease Control at CDC, said that the study "was never clandestine," correctly pointing to 15 published articles in medical and scientific journals over a 30-year span.

The Aftermath

After Heller's story appeared, the Secretary of Health, Education, and Welfare terminated the Tuskegee Study. At that time, CDC estimated that during the study, 28 syphilitics had died of syphilis. The remaining syphilitic subjects then received penicillin.

In 1973, lawyer Fred Gray filed a class-action suit against the federal government on behalf of the Tuskegee subjects. In 1974, the U.S. Government settled out of court. According to the settlement, living syphilitics received $37,500 each; heirs of deceased syphilitics, $15,000 (since children might have had congenital syphilis); heirs of living controls, $16,000; heirs of deceased controls, $5,000. Controls and their descendants received compensation because they and their families had been deprived of antibiotics during the decades of the study. The government also provided free lifetime medical care for Tuskegee subjects, their wives, and their children.

In 1972, and as a direct revelation of the study, the federal government required all institutions that conduct human medical experimentation and receive federal funds to have Institutional Review Boards (IRBs). Today, IRBs must scrutinize written proposals and are the first line of defense against abuses in medical research.

In 1988, 21 of the original 399 syphilitic subjects were still alive, each of whom had had syphilis for at least 62 years.[29] In addition, 41 wives and 19 children had evidence of syphilis and were receiving free medical care.

In 1997, President Clinton met four of the eight living survivors to apologize for the Tuskegee Study, "What the United States did was shameful, and I am sorry."[30] The youngest survivor then was 87, the oldest between 100 and 109.[31] By then, the government had paid $10 million to the study's original 600 members or to their families or heirs, who by then numbered more than 6,000. Because of lack of treatment for syphilis of men in the study, any of these other people might have contracted syphilis.[32]

Perhaps the most pervasive effect of revelation of the study was that African-Americans came to distrust medical experiments, a legacy that medical researchers today must struggle to overcome.

ETHICAL ISSUES

Informed Consent and Deception

In the Tuskegee Study, the subjects did not know they were part of a government study lasting throughout their lives, did not even know what syphilis was, and did not know that they weren't being treated with available drugs. In other words, they had no informed consent, which many critics considered to be ethically outrageous.

R. H. Kampmeier, an emeritus professor of medicine at Vanderbilt Medical School, worked as a syphilologist during the decades of the Study.[33] He argued that a study undertaken in the 1930s could not be faulted for lack of informed consent, which began only after 1966. Would it make sense, he argued, to judge Pasteur unethical because he, too, did not get consent?

Kampmeier cites another landmark study by USPHS in 1943 that examined giving penicillin to 35,000 syphilitics; it did not get consent from subjects. He claims that during the 1930s and 1940s, it was accepted practice for physicians to walk into a patient's room and simply announce they were taking out the patient's gallbladder.

Medical historian and physician Thomas Benedek dismisses the issue of informed consent in the Tuskegee Study as "anachronistic." He agrees that USPHS did not require informed consent until 1966.[34]

While it is true that informed consent in medical experiments was not mandated by court decisions until 1966, the presumption had always been that physicians would "First, do no harm" to their patients. Not obtaining consent for procedures that might benefit subjects differs from procedures that might *harm* subjects.

Finally, and granted that telling patients the truth was not *legally* required before 1966, was it *ethical* for the Tuskegee researchers to lie to their subjects for all those decades? Isn't the truth what one person owes another, especially as doctor and patient?

Racism

The Tuskegee Study took place in Alabama in the deep South and all its subjects were African-American. Under such circumstances, was it only a coincidence that no subjects were white? Would white subjects have been deceived and left untreated the same way?

In his classic work, *Bad Blood*, medical historian James Jones saw the Tuskegee study as a result of pervasive racism in American medicine during the 1930s. How bad was that? To take one example, black students at Tuskegee Institute in the 1930s lived in fear of rural white toughs just outside their campus.

Although studies in nature were important in medicine during the early 1930s, there was no reason why a study in nature of syphilis should use only African-American subjects. On the contrary: some physicians believed then that syphilis ran a different course in different races, and this implied the need for a parallel study of untreated white syphilitics. That no parallel study of white subjects occurred shows that poor black subjects were regarded as expendable.

Media Coverage

In defending the Tuskegee study, Kampmeier objected to the "great hue and cry" in the media in 1972, and to journalists' claim that "treatment was purposefully withheld to evaluate the course of untreated disease." He said about *Time* and *American Medical News*: "In complete disregard of their abysmal ignorance, members of the fourth estate bang out anything on their typewriters that will make headlines."[35]

To begin with the second objection, Kampmeier attacked the media for reporting the damaging aspects of the study, such as the withholding of treatment; but withholding treatment was precisely the intention of the study. The media reported the study accurately.

With regard to the first objection, Kampmeier's description of a "hue and cry" was exaggerated. Indeed, the media botched the story. Coverage shrank within days, and the story moved to the back pages of newspapers, where only short paragraphs followed it.

Yet the Tuskegee Study deserved more attention. True, its issues were complicated and they involved racism at a time when racial turmoil upset Americans. Yet today such a story would receive weeks of nationwide scrutiny, and probably get a Congressional hearing on television.

The relation then between medicine and the media can also be questioned. Before Heller's story broke, the Tuskegee Study had been reported repeatedly in medical journals in at least 17 articles between 1936 and 1972. Researchers did not conceal the study within medicine. Despite this, no professional publication, physician, or editor alerted the nation to the story.

Between 1966 and 1971, one African-American professional at CDC did mail boxes of documents about the study to several national newspapers and magazines.[36] Nothing happened. Why is that?

The answer is important to understanding many issues in medical ethics and to whistle-blowing about corruption. Print and television reporters need an expert to help them understand such complex stories and, equally important, to take responsibility for claims about wrongdoing. Virtually no reporters then or now have the medical background to understand such complicated stories and, without that, cannot risk charging physicians with possible crimes.

A natural tendency also exists to want *someone* else to be the whistle-blower and to bear the brunt of the kind of retaliation that CDC threatened against Peter Buxtun. As a result, merely mailing information or passing it along conversationally is usually not enough for reporters to publicize wrongdoing.

Harm to Subjects

Kampmeier argued that if the Tuskegee Study had never occurred, its subjects would have received no treatment and would have been no worse off. Such a claim can never be proved. If the Tuskegee Study had not occurred, many things might have happened. Another charity might have provided Neosalvarsan. A writer like John Steinbeck might have soon written a novel about syphilis in Macon County, arousing national concern and getting penicillin to people there infected with syphilis.

Withholding Treatment

What harm, if any, resulted to subjects with syphilis from nontreatment? This question might seem even absurd: if subjects were left untreated, of course they must have been harmed! However, the issue is not that simple.

In 1931, penicillin was unavailable, so physicians withheld Neosalvarsan from subjects. Because Neosalvarsan was expensive and cumbersome to administer, even if this study had not occurred, subjects might not have received it. Boeck and Bruusgaard had also undermined claims about the benefits of heavy metals, so harm is difficult to prove. In a review of medical evidence available in 1940, medical historian Benedek concluded that in 1937, untreated syphilitics actually lived longer and better than those partially treated with heavy metals.[37]

Not everyone agrees. UAB professor of internal medicine, Benjamin Friedman, whose career spanned the decades of this study, countered that:

> In the 1940s it was known that patients receiving as few as 20 injections of arsenicals rarely developed symptomatic aortic disease. Since we could not determine in advance which of the latent syphilitics would, after 20 or 30 years, develop symptomatic aortic disease, it was necessary to treat all of them. One cannot maintain that some small number of syphilitics deprived of treatment did not therefore suffer injury.[38]

By 1934 the major professional organization of physicians treating syphilis, the Cooperating Clinical Group, had demonstrated that use of heavy metals improved Bruusgaard's statistics and had recommended that all syphilitics get Neosalvarsan, mercury, and bismuth.[39] Even if many patients could not afford such therapy or complete it, they should have been told about it.

Later during the study, penicillin became available. Although Alexander Fleming discovered penicillin in 1929, his discovery was not appreciated until 1941. Penicillin became available only around 1946, as a result of wartime production and to treat soldiers with syphilis. By 1948, any American could get it.[40]

Kampmeier argued, first, that withholding penicillin in 1946 did not harm subjects. Latent syphilis, he said, is a "chronic, granulomatous, self-limiting disease" and not fatal. Second, proof of penicillin's effectiveness did not come until 1948 and then only for primary syphilis. So third, the Tuskegee subjects by 1948 could no longer have been helped by penicillin; the damage to them from syphilis had already been done.[41]

Benedek disagreed somewhat with Kampmeier. He concluded that giving penicillin to latent syphilitics in 1948 "might have exerted a definitely beneficial effect on the prognosis of only 12.5 percent of the subjects."[42] Still, that would have been 50 subjects who could have been helped.

Effects on Subjects' Families

Virtually all subjects were or had been married and had an average of 5.2 children.[43] Recall that Macon County had a rate of congenital syphilis of 62 percent.

When we consider the subjects' families, wouldn't the men in the study want to know they had syphilis? Even in the latent stage, wouldn't they want to know they could become infectious again? Did the researchers withhold the truth because they thought these men couldn't refrain from sex?

These researchers subjected women and children in Macon County to harm. Either the researchers discounted this harm, or thought it didn't matter compared to their study in nature.

Kant and Motives of Researchers

When physicians at CDC and USPHS debated the Tuskegee Study in 1969, many assumed that if no harm could be proved, nothing unethical had been done. This is also Kampmeier's unstated assumption. Focusing on consequences, however, is only one way to judge morality. We can also adopt, not a consequentialism or utilitarianism, but a Kantian ethics focused on motives and the character of researchers.

Although we cannot prove that Tuskegee subjects were harmed by being left untreated, it may have been only good luck that the study caused no more harm than it did. Why is that?

Because the historical evidence cuts both ways. We cannot use differing historical standards at differing times to excuse lack of informed consent, but not pay attention to what else was believed at the time. Let us put ourselves in the minds of researchers in the late 1940s, *and the crucial fact is, that when penicillin became available, most physicians then believed that penicillin would help latent syphilitics.*

So they believed that subjects would be harmed by not getting penicillin. For all anyone knew in 1948, penicillin could have helped patients with aortic heart disease or would have prevented it.

So in terms of Kantian ethics, the researchers deliberately willed harm on these subjects. They used them as "mere means," as guinea pigs, and could not universalize such behavior as a maxim for all physicians or all people to act on. Not only did they lack what Kant calls a "good will," they had an ill will toward their vulnerable subjects.

It is no good appealing to sophisticated knowledge that came later that the damage from syphilis had already occurred. That was not known then. At the time, researchers must have known they were depriving syphilitics of something likely to help them, or depriving them of something that could help them not pass syphilis on to their female partners. But out of a desire to see the final ravages of syphilis, subjects were not told, and harm was intentionally allowed to occur.

Tuskegee and HIV Prevention in Africa

In 1994, the federally sponsored 076 study proved that giving AZT (zidovudine) during pregnancy cut by two-thirds the risk of transmission of HIV from mother to child.[44] CDC, NIH, and WHO then set out to prevent the 1,600 babies born with HIV every day to HIV-infected mothers in developing countries.

In 1997, Marcia Angell, executive editor of the *New England Journal of Medicine*, claimed that American research in Africa to study AZT resembled the Tuskegee Study because half of pregnant, HIV-infected black women were given placebos. Researchers permitted many babies in their care to be born with preventable HIV infection.[45]

So this study had subjects who were (1) black, (2) female, (3) poor, (4) illiterate, (5) victims of sexually transmitted diseases, and (6) without other available treatment. Like the Tuskegee Study, research was conducted by magisterial but distant governmental agencies. Like the Tuskegee Study, subjects were about as vulnerable as subjects can get, and hence, powerless to reject the study or to go elsewhere. Columnist Ellen Goodman noted that the Tuskegee Study had not ended, but had been merely exported.[46] Public Citizen, a consumer rights organization founded by Ralph Nader and its physicians Sidney Wolfe and Peter Lurie, echoed her charges.[47]

Dr. Angell's comparison of these studies to the Tuskegee Study sparked a firestorm of rebuttals. Researchers retorted that, if the research had not been done, these infected mothers would never have gotten AZT. So the women were no worse off than they had been before.

Angell replied that it had long been established that placebo-controlled studies could not be done on American women. Once AZT had been proven effective in preventing transmission of HIV, it became *the standard of care* for all pregnant, HIV+ women. Angell argued, "If it is unethical to do placebo-controlled trials in America, it should also be unethical to do them in third-world countries."[48]

Apologists for the study, including officials in developing countries, replied that it was ethical imperialism to impose American ethical standards on African countries.[49] Moreover, many local officials were black and had lost children to HIV, so they were not like the white USPHS physicians of the Tuskegee Study.[50]

The sponsoring agencies replied that 300,000 children were infected every year with HIV by perinatal transmission, and that if they could prove—via a placebo-controlled trial—that a shorter regimen could reduce transmission by half—they could save 150,000 thousand children a year. If skeptics such as Angell caused delays of proof, they would cost many children their lives.

Central to the defense of these studies by public health agencies were two more claims: a placebo-controlled trial of HIV-transmission could be done faster and with fewer subjects than an AZT-controlled study, and that once good results were obtained, African and Asian governments would give all pregnant, HIV+ women the new, smaller dosage of AZT.

Researchers also defended themselves procedurally, arguing that review committees in both countries had approved the studies and that, unlike the Alabama men, the women themselves had consented. Subsequent interviews by the *New York Times* cast doubt on how much the women understood, a claim disputed by local health officials in Africa, who said the women had understood.

Angell argued that placebo-controlled studies were not necessary to prove such results, that comparing dosages of AZT to other treatments could prove the same thing. She denied that, given the poverty of such countries, a proven, reduced dosage would later be given to all pregnant women. Even a cheap AZT regimen of $80 exceeded by 11 times the amount spent per year on average on medical care for such African women.

Both sides invoked justice.[51] Here, philosophical medical ethics collided, not factual medicine. Philosophically, on one side resided Jeremy Bentham, utilitarianism, and public health ethics. On the other side resided Immanuel Kant, his axiom that people can never be used as a "mere means," and his belief that ethical principles are not local but universal.

For researchers, the risk-benefit ratio had to be different for poor, illiterate women in backward countries who otherwise would not have gotten treatment. For critics, the same reasoning had led to the Tuskegee Study and to Nazi experiments: "they're going to get it anyway, so we might as well study them to learn something."[52] As Angell retorted, "People can't be used as a means to a noble end.[53]

In 1998, CDC suspended the studies, announcing that the experimental, reduced-dosage treatment had been proven effective in reducing mother-to-child HIV transmission: $80 worth of AZT in the last four weeks of pregnancy cut transmission in half.[54] At this early cessation of the American-sponsored studies, both sides claimed victory.

Meanwhile many thousands of subjects in third-world countries continued to be subjects of HIV-vaccination studies, many of which were placebo-controlled.

Secret Governmental Medical Experiments

During the 1940s, radiation enthralled some physicians. Joseph Hamilton of the University of California at Berkeley injected plutonium into 18 unsuspecting patients diagnosed with cancer. According to Kenneth Scott, a scientist who later investigated these abuses, two patients were mistakenly diagnosed with cancer but nevertheless given "many times the lethal dose of plutonium."[55]

Physicians also studied radioactive isotopes used in diagnosis and research. In the late 1940s at Vanderbilt University, physicians injected 819 pregnant women with radioactive iron in a nutritional study. A study in 1960 found that three of their children died of rare forms of cancer.[56] In 1945, Eda Charlton entered Strong Memorial Hospital in Rochester, New York, with a mild case of hepatitis, and was secretly injected with plutonium-239 to study how her body eliminates radiation. Physicians there secretly followed her for years to observe the effects (she died of a heart attack in 1983).

From World War II to the mid-1970s, physician-researchers subjected over 16,000 American patients to radiation experiments.[57] At least 435 experiments were conducted by the Department of Energy or its predecessors in 21 states. From the 1940s to the 1960s, physicians exposed 1,500 military aviators and submarine crewmen to encapsulated radium on the end of wires inserted high into their nostrils for several minutes.[58] In another experiment, 130 male prisoners were paid $200 to undergo x-ray radiation of their testicles; afterwards, these men got vasectomies. In another, an indigent 36-year-old Texan was given a shot of plutonium in an injured leg, which was then amputated.

In 1995, the President's Committee on Human Radiation Experiments investigated these experiments and concluded that the government should apologize to those who were involuntary subjects of the tests and should compensate people who had been injured.[59]

In 1991 in Operation Dessert Storm, military personnel were forced to take antibiological warfare, experimental vaccines. Federal law stated that soldiers could not refuse such vaccinations under operational conditions. Subsequently, many soldiers became sick. For years afterwards, the Pentagon and Department of Defense denied that their sickness was service-related. Yet the military's own records showed many causes of such sickness, especially all acting in combination: such as sand storms, biological weapons, oil fires, contaminated water, rare microorganisms, the above vaccines, chemical vapors from bombed Iraqi storage ages, unspent rocket fuel, and high levels of stress.[60]

The above cases show a pattern where physicians in the armed services subjected people to experimental risks. In such cases, service men and women can be ordered to take such risks by superiors who are both physicians and higher-ranking officers.

The Krieger Lead Paint Study

In 2001, the federal Office of Protection from Research Risks (OPRR) halted all federally funded research at Johns Hopkins Medical School after Ellen Roche died in a study of a drug to prevent asthma. When she volunteered for the study, Ellen was healthy; soon, she was dead.

After its research was halted, a physician from Hopkins on television denounced suspension of Hopkins' research monies, claiming Hopkins had only killed one person in many decades of medical research and that lives would be lost from such a suspension because of delayed cures.

Normally, when a hospital kills someone, its spokesperson should go on television to say it's sorry, not to complain about being disciplined. So in this case, lack of remorse motivated reporters to dig further, and they uncovered interesting details about the workings of Hopkins' IRB and the Krieger case.

The Krieger case was a study by a branch of Johns Hopkins Medical School that examined retardation in children from lead paint, and which six of seven judges on Maryland's highest court likened to the Tuskegee Study.[61] The study, conducted in the mid-1990s by Hopkins's Kennedy Krieger Institute, recruited 108 poor, black families to live in East Baltimore in houses with lead paint.

Ingesting lead-based paint is a known cause of mental retardation in small children. According to the Krieger Institute, the study sought cheaper ways to reduce lead contamination in houses, so landlords in East Baltimore would not abandon them.

Did the parents understand the nature of the study? Did they understand the risk to their children by living in these houses? "It can be argued that the researchers intended that the children be the canaries in the mines but never clearly told the parents," one critic said.[62] Moreover,

> Maryland Court of Appeals Judge Dale R. Cathell, who wrote last week's scathing opinion, said the board [had] instructed Kennedy Krieger researchers to write consent forms for study participants that skirted federal regulations requiring disclosure about risks.
>
> The Court of Appeals ruling ordered trials to be held in lawsuits filed against Kennedy Krieger by two women, Viola Hughes and Catina Higgins, whose children were involved in the study. Hughes's daughter now suffers from learning disabilities and cognitive impairments, both of which are often associated with lead poisoning. . . . Higgins says researchers withheld tests results from her that showed high levels of lead contamination.

Kennedy Krieger is a major institution in the study of lead paint abatement. Marc Farfel, who conducted the study, said today that it identified more effective ways to remove lead hazards and prompted legislation forcing landlords to remove those hazards.[63]

Amazingly, an investigation by OPRR revealed that the IRB at Johns Hopkins, which supposedly had reviewed and discussed the ethics of the Krieger Study and all other research at the medical school, had rarely met face-to-face.

The Krieger Study resembled the Tuskegee Study in that poor black people were deliberately recruited to a study where physicians foresaw harm to subjects. Researchers rationalized the harm by saying that if the study had not occurred, the subjects would have lived in such housing. Revelation of the Krieger Study further damaged already bad relations between Baltimore African-Americans and Hopkins.

The Death of Jesse Gelsinger

In 1999, the death of teenager Jesse Gelsinger from gene therapy, like revelations of the Tuskegee Study or Gennarelli's head-injuries on baboons, changed regulation of American medical research.

In 1999 in Tucson, Arizona, 17-year-old Jesse Gelsinger worked as clerk and rode a motorcycle on weekends. He heard about experimental gene therapy at the University of Pennsylvania for his inherited disorder, ornithine transcarbamylase deficiency (OTC).

In the genetic disease OTC, the liver doesn't properly cleanse blood of ammonia (produced in normal metabolism) resulting in toxic levels. Many OTC newborns die around birth; half don't live to age five. A new regimen of drugs and diet enabled Jesse to live to be a teenager, but without a cure, he would eventually die.

Jesse entered the study as a healthy research volunteer. A friend said he "wanted to prove he was a man."[64] Penn researchers claim Jesse was informed that the experiment wouldn't help him, and told him that it might help OTC babies. His father said Jesse wanted "to help save lives."

But why weren't studies done on dying OTC patients? Answer: Because OTC babies are born dying, their parents are so desperate they will consent to anything, no matter how dangerous the experiment.

So Penn researcher James Wilson sought adults with OTC whose livers were still functioning. He wanted to inject into them an adenovirus that contained copies of the gene lacking in OTC patients. Adenoviruses are quite common and can transmit genes to patients with genetic diseases.

What actually happened when Dr. Wilson injected his adenovirus into Jesse is quite grim:

> Four days after scientists infused trillions of genetically engineered viruses into Jesse Gelsinger's liver . . . the 18-year-old lay dying in a hospital bed at the University of Pennsylvania. His liver had failed, and the teenager's blood was thickening like jelly and clogging key vessels while his kidneys, brain, and other organs shut down.[65]

The wrongful death lawsuit claimed that Wilson knew the virus had injured other OTC adults and that Wilson failed to use simple, direct language to explain this dangerous study to the Gelsingers. As Penn bioethicist Arthur Caplan said,

> Not only is it sad that Jesse Gelsinger died, there was never a chance that anybody would benefit from these treatments. They are safety studies. They are not therapeutic in goal. If I gave it to you, we would try to see if you died, too, and if you did, OK.
>
> If you cured anybody, you'd publish it in a religious journal. It would be a miracle. All you're doing is you're saying, I've got this vector. I want to see if it can deliver the gene where I want it to go without killing or hurting or having any side effects.[66]

Doctor Wilson also had a financial conflict of interest from his biotech company, Genovo, which owned a patent on the adenovirus, should it prove therapeutic. Biogen, Inc. had paid Genovo $37 million for rights to market its genetic therapies.

Wilson denies that money influenced his decisions. He claims his main desire was to be the first to cure a genetic disease.[67]

Wilson reported to the FDA only 39 of 700 problems about the virus, although the law required reporting all of them. In 2000, researchers concluded that adenoviruses should only be used as a last resort, not on healthy volunteers. They curtailed gene therapy until it could be proved safe.

After an investigation of Wilson's research, the NIH in 2000 suspended medical research at Penn. After a Congressional hearing into Jesse's death, the NIH vowed to better monitor medical research. As a result, it suspended medical research at the University of Colorado Medical Center, the University of North Carolina, Johns Hopkins Hospitals, and the University of Alabama at Birmingham. The Gelsinger family settled out of court with Penn for undisclosed monies. After improving their regulation of medical research and conflicts of interest, these medical centers regained their grants, although Wilson's protocols were stopped.

Financial Conflicts and 21st Century Research

The Bayh-Dole Act of 1980 erased an ethical bright line between academic and corporate medicine and allowed universities and their researchers to patent and reap royalties together. Since then, scandals keep recurring in medical research about money.

Twenty-five years later, pharmaceutical companies fund most research into drugs and devices at universities; they do not fund independent peer review of their new drugs and do not publicize bad results. By indirectly paying physicians to test new drugs and by financially encouraging physicians to recruit patients for experiments, drug companies cause physicians to choose their drug and not the best drug for their patients.

In 1998, a study by the Department of Health and Human Services concluded that IRBs could no longer handle the job of protecting subjects from abuses in medical experimentation.[68] It found that IRBs were underfunded, overworked, and that the volume of work expected of volunteers could not be accurately and conscientiously performed. Another study in 2002 by the Institute of Medicine reached similar conclusions.[69] Since then, several medical research centers improved their structures for reviewing research, although financial conflicts continue.

Several scandals erupted in the 1990s wherein a few physicians appeared to have taken millions of dollars from drug companies for dubious research.[70] Some doctors in Georgia allegedly made $4 million over seven years from aggressively soliciting people with schizophrenia for drug trials; they made another $6 million over the same period from testing other drugs.[71]

Some physicians who worked for drug companies made an extra $100,000 a year flying around the country to give talks to physicians to promote a drug for a pharmaceutical company.

Today, all medical journals continue to take expensive ads from drug companies and almost all medical practices allow drug representatives to buy them and their staffs expensive daily lunches or dinners. Drug companies give these gifts because they work. In many states, drug companies can monitor how much of their drugs are prescribed each month by a particular physician and adjust their gifts accordingly. Learning to take free stuff from drug companies begins in medical school, when students learn to expect free food at lunch paid for by drug companies. Everyone ignores the corrupting influence of taking these gifts on their later decisions about prescribing drugs to patients.

FURTHER READING AND RESOURCES

Thomas Benedek, "The 'Tuskegee Study' of Untreated Syphilis: Analysis of Moral Aspects versus Methodological Aspects," *Journal of Chronic Diseases*, vol. 31, 1978.

Alexee Deep, "Placebo-Controlled Zidovine Trials in the Developing World," *Princeton Journal of Bioethics*, vol. 1, no. 2, Fall, 1998, pp. 21–39.

James Jones, *Bad Blood*, Free Press, New York, 1981.

CHAPTER 12

Surgeons' Desire for Fame: The Ethics of Heart, Hand, and Face Transplants and Separating Conjoined Twins

The desire for fame motivates many surgeons. To not only be brilliant but to be so in a way that benefits humanity is to achieve accolades and prizes. But the ethical cost of this desire is high. For most breakthroughs, many patients suffered, usually without understanding what lay ahead of them.

This chapter describes Christiaan Barnard's first heart transplant, William DeVries's implantation of an artificial heart, Jean-Michel Dubernard's first hand and, later, first face transplant, and the separation by surgeons such as Ben Carson of Johns Hopkins of conjoined twins. It also discusses the dismal history before cyclosporin of organ transplants, the sad history of artificial hearts, and for patients, quality of life, costs, prevention, and selection. The overarching prism of the chapter is the cost and benefits to patients of surgeons' desire for fame.

THE FIRST HEART TRANSPLANT

When he performed the first heart transplant on December 3, 1967, Christiaan Barnard was 44. He had grown up poor in South Africa and attended medical school there.

Barnard trained between 1955 and 1957 under surgeon Owen Wangansteen in Minneapolis-St. Paul. When Barnard returned to South Africa in 1967, Wangansteen gave him a heart-lung machine. Did Wangansteen expect Barnard to transplant a heart? Transplant surgeon Thomas Starzl says that everyone expected Barnard to transplant kidneys, not hearts.[1] Until surgeons overcame the problem of immune rejection of the foreign heart, no one expected a heart to be transplanted.

After researching heart transplantation in animals for a decade, Stanford University's Norman Shumway announced on November 20, 1967 that he was now ready to transplant the first human heart and awaited a suitable candidate and donor.[2] Two weeks later, the unknown surgeon Barnard would best him for this first.

In Cape Town, Barnard had secretly decided to try to transplant a human heart. He yearned for international fame. With his physician-brother Marius, he quietly assembled a team at Groote Schuur to perform the first heart transplant.

In 1967, Louis Washkansky was about as sick as a cardiac patient can be and still live. He had diabetes, coronary artery disease, and congestive heart failure; his flabby heart extended across the inside of his large chest, from wall to wall.

Washkansky, a.k.a. "Washy," as a young man had been a weightlifter and amateur boxer. A big, intelligent man with a ferocious desire to live, he had an exuberant, macho personality and liked to flirt with nurses.

Knowing that death approached and that his last two years had been hellish, when approached about the transplant, Washy did not hesitate. Barnard told his patient, "We can put a normal heart into you, after taking out your heart that's no longer good, and there's a chance you can get back to normal life." To that, Louis replied, "So they told me. So I'm ready to go ahead."

After obtaining Washy's permission to seek a heart to transplant, Barnard waited three weeks for a donor. Meanwhile, Washy developed fulminant pulmonary edema—a sign of imminent death—and Barnard feared his chance would pass.

On December 2, 1967, as she walked with her mother to a bakery a half mile below Groote Schuur Hospital, a speeding car smashed into 25-year-old Denise Ann Darvall. The accident injured her head, and a few minutes later, an ambulance took her up to the hospital's emergency room. By coincidence, at this moment Ann Washkansky was driving up the mountain to visit her husband when she saw a crowd gathered around an automobile accident.

Shortly after Denise's arrival, Barnard spoke to Edward Darvall, who had just learned of the death of his daughter. "We have a man in the hospital here, and we can save his life if you give us permission to use your daughter's heart. . . ." Edward replied simply and trustingly, "If you can't save my daughter, try and save this man."

Barnard summoned his transplant team. As the story is told, the car of one physician broke down, but he ran up the mountain to the hospital, arriving breathless and in pajamas. The operation took place during the early hours of December 3, 1967.

Denise Darvall was declared dead after her heart had stopped beating; surgeons then opened her body, preparing it for Barnard's excision. In an adjacent room, surgeons gave Washkansky drugs to produce paralysis and prevent spontaneous breathing, and placed him on the heart-lung machine.

At this point, everything almost failed. Washkansky's femoral artery, where a tube was attached, had been narrowed by buildup of cholesterol and the machine couldn't force blood into his heart. The pressure on the tube climbed to 290, just below the point where the lines would blow, spilling liters of blood over the room. Frantically, Barnard and other surgeons reattached the line directly to Washkansky's aorta, and gradually the pressure dropped.

Barnard then walked to the next room and excised Denise Darvall's heart, leaving part of the wall attached to it like the lid of a jack-o-lantern. He put her heart into a basin of chilled fluid and walked 31 steps back to Washkansky's operating room, where he gave it to a nurse to hold. Barnard then cut out Washkansky's flabby heart. Peering down into Washkansky's empty chest cavity, he said, "This really is the point of no return."[3]

He next sewed Denise Darvall's heart with its attached wall into Washkansky's chest, where it looked small. After some false starts, the new heart started to beat. After working all night, the surgeons finished the operation at 7 A.M. on December 3rd. An hour later, Washy regained consciousness and tried to talk. Thirty-six hours later, he ate a soft-boiled egg.

He then had five rough days, when his urine output, enzymes, and heart rate were problematic. Also worried about immunological rejection of the heart, Barnard's team flooded Washkansky with gamma ray radiation and administered prednisone and azathioprine, but Louis didn't tolerate them well. By day five, he said, the constant tests were "killing me. I can't sleep. I can't do anything. They're at me all the time with pins and needles. It's driving me crazy."[4]

On the sixth day, Louis received steroids to prevent rejection, and this began five good days when he laughed, visited with his family, and wanted to go home. At this time, Barnard told a press conference that if his patient's progress held, he would "have him home in three weeks."[5]

In retrospect, these five days were the eye of the hurricane: soon Washkansky's body would reject the new heart. As this rejection process started, he began to feel, as he said, "terrible" and he suffered from constant pain in the shoulders; dark circles formed under his eyes; his heart and breathing rates climbed; on the 13th day, a shadow of unknown origin could be seen on his lung x-ray. Moreover, his personality changed. This vibrant, forceful man became sullen and irritable.

In addition to the threat of rejection, dangers of infection loomed. At the time, most post-transplant symptoms could indicate either rejection or infection, and treatment of one problem could exacerbate the other. So Barnard waited for a definitive diagnosis, even if waiting risked his patient's death.

By the 14th day, Washkansky felt he was dying. He couldn't eat. He lost bowel control. He had such severe pain in his chest that he preferred to lie in his own feces than try to move. Barnard said that he was "constrained" to insert a nasogastric tube to feed his patient, but Washkansky didn't want it. To him, it didn't look as though he would ever be normal again; he had lost his dignity and hence his will to live.

On day 15, mottled patches appeared on Washkansky's legs, indicating circulatory failure. He breathed with difficulty, and X-rays showed ominous patches on his lungs. As he gasped for breath, Barnard decided to place him on a respirator. Washkansky resisted. He had been on the respirator when he first woke up after the operation, and he knew that reconnecting it meant giving up speech. He also felt that he was near death.

Barnard disagreed; on December 18, he told Washkansky that there was "a chance" to be home by Christmas. Washkansky replied, "No, not now." His bed was in a sterile tent, and despite his extreme weakness, he grabbed its sides to prevent Barnard from entering to reopen his tracheotomy hole.

As Barnard entered, Washkansky persisted, saying, "No, Doc."

Barnard replied, "Yes, Louis," and put him on the respirator.[6] Washkansky never spoke again. Such is the way of surgeons who, when they want to achieve a breakthrough, push patients.

On December 19, new X-rays now showed that bilateral pneumonia—klebsiella and pseudomonas—had infiltrated Washkansky's lungs. Earlier treatment with penicillin had killed one organism but allowed others to grow. Immune suppressants had also allowed all these organisms to flourish.

On December 20, 17 days after the operation, Washy received 40 percent oxygen; then, as his breathing worsened, 100 percent. By day 18, infection overran his lungs and he began to suffocate.

After two hours of Washkansky's dying gasps, the transplanted heart went into wild fibrillation from lack of oxygen and stopped beating. Even then, Barnard would not give up; he rushed a team together to put him on a heart-lung machine. At this point, his brother Marius argued passionately that it was "madness" to continue because Washkansky was "clinically lost." Reluctantly, Barnard agreed. On December 21, after having lived 18 days with a transplanted heart, Louis Washkansky died.

The next morning, Barnard watched the postmortem, which showed that lobar pneumonia had destroyed the lungs (so the heart-lung machine would have been useless). The heart and Barnard's surgery were perfect.

Barnard went on to transplant Phillip Blaiberg, who lived several months. Considered a real success, Blaiberg walked out of the hospital on his own, the minimal criterion for most surgeons later of any quality of life at all.

Fame Cometh

Perhaps no physician before or after would ever get the kind of saturation coverage by television, magazines, and newspapers that Barnard now got. Long before "superstar" was coined, Christiaan Barnard was one. When he divorced his first wife after 20 years of marriage, she told reporters, "He was more famous than the Beatles and he loved it."[7]

In 1968, Christiaan Barnard may have been the most famous person in the world. His handsome face smiled from the cover of *Time* magazine, he appeared on television in England, and American President Lyndon Johnson entertained him.

He looked younger than his age, was tall, in good physical shape, witty, worldly, ambitious, and lusty. In his two autobiographies, he admits that fame went to his head and brags about bedding beautiful women, including the actress Gina Lollobrigida. He admits that all this ruined his first, second, and third marriages.[8]

After a decade, he developed crippling arthritis and could no longer operate. In 1984, he took $4 million for saying in ads that a facial cream named Glygel reverses aging in skin (it doesn't), for which dermatologists derided him. In 2001 Barnard died of an asthma attack, alone at age 78, at a swimming pool on vacation in Malta, still a famous person.

Barnard's fame influenced surgeons far more than his surgery. For the first time, hordes of journalists followed a physician around like a movie star! Beautiful women seduced him and everyone wanted to be seen with him.

In Plato's *Republic*, Socrates relates the story of the Ring of Gyges, a ring which made its wearer invisible (like the modern film *Hollow Man*). When Gyges found it, he killed the king, married his beautiful wife, and became king himself.

The moral of Socrates's story is that when luck gives a person the opportunity to do anything he wants, that person's true character emerges. In Gyges's case and in Barnard's case, that character was not admirable.

The Post-Transplant Era: "When Surgery Went Nuts"

Following Barnard's success with Blaiberg, surgeons around the world went wild trying to transplant hearts. Magazines called 1968 the "Year of the Transplant." During 1968, 105 hearts were transplanted. After one year, of the 105 heart-transplant patients, 19 had died on the operating table, 24 had lived for three months, two had lived for 6 to 11 months, and only one had lived for almost a year. Of 55 liver transplants in 1968 and early 1969 (the 15 months after Barnard's landmark operation), 50 of the 55 patients failed to live even six months. Almost all these early transplants failed because the immune system rejected the organs.

Most reporters also missed the fact in 1968 that 25 percent of transplant recipients became temporarily psychotic. Massive dosages of immunosuppressive drugs produced initial euphoria, followed by catatonia, severe depression, hysterical crying, and even permanent psychosis. Few deaths could be more distasteful than as a psychotic patient in a post-operation bed in a hospital.

One of the great figures of medicine, Francis Moore, says that the year 1968 saw "epidemics" of chauvinism and of surgeons' egos: "It was the only example I know in the history of transplant medicine where everyone went nuts."[9] Nobel Prize winner (1954) Andre Courmand of Columbia University called Barnard's operation a mere stunt: "Merely demonstrating that it is technically feasible" to transplant a human heart, he said, was unethical.[10] Physician Norman Staub said Barnard's operation was "grandstanding," a blatant grab for fame.[11]

Many cardiac surgeons criticized heart transplantation with reason. In animals or humans, heart transplants rarely lasted more than a month, let alone years, and the death rate in early heart transplants appalled knowledgeable observers. While 1968 may have been the "Year of the Transplant," the following two years were the years of the high-tech last gasp.

Because of poor results, the Montreal Heart Institute in 1969 suspended heart transplants, followed by suspensions at Harvard and Pittsburgh. Threatened with Congressional investigation and oversight, by 1970 almost all surgeons had stopped transplanting.

BARNEY CLARK'S ARTIFICIAL HEART

Barney Clark practiced dentistry in Utah for decades. A Latter-Day Saint, for 30 years he smoked cigarettes.

In 1970 at age 49, he felt unwell. Eight years later, he was diagnosed with emphysema, an incurable, obstructive lung disease, and cardiomyopathy, a disease where the muscles of the heart weaken and quit pumping blood. Too late, he quit smoking.

Over the next four years, powerful drugs dilated his blood vessels and kept him alive, but by November, 1982, he was dying. Initially scoffing at an artificial heart, approaching death gave him a new perspective and he decided to go for it.

At the University of Utah in Salt Lake City, physician Willem Kolff had been working on an artificial heart for two decades. In many ways, Kolff symbolizes the pros and cons of the desire to achieve a medical breakthrough.

In 1943, Kolff invented the first hemodialysis machine in the Netherlands. He converted a fuel pump from an automobile to force blood through a semipermeable membrane to clean it before it returned to the body. His first patient, a woman who had belonged to the Nazi party during World War II, lived a few days. Unlike modern dialysis machines, his machine could not sustain patients indefinitely because to use it each time, physicians had to make new connections between arteries and veins for its cannulas. Only in 1960, when Belding Scribner of Washington invented a permanent indwelling shunt, could dialysis sustain patients for years.

Despite the crudity of his machine, Kolff was lauded for decades as a genius, as a man of vision, as brave, and as one who pushed back the frontiers of medicine. Even though his had been a crude breakthrough, and with little elegant scientific understanding behind it, it had brought him fame, and many honorary doctorates and awards, including the Lasker Award for medical research. Some dubbed him the "Father of Artificial Organs." At Utah, he got his own research lab and didn't need to see patients to make a living. No wonder physicians emulated him.

Now 40 years after inventing the dialysis machine, Kolff in 1985 had paired with Robert Jarvik, an ambitious young medical student whom Kolff had helped get into Utah's medical school. After medical graduation, Jarvik directly went to work in Kolff's lab, never did an internship or residency, and never directly cared for patients. Jarvik modestly named the first artificial heart after himself.

The surgeon who implanted the Jarvik-7 was 36-year-old William DeVries, a tall, blonde-haired Nordic man with a lean, tanned face. Because of his rugged good looks and macho daring in surgery, some American reporters lionized him as a surgical John Wayne.

Like Christiaan Barnard, DeVries wanted to make surgical history and to place Utah on the world's medical map. Jarvik, Kolff and DeVries worked hard to go beyond the limits of surgical-biomedical engineering, all motivated by the desire to achieve a first.

The Implant

In a biological heart, blood is pumped by the powerful lower parts, the two ventricles. The Jarvik-7 consisted of molded polyurethane with two chambers of plastic and aluminum holding an inner diaphragm. A wall of thin membrane separated the two chambers, through which the diaphragm's contraction forced blood. An air compressor moved the diaphragm, brought by 6-foot tubes inserted through the upper abdomen. The compressor weighed 375 pounds and rolled around on wheels on a large metal cart.

The Jarvik-7 contained the same commercial valves used by heart surgeons, and, as in a natural heart, there were four of them (analogous to mitral, tricuspid, etc.). Someone pressing his ear to Barney Clark's chest could hear their clicking sounds as they opened and closed against the walls of the Jarvik-7.

DeVries operated on Barney Clark on December 1, 1982, almost 15 years to the day after Washkansky's transplant. On his way to the operating room, Clark joked, "There would be a lot of long faces around here if I backed out now."[12]

Upon opening the chest, DeVries found a flabby, enlarged heart: Twice the size of a normal heart, it merely quivered and didn't contract: one physician there described it as looking like "a soft, overripe zucchini squash." DeVries first cut away the lower part of the heart, the two ventricles; then he stitched two Dacron cuffs to the intact upper part, the atria. He then connected these Dacron cuffs with Velcro fasteners to the plastic ventricles of the Jarvik-7. However, the patient's atrial walls were paper-thin, so when DeVries snapped the Velcro fasteners, the pressure ripped out the atrial stitches; the cuffs had to be re-stitched into a new section of heart wall and the fasteners gently snapped into place.

The cuffs then held, but when DeVries turned on the Jarvik-7, it didn't pump blood out of its left ventricle. Frustrated, DeVries tried for an hour to get it to work. Three times he opened the ventricle by hand, each time risking introduction of air into the blood and a stroke. At one point, DeVries reportedly exclaimed, "Please, please, please work this time!"[13]

DeVries finally replaced the faulty Jarvik-7 with parts from another one and got the rebuilt machine working, two hours after it was supposed to have started.

The operation, having taken all night, concluded about 7 A.M. on December 2. When the anesthesia wore off a few hours later, DeVries watched anxiously as Barney Clark opened his eyes. If the patient had missed a bad stroke, he would be able to move his extremities. Clark did so and everyone felt relieved.

Later that day at a press conference, university physicians falsely described the operation as a "dazzling technical achievement," something "as exciting and thrilling as has ever been accomplished in medicine"; hospital administrators modestly called it "one of the most dramatic stories in medical history."

The conditions of patients after major heart surgery shock visitors, and this held for Una Loy Clark. She saw that Barney had a hole in his throat through which a breathing tube ran, a feeding tube running into his stomach, a bladder catheter, and the two hoses connecting the Jarvik-7 thumping through his upper abdomen to the 375-pound air compressor at his bedside.

Like Louis Washkansky, after the operation, Clark felt horrible. Though he had not suffered a massive stroke, he experienced intensive care psychosis and was confused, delirious, amnesiac, and at times, unconscious.

On December 4, DeVries operated to repair ruptured air sacs in Clark's lungs. On December 6, Clark felt better and asked DeVries how he was doing. DeVries replied, "Just fine." Seconds later, Clark had seizures—involuntary shuddering from head to toe—perhaps caused by the dramatic increase in blood flow from the Jarvik-7. DeVries injected muscle tranquilizers and anticonvulsants. Clark lost consciousness for the next several hours and his seizures continued, though gradually the quivering became confined to his left leg and left arm. At this point, he probably had some small strokes. Throughout the next months, he was confused.

During the following days, Clark wanted to die and once asked DeVries directly, "Why don't you just let me die?"[14] Such a reaction is not uncommon after traumatic surgery and often passes. His lack of energy, difficulty in breathing, and stupor depressed Clark; he told a psychiatrist several times, "My mind is shot."

On December 14 one of the $800 welded commercial valves broke inside the Jarvik-7 Clark's blood pressure dropped dramatically, threatening his life, and DeVries had to operate again to replace the valve.

Nineteen days after the operation, Clark temporarily improved, and DeVries hinted he might eventually go home. Instead, complication after complication began. Heparin, a blood thinner, was administered to prevent clots, but it caused severe bleeding. On January 18, DeVries surgically sealed a persistent, severe nosebleed. Clark's underlying emphysema created pneumothorax, escape of air from lungs into the chest cavity, requiring DeVries to operate yet again to relieve pressure on his weak lungs.

From January to March, Clark complained of conditions caused by this emphysema. He never could get a good breath because he was suffocating, a situation unrelated to the Jarvik-7. On February 14, he left the surgical ICU for a private room, but because he needed a respirator, he returned on February 15, and he was on it for the next nine days.

On February 24, he returned to a private room and had a good week. On March 1, DeVries filmed several interviews with Clark. Humana Hospital edited one of these and released a short clip of it to the public on March 2. According to the cardiologist Thomas Preston, this clip "came from an extensive interview in which, encouraged by Dr. DeVries, Clark issued a semblance of a positive statement."[15]

Although the clip showed his best moment, even then, Barney Clark, tethered to a huge machine, in pain, and not fully alert, looked grumpy and uncomfortable. Prompted by DeVries, he claimed to be glad to be alive and not sorry to have undergone the operation.

The next day he developed severe nausea and aspirated vomit, which led to pneumonia. He went downhill rapidly. By March 21, the beginning of the end, his kidneys failed and he ran a high fever.

On March 23, 1983, having lived 112 days with an artificial heart, Barney Clark died. Inside his body, after someone "called" the death, the Jarvik-7 continued to pump. Asked if she wanted to be present when DeVries turned off the Jarvik-7, Una Loy Clark said, "He's already dead," and left the room.[16]

Following Clark's death, public opinion varied. Some people called the operation "one of the boldest human experiments ever attempted"; others concluded that it had failed to prove its worth, and that even if it had returned Clark to normal, its costs were exorbitant.

The university's IRB and the FDA postponed any further implants until more data could be studied. Kolff defended the project: "A number of doctors were opposed to the artificial kidney and wrote articles against it. I decided not to respond at all. . . . I still have the same policy now for people [who] tell us that the artificial heart has no future."

DeVries surprisingly commented: "After the first two days, 95 percent of the issues we were dealing with concerned ethics, moral value judgments, communications with the press—problems I had never thought about."[17]

A few weeks after Barney Clark died, the hospital revealed that it had not disclosed that a valve had broken and killed Ted E. Bear, a 220-pound ram who had lived 297 days with a Jarvik-7. Heart surgeons understood the import of this revelation: even if Clark had lived a few more months, breaking valves would have killed him.

Unlike hemodialysis, in which the machine can fail and the patient lives on by getting another machine, if patients leave the hospital and the Jarvik-7 fails, they immediately die. The challenge of creating a totally implantable artificial heart, such that patients could pass the "walk-on-their-own-out-of-the-hospital" test, is that the mechanical heart needs to be flawless, subject to no breakdowns, interruptions, or failures. Otherwise, the patients immediately die.

Post–Barney Clark: Not Fame but Infamy

After Barney Clark died, the FDA allowed DeVries three more such operations. At Humana, on November 25, 1984, nearly two years after Barney Clark's operation, DeVries implanted a second Jarvik-7 into William Schroeder.

"Bionic Bill," age 51, was not only younger than Barney Clark but also much healthier and had no emphysema. Not surprisingly, he lived much longer, 21 months. But his quality of life was poor. Only 19 days after his operation, he suffered a stroke from a clot formed by the Jarvik-7. Schroeder then had a cascade of strokes, repeated bouts of endocarditis, and eventually underwent a tracheotomy. On August 6, 1986, he died of suffocation.

On February 17, 1985, Murray Haydon became the third recipient of a Jarvik-7. On the 17th day after the implant, he started to suffocate and also had a tracheotomy. He then experienced various infections, and he lived for 10 months. After he died, an autopsy revealed that a hole from a catheter in part of his natural heart wall had not healed, and so blood had poured into his lungs.

The fourth recipient, Jack Burcham, had an awful death. Going into surgery on April 16, 1985, Jack thought he had nothing to lose by going for it, but during the operation, DeVries made the amazing discovery that the Jarvik-7 *wouldn't fit* inside Jack's chest. When Jack Burcham left the operating room, "his chest, draped with sterile dressing. . . [was] only partly closed around the device."[18]

An autopsy showed that large blood clots had clogged the valve openings in his artificial heart. Afterwards, DeVries admitted that the surgery had shortened Burcham's life.[19] Critics wondered how any surgeon could not, before removing a beating heart, measure the chest cavity to make sure the Jarvik-7 would fit inside.

Three years later in 1988, after a long dispute, William DeVries left Humana Heart Institute, claiming that he was unhappy with its red tape. After divorcing his wife of 24 years, he then moved to Humana Hospital in Louisville, Kentucky, a for-profit center where he said he would be given a freer hand and three times his former salary.

Over the next four years, he joined and left three different surgery practices around Louisville before starting a risky solo practice in 1992. Because they saw only miserable outcomes, grandstanding, and obliviousness to clinical realities, physicians didn't refer patients to DeVries. For some time, he continued to claim that the Jarvik-7 could be successful, but he was a voice in the wilderness. The collective moral decision of physicians to stop referring patients to him effectively stopped him from implanting artificial hearts.

After Barney Clark's death, Robert Jarvik, like Christiaan Barnard, sought and enjoyed fame. He modeled Hathaway shirts in ads and gave interviews to *Playboy*, with whom he discussed his sex life. In 1988, he divorced his wife of many years and, after having known her for only five days, married the columnist who calls herself Marilyn Vos Savant ("Marilyn the wise" in French). Billing themselves sometimes as "the world's smartest couple," Jarvik and Vos Savant amazingly claimed that their children from previous marriages were their children "only in the biological sense." Marilyn once added, "I don't consider either of us to have children."[20]

In 2006, Jarvik reappeared in television ads for Lipitor, rowing across the screen. In intervening years, he had founded Jarvik Heart, a small company developing not an artificial heart but a cardiac pump.[21]

William DeVries struggled as a normal cardiac surgeon between 1992 and 1999, when he took early retirement. After the bombing of the World Trade Center in 2001, he reinvented himself, joined the Army Reserve and entered the Army Medical Department Basic Officer course, graduating in 2002 as one of the oldest officers to do so at age 58.[22] Today he works as a cardiac surgeon out of the 324th Combat Support Unit south of Miami, Fla.

ETHICAL ISSUES

The Desire to Be First and to Be Famous

In 1967, surgeon Norman Shumway at Stanford University Hospital in California had trained the longest and most rigorously to ensure good first results. After Barnard jumped the gun, Shumway transplanted the first heart in America. Earlier, because the underlying medical problems had not been solved, Stanford's research ethics committee may have stayed Shumway's hand.[23]

A dozen heart surgeons around the world could have done what Barnard did. Isn't it arbitrary to glorify the surgeon who did the first heart transplant but ignore the great heart surgeons who laid the foundation and who could have done the transplant but whose integrity held them back?

Soon after Barnard's operation, Brooklyn surgeon Adrian Kantrowitz transplanted a heart into a newborn. Kantrowitz needed an anencephalic infant as a source of a heart and only found one two days after Barnard's operation. If he had found it sooner, Kantrowitz would be known today.

Reporters describe breakthrough surgeons as "brave," "brilliant" and "dedicated," but rarely do they report on those who almost were first or those who built the framework for the breakthrough. Rarely do reporters explain how many patients suffered before surgeons obtained good results, or how hard the surgeon pushed these patients.

One factor in being first is the media, which feeds public hunger for medical breakthroughs. On the journalistic side, this hunger leads to inaccuracy and sensationalism. On the medical side, this hunger leads to haste and imprudence. In Brazil, a surgeon so raced to do the first heart transplant there that the first patient only learned of the heart transplant when he woke up with another heart inside him.

Barnard wanted fame and seemed to relish talking to reporters. He held daily briefings. When leaving the hospital, he paused for photographers and shook the hands of waiting South Africans. For access to himself and Washkansky, he took money from American journalists. He justified doing so to raise money to benefit future patients.

Although Barnard wouldn't allow Washy's wife to touch Washy after the operation, citing dangers of infection, such dangers seemed to vanish when he allowed a film crew to tape the first conversation between Washkansky and his son inside the hospital room.

Reporters understandably focused on the symbolism of the operation: a heart that once lived inside one human now pumped inside another human body. But this symbolism and Barnard's resulting fame blinded them to the awful clinical realities. Most reporters had too little medical background to understand what was occurring, and the public wanted medical miracles, not messy clinical details.

Officially criticizing the media circus DeVries first told the media about the operation. But with Barney Clark, the media had changed since Barnard's operation 15 years before and were more skeptical. At one point, when told there would be no further briefings, reporters exploded. The hospital later relented, but as weeks went by reporters became angry and as the hospital kept trying to put the best spin on the facts.

What was going on? DeVries and the University of Utah had encouraged hundreds of television and print reporters to follow the operation, but when it didn't turn out well, tried to stonewall them. The desire for fame conflicted with the desire to tell the truth.

Medically, is it ethical to try to achieve a "first" when the essential, underlying problem remains unsolved?

In Barnard's case, he could not selectively suppress the immune system's rejection of a transplanted heart. Moreover, the drugs that suppressed the immune system left the body vulnerable to infection.

After Barnard's operation, in trying to be first in their area, surgeons hoarded possible donors and did not share them with other surgeons, even if they better tissue-matched a patient at another hospital. Everyone in the 1970s needed a system that matched donor organs and patients, but the United Network for Organ Sharing (UNOS) did not begin for another decade.

The artificial heart presented medical problems similar to that of heart transplants before cyclosporin in that poor trade-offs for the patient existed in both cases. Preventively treating one kind of problem worsened another.

With transplants, surgeons fought infections with antibiotics and by holding off immunosuppressive drugs, but thereby increased chances of rejection of the foreign heart. If they gave immunosuppressive drugs, infections flourished. With artificial hearts, blood clots (thrombi) formed on joints and surfaces of mechanical surfaces. When such clots break free (embolism), they travel in the blood to the small vessels in the brain, lodge there, and cause brain damage (strokes). Blood-thinning medications such as Heparin reduced or prevented clots, but when given to post-operation patients such as Barney Clark, the patients bled out of their sutures.

In 1988, three heart experts reviewed DeVries's surgeries and concluded:

> At the time of the device implantation or at autopsy, thrombi have frequently been identified as components of the mechanical heart. Prolonged, although temporary, use of prosthesis, similar to a permanent heart substitution, only provides time to increase the number of thromboembolic events and to allow further establishment of infection.[24]

In effect, they had written the epitaph of the artificial heart.

Concerns about Donors: Criteria of Death

In 1968 and after Barnard's operation, cardiac surgeon Werner Forssmann pub-licly criticized Barnard for taking a beating heart out of one patient to transplant it into another.[25] For Forssmann, before it became a candidate for transplantation, a heart should stop. Because of similar concerns, Japan banned heart transplants for many decades.

Although Barnard did not discuss this with Edward Darvall, he must have been concerned about whether Denise Darvall's death would be accepted. Critics would scrutinize him for any sign of Dr. Frankensteinian overeagerness.

Louis Washkansky needed a heart in the best possible condition, and if Barnard had waited too long before excising Denise Darvall's heart, he might have lost it. Barnard's brother Marius, who was also a surgeon, wanted to remove Denise's heart before it stopped beating. Instead, Christiaan Barnard waited until Denise's heart had stopped beating, and then waited another three minutes, all to be certain it wouldn't resume beating spontaneously.

As Denise Darvall had a healthy heart, why did her heart stop at all? The answer is that Barnard placed her on a respirator and caused her heart to stop by turning the respirator off; this stoppage damaged the heart slightly and was done to deflect anticipated criticism. As the surgeon Thomas Starzl explained much later:

> [Standards of brain death] were not in effect during the operation and would not be until 1968. Rather than trying to maintain a strong heartbeat and good circula-tion in the cadaver donors, the legal requirement before the end of 1968 was the opposite. Because all such donors were incapable of breathing if the brain actual-ly had been destroyed, they were supported by ventilators. The steps to donation began with disconnection of the ventilator, which the public called "pulling the plug." During the 5 to 10 minutes before the heart stopped and death was pro-nounced, the organs to be transplanted were variably damaged by oxygen star-vation and the gradually failing and ultimately absent circulation.[26]

Because of ethical considerations, recipients like Louis Washkansky received damaged hearts that could have been supplied in better condition. On the other hand, most transplant surgeons at the time realized that they had little choice in this matter. For one thing, moral caution coincided with their professional interests. Transplant surgery depended entirely on altruistic, voluntary donations, and any suspicious or doubtful procedures would sabotage donations.

Responding to this emergency, Harvard appointed a committee to decide when beating hearts could be ethically removed from head-damaged patients. This committee gave birth to the famous *Harvard Criteria of Brain Death,* discussed in the chapter on comas, which required all the brain to be nonfunctioning.

Even as late as 1985, a Gallup poll showed that 44 percent of Americans hadn't signed organ cards because they feared being declared dead prematurely. In the United States today, by law in all states, physicians who declare a potential organ donor brain-dead may not belong to the surgical transplant team.

Quality of Life

An important ethical issue concerned the resulting quality of life for the recipients. In both cases, it was poor.

Barnard and DeVries correctly emphasized that for the first case, the question was not how long the patient could live, but whether. That a heart *could* be transplanted, or that an artificial heart *could* run a human body, counted as an achievement.

But then reflection set in. Did Washy have 17 days worth living? Did Clark have 112? Or was it merely, as the *New York Times* said, "112 days of dying"?[27] The same *Times* dubbed research on the artificial heart, "The Dracula of Medical Technology," a phrase which stuck.[28]

In the early 1980s, cyclosporin, a drug that selectively blocks immune rejection of foreign tissue, was discovered and revolutionized organ transplants. Thereafter, the number of organ transplants soared dramatically.

Today, 75 percent of heart transplant patients survive for at least three years and more than 61,000 heart transplants have been performed in America. American surgeons in 2005 performed over 2,100 hearts transplants.[29] Dirk van Zyl, Barnard's sixth heart transplant patient, died in 1996 of diabetes unrelated to his transplant, the longest-living heart transplant recipient at 23 years. Sara Remington, the first infant in the world to receive a heart transplant in 1984, survived to reach her 13th birthday.

Even today, life after a heart transplant is often not the miracle reported in popular media. Taking cyclosporin for life often causes cancer, and many recipients are in and out of hospitals for complications.

For recipients of the artificial heart after Barney Clark, quality of life was, frankly, terrible. The unfolding story of their misery continues the sad story of the artificial heart.

Hand Transplants and the Desire to Be First

In 1998, surgeon Jean-Michel Dubernard performed the first hand transplant in France. The source of the hand was a 41-year-old man who had died in a motorcycle accident, and the recipient was 48-year-old New Zealander, Clint Hallam.

A year later, Louisville's Jewish Hospital did the first hand transplant in America on 38-year-old Matthew Scott, who lost his hand to a firecracker.

Before these hand transplants, doctors debated whether transplanting a non-vital organ was ethical. Unlike heart and liver transplants, a hand transplant was not necessary for survival, and the recipient had to take antirejection drugs for life, increasing risks of later cancer.

In 2001, Clint Hallam demanded that his transplanted hand be amputated. He claimed that he only felt pain and had no normal feeling in his hand. Because they gave him diarrhea and influenza, Hallam had not taken antirejection drugs. He also did not undergo physical therapy.

In contrast, Mathew Scott began to feel cold and heat in his palm and within a few months, nerve growth had reached his wrist. He could write his name, tie his shoelaces, and wears a new wedding ring on the new hand. In January 2006, Scott had his hand six years.

In another case, which should have been front-page news in ethics, surgeons in South Africa considered but declined to try to be first to transplant fingers in children.[30] Citing the significant dangers of taking immunosuppressive drugs over many decades, which include cancer, hypertension, opportunistic infections, and diabetes, the surgeons decided that the children might be able to adapt easier and live better without the transplanted digits.

By 2006, surgeons around the world had completed 30 hand-forearm transplants, including three in Lyon, France.[31] Double amputees reported the best psychological results. All patients survived and after two years, none had rejected their new limbs. All had to endure immunosuppressant therapy, including steroids. Despite taking these medications, 12 had acute rejection episodes.[32]

Face Transplants and the Desire to Be First

In May 2005, Isabelle Dinoire, an unemployed, divorced mother of two teenage daughters living in government housing in Northern France, came home from a day of "lots of personal worries" and took sleeping pills to forget about her distress.[33] Dinoire probably was attempting suicide. These pills caused her to pass out, and as she was losing consciousness, her head hit a piece of furniture.

In a situation eerily like that of Shumway and Christiaan Barnard in 1967, American surgeon Maria Seimionow of the Cleveland Clinic had been preparing for 20 years to do a face transplant and only the month before had been given permission by the IRB of her hospital.[34] In London, surgeon Peter Butler had also gained permission to start evaluating patients for a face transplant.

While Dinoire was unconscious, her newly acquired black Labrador retriever bit off her nose, chin, mouth, and supporting facial muscles and tissue, allegedly trying to wake her up (the dog later was inadvertently destroyed). Soon Dinoire would receive the world's first face transplant, consisting of a brain-dead cadaver's chin, nose, and mouth in a triangular flap.

Many unresolved questions surround her actions: What drugs did she take? They must have been powerful, if a dog's mauling didn't wake her up. Did she try to kill herself? (The transplant surgeon denies it.) When her coma occurred, where were her teenage daughters? Why did the dog attack her?

After the mauling, and according to her transplant surgeon, Dinoire's wounds were so severe that she had difficulty eating. Her surgeons claimed that food fell out of the area where her mouth had been.

Other questions surround selection of her for the transplant. Was this case like Barney Clark's? In other words, "She's got nothing to lose, so why not try it?" A rival transplant surgeon in Paris accused Dubernard of bypassing established ethical and legal guidelines for doing transplants.[35]

Dinoire awoke with a severely disfigured face: "When I woke up, I tried to light a cigarette and didn't understand why it wouldn't stay between my lips. That's when I saw the pool of blood and the dog beside it."[36] According to the doctors' records, when she arrived at the hospital, her lips were gone, along with her chin and much of her nose, which left her teeth and part of her lower jawbone exposed.

After the attack, Isabelle could not move many of the muscles in her face, and she could barely speak or eat. At the university hospital in Amiens, Dr. Devauchelle, the head of maxillofacial surgery, despite the fact that Ms. Dinoire smoked, used depressant drugs, and seemed mentally unstable, decided to transplant a new face onto hers.[37]

Several months passed between the mauling and the face transplant. During this time, Ms. Dinoire returned home and could carry groceries to her apartment. When outside, she wore a surgical mask. Without the mask, as she tried to talk, people could see her jawbone move. Surgeons said they could not reconstruct her former face, a gaping wound.

When asked about the face transplant, Ms. Dinoire consented. A French national ethics committee dismissed it: "the very notion of informed consent [in this case] is an illusion" in such cases.[38]

Dr. Devauchelle had already identified a potential candidate in a hospital in Lille, Maryline St. Aubert, who had committed suicide by hanging and who was brain-dead. Devauchelle claimed later that he did not know that St. Aubert had hanged herself, because the hanging might have damaged her facial veins. Devauchelle cut a triangle of facial tissue from St. Aubert, put it on ice, and later attached it to Dinoire's disfigured face.

Following the surgery, Devauchelle turned over Dinoire's post-operation care to Dr. Jean-Michel Dubernard, the French surgeon who performed the first successful double hand transplant in 2004 on Clint Hallam. "There's a big brain behind him and steely will that is willing to confront massive criticism," said Thomas Starzl, who performed the world's first liver transplant.[39]

Dubernard, a former deputy mayor of Lyon, also served as an elected Deputy in the French National Assembly. A self-described workaholic and chain-smoker, Dubernard commutes from Lyon two days a week to work in the French Parliament and on other days does medicine in Lyon. Under French law, he faces mandatory retirement in 2008. Like Christiaan Barnard, he confesses to loving international publicity.

Through a steady treatment of immunosuppressants, Dubernard ensured that Dinoire's immune system did not reject the new skin. After a week, Dinoire could speak and could drink water from a glass.

Ethical criticisms focused on, first, the fact that Dinoire had to take immuno-suppressant drugs for life. Already in late 2005, surgeons had to give her increased dosages to prevent her body's attempt to reject her new face. As we know, such drugs increase Dinoire's risk later of cancer, diabetes, and other medical problems. Estimates predict that 10 percent of such grafts will fail the first year and 30 to 50 percent within three to five years, so candidates must be prepared for failure. Because transplanted skin triggers more fierce rejection than any other organ, facial transplantation carries great risk of rejection and more risk of cancer from taking immunosuppressant drugs at higher levels.

Second, ethical criticism focused on selection of Dinoire, a mentally unstable smoker. Would she adhere to rigorous post-transplant regimens? If her face sloughed off in the worst case, did she possess the mental health to continue living?

Third, did the French physicians rush Dinoire into surgery merely to be first? Did they fear the American and English surgeons getting there first? They seemed to care little for protocol.

In early 2006, Dinoire resumed smoking, which jeopardized the healing and stability of her transplant by constricting blood vessels and increasing chances of infection. On the other hand, many of the French smoke and consider smoking a nonissue.

In July 2006, surgeons disclosed that the donor's face lacked a key nerve that controlled the lower portion of her face. They also indicated just how worried they were about Dinoire's mental state: prior to the operation, three local psychiatrists approved Dinoire for the operation, and a fourth independent psychiatrist also had to agree.[40] After the operation, Dinoire had daily psychological evaluations for a month, which then tapered to twice a week.

Later in 2006, Chinese surgeons in Xian attempted a copycat operation, trans-planting two-thirds of face of a man mauled by a bear in a 14-hour operation.[41] When the operation occurred, the patient had been living for two years as a recluse.

Two years later, Dinoire fared better than expected and had not rejected her face.[42] She had gone out in public with her psychiatrist, attracting little notice in Lyon.

Back at the Cleveland Clinic in America, Dubernard's rival, surgeon Maria Seimionow, emphasized, "First, do no harm." She says, "The thing I'm worried about is, if it fails, what I'm going to be left with." London surgeon Butler said, "My main concern is not to harm the patient."

Seimionow's protocol requires good health, good personality and good fami-ly support, none of which Dinoire seems to have had.

The major worry beside rejection is the risk of cancer, deadly infection, or other lethal disease from taking steroids and immonosuppressant drugs for many decades. Who can evaluate whether a chance of normalcy is worth risking an early death from one of the above? Seimionow answers: only the disfigured patient can make such a judgment.

Finally, one wonders what the French surgeons will do if, one day in years to come, Dinoire's face sloughs off. Will she be able to withstand it psychologically? Have they prepared her for this possibility, or have they gambled all on success?

Once More into the Breach: Artificial Hearts Today

In 2001, Abiomed of Massachusetts obtained permission to implant three of its totally implantable titanium artificial hearts, called AbioCor, in patients at Jewish Hospital in Louisville (DeVries was not involved). Two others were implanted at the Texas Heart Institute in Houston, and one each at UCLA Medical Center and Hahnemann University Hospital in Philadelphia. Abiomed's criteria of success were minimal: they wanted to prove, for dying patients with less than 30 days to live, that they could extend life to 60 days.

Robert Tools received the first AbioCor in 2001 and lived 151 days. Three other patients lived for 92, 78, and 32 days, and another died on the operating table. The biggest success was Tom Christerson, who lived 17 months, the record.

By March of 2005, Abiomed had tested 14 patients, two of whom died immediately, the rest of whom lived for an average of five months. The widow of one, James Quinn, sued because her husband and she went through two months of hellish dying, constantly worried about who would pay for round-the-clock nursing care.[43] Abiomed asked a panel of physicians advising the Food and Drug Administration to let it implant more at a cost of $250,000 each, but the panel balked.[44]

In October 2004, a rival company, SynCardia of Tucson, AZ, won approval for a trial of its CardioWest mechanical heart, a direct descendant of the Jarvik-7.[45] Approval was not as a substitute for heart transplants, but as a temporary bridge to transplant for patients on waiting lists.

In 2001, Norman Shumway doubted whether artificial hearts would ever be successful. "An artificial heart is a tremendously difficult problem because the human body is living tissue. . . . [The body] always is going to be opposed to plastic materials."[46]

A final problem with artificial hearts deserves mention. Unlike dialysis machines or pacemakers, once implanted, artificial hearts must work perfectly forever, with no margin of error. When artificial hearts fail, loss of blood to the brain kills patients within 15 minutes. Can any machine achieve such perfection?

Expensive Rescue versus Cheap Prevention

In 2002, a heart transplant cost about $210,000, and bills for immunosuppressants for the rest of the patient's life were $15,000 a year.[47] Eighty percent of commercial insurers and 97 percent of Blue Cross Blue Shield plans covered heart transplants. Medicaid programs in most states also covered them.

In 1999, about 2,200 hearts were transplanted in America, plus 4,700 livers and over 12,000 kidneys. Remarkably, about 900 lung transplants were also done that year.

What about costs? Was the program cost-effective? How much is one more day of longer life worth? Is every life worth the same amount? What's the opportunity cost of spending so much money this way?

Artificial hearts could cost society dearly. NIH invested over $8 million in research leading up to the Utah project and over $200 million nationally in similar projects between 1964 and 1982. Was this the best way to spend limited funds? Should such expenditures be continued? If artificial hearts were successful, could society afford to pay for them? The now-defunct Office of Technology Assessment estimated in 1990 that 60,000 Americans might use artificial hearts, at a cost to Medicare of $5.5 billion a year.[48]

All of which is a lot of money and effort to rescue a damaged heart. Glamorous, high-tech operations are dramatic, but might not the money spent do more good for more people if spent to prevent smoking, promote exercise, and create healthier hearts?

The *Progressive* magazine complained that a "medical establishment grown fat on chemicals and technological wizardry is not willing to empower people so they can prevent illness."[49] *Progressive* argued that artificial hearts would benefit only the small number of cardiac patients who could afford them and hence were "qualitatively different from the basic advances in immunology which have saved million of lives, even among populations not directly treated."

Saving bad hearts illustrates again the rule of rescue. Our society cares more about saving an identifiable life than about preventing future deaths from heart failure.

One way to prevent such deaths is to tax cigarettes out of existence. Around 2002, New York and Washington put high state sales taxes on tobacco. A pack of cigarettes there from a vending machine (often used by teenagers to get cigarettes) costs over $8. Such taxes discourage smoking in people when they are young —just when cigarette companies want them to become addicted for life, as happened to Barney Clark.

Patients: Informed Consent

How much does a candidate for a new kind of transplantation understand about its experimental nature? How much can such candidates understand, given that they are seriously ill and desperate? In their situation, how is *informed* consent obtained?

The media paint a sunny picture of organ transplants, typically citing only one-year survival rates. Within surgery, transplants have grown from being merely *experimental* to being *therapeutic*.

Nevertheless, laypeople believe that healthy transplanted organs will function for a lifetime. The reality is different. If the recipient lives long enough, almost all recipients will reject their organs. One-third to one-half of recipients reject their heart transplants after five years. Kidney transplants began in 1951 and today are closest to being truly therapeutic rather than experimental; but even so, over 50 percent of transplanted kidneys are rejected after 10 years.

To prevent rejection, surgeons prescribe continuous cyclosporin, which over years often causes malignant lymphoma and which often destroys kidneys, the liver, or the brain. Cyclosporin also makes women grow facial hair. After several years, its efficacy fades.

Medical sociologists Renée Fox and Judith Swazey, participant-observers for over 40 years to organ transplantation, came to some dismal conclusions. They argue that the reclassification of organ transplants in the 1990s as "therapeutic" was done not because of medical evidence but to make transplants eligible for reimbursement and to obtain publicity in order to increase the number of donors. They add:

> In the context of the growing organ shortage "crisis," the theme of organ transplantation as gift of life was framed and addressed primarily as a social policy problem of supply and demand. Exhortations to "make a miracle" happen through organ donation were accompanied by a structured forgetting of some of the darker emotional and existential implications of what it involved.[50]

After miserable results from heart surgery, one wonders about the relationships between surgeon and patient. An ethics of care highlights the poignancy of such relationships. Does the patient blame the surgeon for failure? Does the research surgeon grow hardened? Surgeon P. M. Clark eloquently expresses such feelings:

> It is sometimes hard to meet the eyes of patients who have improved enough to have been moved to the regular post-op floor and finally become alert enough to communicate their despair and disappointment. . . . Often, after entering the experience with great hope, patients for whom transplantation has been a series of setbacks clearly articulate their feelings of betrayal: "No one ever told me it could be like this."[51]

Certainly they were told that there would be no guarantees, and that it would be hard, and that there would be setbacks, but probably not how hard, or what some of the worst-case scenarios could be. When they were told, "You have to have a transplant or you're going to die," they were left a slim margin to make decisions.

Fox and Swazey report that many patients and families never imagined that "it could be as bad as this." This remark recalls bioethicist Margaret Battin's call at the end of life to not present the choice between "Do you want a chance to live or do you want to die?" but to inform patients that they will die eventually and that surgery may bring about the "worst death," whereas forgoing surgery may bring the "least-worst death."

Growth of Left Ventricle Assist Devices: More Rescue?

In 1998, the FDA allowed cardiac surgeons to insert left ventricle assist devices (LVADs) into patients as bridges to heart transplants. Being on the pump gave patients 408 days of life compared to 150 on drugs. In 2001, average first-year costs were $222,000.[52]

In a trial at 20 American cardiac transplantation centers, patients ineligible for a transplant and put on the "HeartMate" LVAD lived 250 days longer than those in a control group. Nearly a fourth of patients lived for two years (and presumably, would've otherwise died within a few months). The beauty of HeartMate is that, if the machine fails, the patient's original heart continues pumping, keeping him alive.

Although the FDA may approve the HeartMate for a limited class of patients, most insurance companies do not pay for it. Over 100,000 Americans a year could use a HeartMate. Each time a surgeon puts a patient on an LVAD, he or she commits a quarter million dollars' of society's resources. If use of such devices soars, Heartmate's costs could also skyrocket and for limited benefit.

With the lack of any great progress on artificial hearts between Barney Clark's 1982 operation and the FDA panel's decision above in 2005, "the workhorse of mechanical support for patients with heart failure today is the left ventricle assist device, which piggybacks onto the native heart, pumping blood directly out of the left ventricle into the aorta."[53] These have been bridge therapy and "final destination" for about 7,000 people.

One wonders about LVADs as a final destination. Is this a good way to live? Can the quarter million North Americans who die each year of heart failure each have an LVAD? At what cost? Or is giving a few thousand an LVAD a case for each person of the rule of rescue, perhaps with hope of a lucky match and donated heart?

Conclusion

Norman Shumway died at age 83 in February 2006, regarded inside surgery as the true "father of heart transplant surgery," but whose passing otherwise attracted little notice from the media. In life, Shumway was humble and did not like to mention his accomplishments, but at his passing, doctors called him "one of the 20th century's true pioneers in cardiac surgery." Philip Pizzo, MD, dean of Stanford School of Medicine, said of Shumway that "he developed one of the world's most distinguished departments of cardiothoracic surgery at Stanford, trained leaders who now guide this field throughout the world and created a record of accomplishment that few will ever rival. His impact will be long-lived and his name long-remembered."[54] Let us hope.

FURTHER READING AND RESOURCES

Robert M. Arnold, Stuart Youngner, and Renie Shapiro, eds., *Procuring Organs for Transplants: The Debate over Non-Heart Beating Cadaver Protocols*, Johns Hopkins University Press, Baltimore, MD., 1995.

Christiaan Barnard and Curtiss Bill Pepper, *One Life*, Macmillan, New York, 1969.

Renée Fox and Judith Swazey, *The Courage to Fail: A Social View of Organ Transplants and Dialysis*, 2d ed. rev., University of Chicago Press, Chicago, IL, 1978.

Thomas Starzl, *The Puzzle People: Memoirs of a Transplant Surgeon*, Pittsburgh University Press, Pittsburgh, PA , 1992.

CHAPTER 13

Allocation of Artificial and Transplantable Organs

The God Committee

Many times every day in American medicine, someone decides who gets limited, expensive medical resources and who does not. Sometimes individual physicians do so by admitting patients; sometimes hospital administrators do so by setting criteria for organ transplants; more frequently, government and insurance administrators do so by deciding what they will cover. Each of these decisions raises questions about fairness.

This question becomes complicated when conjoined to a related question about who *deserves* a scarce resource, and specifically, whether bad decisions about personal health justify denial of the resource. Should smokers with emphysema be eligible for lung transplants? Alcoholics for liver transplants?

This chapter's classic case describes the famous God Committee in Seattle in the 1960s that decided which patients in renal failure would receive dialysis. The chapter also discusses issues of distributive justice concerning who gets an organ transplant.

BACKGROUND

An Artificial Kidney: Hemodialysis

The kidneys remove toxins accumulated by normal cellular metabolism in the blood. When both kidneys fail, unless the cleansing function of the kidneys is replaced, toxins accumulate to a lethal level.

Hemodialysis (literally "tearing blood apart") substitutes for the kidneys: It removes blood from the body and sends it through cannulas (tubes), where a semipermeable membrane absorbs toxins by osmosis to a surrounding solution; then the cleansed blood is returned to the body. Patients in renal failure must undergo hemodialysis (more simply, "dialysis") for several hours, two or three times a week.

The process by no means cures kidney (renal) failure. It leaves patients tired and cranky, with lives revolving around appointments. Most patients want to get a kidney transplant to get off dialysis.

Dutch physician Willem Kolff invented the hemodialysis machine in the Netherlands in 1943 and later worked on artificial hearts with Robert Jarvik. Kolff converted an automobile's fuel pump to force blood to and from the body for cleansing. Unfortunately, each session of dialysis required surgeons to reconnect cannulas to arteries and veins. Because an artery or vein could only be used once, surgeons soon exhausted all sites.

In 1960, Belding Scribner in Seattle invented the permanent indwelling shunt, a piece of tubing permanently attached to one vein and one artery, which allowed blood to flow continuously. The shunt could be shut off between dialyses, like a spigot.

For the first month, Scribner did not realize that the combination of a workable dialysis machine and a permanent shunt meant that he and Kolff had created an artificial kidney that could sustain life indefinitely.

This breakthrough led to something wonderful: thousands of dying patients would now live. It also led to a new ethical issue: if no way could be found to dialyze them, many others would die. Given the scarcity of machines, some criteria of distributive justice had to be employed to select who would live and who would die.

Supply and Demand of Donated Organs

Problems of distributive justice often arise in allocating solid organs. Over the past decades, the number of available organs for donation has never matched demand: the number from cadavers hovers around 4,000 a year. Second, the need for transplantable organs has steadily increased, especially as more Americans on dialysis desire kidney transplants. The new source of organs has been live donations from friends and relatives. In 2003, more transplantable kidneys came from such donors than from cadavers, a milestone.

Less than 20 percent of American adults agree to be organ donors. Young adults notoriously do not think about death and resist signing donor cards. Some people resist the idea of desecrating a corpse by removing organs.

Some African-Americans refuse to sign donor cards because they consider themselves more likely to be declared dead prematurely. In 1968 in the case of African-American Bruce Tucker in Richmond, VA, before the Harvard brain-death criteria, a jury almost convicted surgeons of murder when they transplanted Tucker's heart after he sustained massive head trauma. Tucker's family pressed charges because they had not consented, and because, when Tucker's heart was removed, he was not legally dead.[1]

Of course, a family may donate organs of a brain dead relative in the absence of a signed donor card. Even if the brain dead patient has a signed card, if the family refuses, American surgeons generally do not take organs because they fear lawsuits and bad publicity.

Confusion over the definition of brain death decreases organ donation. For this reason, America has not moved beyond the conservative Harvard criteria of brain death to broader criteria that could include, say, patients with PVS of five years' duration.

For successful transplants, physicians must keep the cadaver's organs in good condition. For their own well-being, victims of head trauma should be kept as dry (internally) as possible, whereas transplant surgeons need well-hydrated organs. As discussed in this chapter about the Pittsburgh Protocol, what's best for the organs may not be what's best for trauma patients.

Young, healthy adults constitute the best sources of good organs; in practice, this means people killed in motor vehicle crashes. In his first efforts, Dr. Kevorkian worked to allow prisoners on death row to donate organs before execution, but most of them would have had unsuitable organs due to age, abuses of alcohol or other drugs, cancer, or hepatitis B or C.

Today, surgeons will consider transplanting organs with hepatitis in young recipients and if the organs look good in other respects. They reason that it's better to continue living with hepatitis than to die.

Preventing car accidents reduces the number of donatable organs: restraints and seats for infants and children, helmets for motorcyclists, a legal drinking age of 21, lower speed limits, and laws and social pressure against drunk driving all reduced deaths among Americans under 40—the age group most likely to have donatable organs. When one state recently allowed motorcyclists not to wear helmets, the number of organs from "motorcycle cadavers" soared.

Given the increasing need for organs and their persistent scarcity, it is not surprising that each year over 4,000 Americans die waiting for an organ. This continuing tragedy has created many proposals for expanding available organs, each with some ethical controversy, such as that surrounding the Pittsburgh protocol.

At least 14 European countries follow France and *presume consent*: a dead person is presumed to be a donor unless he specifically declines in writing to a national agency. Presumed consent has not been tried in America, where mistrust of doctors already prevents donation and where physicians fear lawsuits.

Mandated choice requires adults, in obtaining a driver's license, to indicate whether they want to be organ donors. Most American states require this choice.

The God Committee

When Belding Scribner developed his shunt, inpatient dialysis cost $20,000 a year. As an experimental treatment, insurance companies refused to pay for it. To hold down costs, such companies do not cover the experimental treatments until they are proven therapeutic. So Scribner's Swedish Hospital dialyzed its first patients without charge.

Swedish Hospital soon told Scribner he could admit no more dialysis patients. By then, Scribner had a year's experience and decided that patients could undergo dialysis outside the hospital in clinics staffed by nurses. In 1963, Swedish Hospital started an outpatient dialysis center.

That center could serve 17 patients, but many more patients were eligible. From its beginning, the ethical problem flared of *who shall live when not all can*?[2]

Instead of leaving the problem of distributive justice to physicians, Swedish Hospital, Scribner, and King's County Medical Society took the unusual step of creating an Admissions and Policy committee to decide who would get a dialysis machine. Scribner wrote in 1972, "As I recall that period, all of us who were involved felt that we had found a fairly reasonable and simple solution to an impossibly difficult problem by letting a committee of responsible members of the community choose which patients [would receive treatment]."[3]

The intent of creating this committee was to take the burden of decision off physicians, since a physician would naturally want her patients to be accepted.[4] The committee of seven members represented the community: a minister, a lawyer, a housewife, a labor leader, a state government official, a banker, and a surgeon. Two physicians familiar with dialysis served as advisers and screened applicants for medical unsuitability. The committee worked anonymously and never met candidates.

The committee first limited candidates to residents of the state of Washington who were under age 45; candidates had to be able to afford dialysis or have insurance that covered it. Almost immediately too many patients applied and additional criteria became necessary. The committee then considered a candidate's employment, children, education, motivation, achievements, and promise of helping others.

The committee eventually asked for analyses of a candidate's ability to tolerate anxiety and ability to manage his medical care independently; it considered whether a candidate had previously used symptoms to get attention. In its deliberations, it evaluated the personality and personal merit of the candidate and the family's support for a patient on chronic dialysis. So elderly curmudgeons without siblings or children fared badly.

Shana Alexander Publicizes the God Committee and Starts Bioethics

It should be noted that the God Committee struggled with issues of distributive justice long before bioethics became a field. In 1962, no philosophers had written about ethical issues of allocating organs; indeed, no one had written about bioethics at all.[5] At least, they had not in the modern sense in which different values and cases are analyzed to find a just public policy. The major previous writings were in Catholic medical ethics.

In May, 1962, Dr. Scribner took a patient to Atlantic City for a newspaper convention to lobby publicly for more dialysis machines. In the process, he described the God Committee to reporters, and it was his account of that committee, rather than his appeal for more machines, that made the front page of the *New York Times* the next day.[6]

Life magazine assigned its first woman reporter, Shana Alexander, to write the story of this committee, and she spent three months in Seattle doing so. Her article appeared in November 1962 and carried the phrase, "God committee."[7] She described the committee as playing a godlike role in deciding who would live and who would die. She described in detail the committee's criteria, which came to be called *social worth criteria*, or criteria about a person's worth to society.

In the spring of 1963, the *Seattle Times* ran on its front page a picture of nine of the center's dialysis patients, who would die if funding stopped for their machines, with the heading, "Will These People Have to Die?"[8] As a result, the Boeing Corporation and the U. S. Public Health Service offered temporary financial support.

In 1965, television reporter Edwin Newman narrated an NBC documentary on the God Committee, *Who Shall Live?* That year, Congress had added to Social Security two national medical programs—Medicare for the elderly and Medicaid for the indigent, but dialysis was not yet covered under either of them. In the documentary, a congressman asked why, if the United States could have a space program, it couldn't have a dialysis program to save lives. National interest grew about the story, and indirectly about bioethics.

The media mattered greatly in this case. Shana Alexander said that when Scribner went to Atlantic City, he had been "angling" to get the story into the magazine with the largest circulation. Medical sociologist Judith Swazey agrees that Scribner set out to get publicity.[9]

Thirty years later, Scribner said that he had been "totally naive" about the kind of national publicity that he created; he also said that he had taken "a lot of flak" about the committee's existence, especially from an early article in *UCLA Law Review*.[10] He claimed that he had had nothing to do with the committee, which had been created and supervised by the King's County Medical Association. He also said he "hated the goddamn committee" and when he had a dying patient who wasn't selected, did everything possible to circumvent it.

The story about his work in the *Seattle Times* could not have been written without the initiation and cooperation of Scribner and other physicians at Seattle hospitals. These physicians manipulated *The Seattle Times*, *Life*, and NBC News to obtain funds for their patients. Their success began a pattern of using the media when patients needed organ transplants, a pattern that came to be called the *rule of rescue*.

The End-Stage Renal Disease Act (ESRDA)

The God Committee continued to select and reject candidates for dialysis for nearly a decade. By 1971, many stories had dramatized the plight of patients in renal failure, and that year Shep Glazer, the president of the American Association of Kidney Patients, testified before Congress. As the story goes (it may be exaggerated), Glazer dialyzed himself before the House Ways and Means Committee, disconnected a tube from the machine, let his blood flow onto the floor, and said, "If you don't fund more machines, you'll have this blood on your hands."

In 1972, Congress legislated for Americans a one-organ right to medical care. The *End-Stage Renal Disease Act (ESRDA)* mandated the federal government to pay for a dialysis machine for any American who needed one. Faced with the problem of distributive justice, of deciding which patients should be funded and how to select them, Congress took the easy way out and funded all patients. It decided not to decide.

Congress passed the ESRDA in a session lasting only 30 minutes. The impetus came from a coalition of kidney patients, lobbyists for some physicians, concerns over high rates of kidney failure in people of color, and concerns that too much money was being spent on space and the war in Vietnam but too little on dying people who might be saved.

By making dialysis available to all patients, the ESRDA ended the problem of allocating machines and thus ended the need for the God Committee.

In retrospect, the ESRDA was hastily conceived, and it set an unfortunate precedent. Other groups, such as hemophiliacs, pressed for similar coverage. No one accurately predicted the long-term costs to society.

Advocates of funding for dialysis predicted that, as more machines were produced, costs would drop. Their prediction is a textbook lesson in how classical supply and demand fails to work in medical finance. Senator Vance Hartke of Indiana predicted that although the ESRDA would cost $100 million the first year, its cost would drop sharply because of increased efficiencies in production. Willem Kolff said that his machines could be mass-produced for $200 each.

But under *cost-plus reimbursement*, in effect for hospitals during the 1970s and 1980s, hospitals could buy as many dialysis machines as they wanted and pass the cost "plus" a percentage of profit on to Medicare. So they had no incentive to buy $200 machines, but did to buy $20,000 machines. The larger the cost, the greater their profits.

In 1983 and in efforts to rein in out-of-control costs, reimbursement by *Diagnostically Related Groups (DRGs)* units replaced cost-plus funding. Hospitals still found a way around DRGs and costs continued to soar. As yet another way to control costs, *managed care* started in the 1990s.

By 2006, instead of costing a few hundred million dollars, the 330,000 Americans on dialysis in the ESRDA cost Medicare $16 billion a year. This yearly figure was 160 times higher than Hartke's prediction, and Senator Hartke had predicted costs to fall dramatically, possibly a thousand times higher. When people started talking about funding Kolff's artificial hearts in the mid-1980s, people remembered these incorrect estimates.

Under the ESRDA, Congress also reimbursed kidney transplants. After the development of cyclosporin, the number of successful renal transplants jumped from 3,730 in 1975 to 9,000 in 1986 and to 15,000 in 2003.[11] In addition to the question whether every dying kidney patient should undergo dialysis, this development raised a new question: should every kidney dialysis patient have a kidney transplant? If so, where would the organs come from?

One thing is certain: what drove the expansion of people on dialysis and people getting kidney transplants was the fact that federal funds paid for all treatments for the kidney, a situation that existed for no other organ or disease. In contrast, during the last decades, over 40 million Americans lacked basic medical coverage. At the same time, any American suffering kidney failure had all medical expenses covered and, frequently, could go on disability.

The Birth of Bioethics

For reasons mixed and complex, Belding Scribner did something that went against a medical practice that went back centuries: he made public a moral dilemma which hitherto had been discussed only privately among physicians. Bringing this issue to the public's attention created controversy within medicine. As in Karen Quinlan's case, physicians felt that such ethical issues should be handled quietly within the profession.

By making this move, Scribner began a new process—the education of the American public about the many ethical problems in medicine. Different moral opinions about medicine's problems now began to be expressed publicly by scholars. With these articles and soon, with new courses, the new interdisciplinary field of bioethics began.

ETHICAL ISSUES

Social Worth

As we have seen, the God Committee took "social worth" into account (although the committee itself did not use this phrase). Medical sociologists Renée Fox and Judith Swazey, who spent 40 years studying artificial kidneys and transplantation, reviewed the minutes of the committee's meetings and criticized its criteria of social worth as follows:

> Within these very general criteria, the specific, often unarticulated indicators that were used reflected the middle-class American value system shared by the selection panel. A person "worthy" of having his life saved by a scarce, expensive treatment like chronic dialysis was one judged to have qualities such as decency and responsibility. Any history of social deviance, such as a prison record, any suggestion that a person's married life was not intact and scandal-free, were strong contraindications to selection. The preferred candidate was a person who had demonstrated achievement through hard work and success at his job, who went to church, joined groups, and was actively involved in community affairs.[12]

Some critics have argued that social worth should never have been a criterion because any such standard implies that some people are worth more than others; therefore, it is inherently unjust. Immanuel Kant argued that every human should be treated as an "end in himself" with absolute moral worth. To judge that one human was more deserving than another is to treat some wrongly as a "mere means." How then would Kant treat everyone the same? The key question is what rule or maxim could be universalized. For Kant, that would be impartial, random selection by lot, say, by drawing straws.

Two severe critics of the God Committee, a psychiatrist and a lawyer, also raked it over the coals for its criteria of social worth:

> [*Life*] magazine paints a disturbing picture of the bourgeoisie sparing the bourgeoisie, of the Seattle committee measuring persons in accordance with its own middle-class suburban value system: scouts, Sunday school, Red Cross. This rules out creative conformists, who rub the bourgeoisie the wrong way but who historically have contributed so much to the making of America. The Pacific Northwest is no place for a Henry David Thoreau with bad kidneys.[13]

Boston University law professor George Annas criticized the Seattle Committee for preferring housewives over prostitutes, working men over "playboys," and scientists over poets.[14] Annas argued that some criteria of social worth can be just at some stage of the selection process, but these criteria must be made public. If the rule is going to be "always prefer housewives to prostitutes," this should be explicit. Secret rules allow discrimination based on race, sex, class, wealth, or other arbitrary qualities.

In fairness to the God Committee, we should note that dialysis at home had become an official goal, because six patients could be supported at home at the same cost as a single patient in the hospital. That being the case, at least two aspects of social worth became paramount: the psychological support of the patient's family and the patient's own attitude. A passive, uncooperative patient can be handled adequately in a hospital setting, but not at home.

Self-Inflicted Injuries

Fox and Swazey described the famous case of a half-Sioux, Ernie Crowfeather. A small time criminal and a charmer, he received dialysis for 30 months but refused to follow the regimen, hated his quality of life, drank, imposed his childlike needs on the staff, and finally turned down further therapy and died.[15] In selecting Crowfeather, Scribner and other physicians actually went around the God Committee.[16]

Liver transplants also raise the issue of self-inflicted injuries. By far the most expensive organ to transplant, transplanting a liver calls for a highly skilled team and takes a long time. The most common cause of liver destruction, or end-stage liver disease (ESLD), is alcoholism. When alcohol is a factor, the condition is actually called *alcohol-related end-stage liver disease (ARESLD)*.

In the 1990s, physicians debated whether patients with ARESLD should be equally eligible for liver transplants. This is partly a medical issue, since it can be analyzed in terms of which patients will benefit most from such a transplant, but it also concerns social worth. Is a nondrinker more deserving of a donor liver? Can someone with ARESLD be blamed for the loss of his liver? Would a drinker keep on drinking, thereby destroying the new liver, or would drinkers be transformed by receiving the gift of life?

With ARESLD, this question is complicated by disagreement over whether alcoholism is a disease or a chosen behavior. The disease model of alcoholism has prevailed for some time, but has recently been attacked by philosopher Herbert Fingarette.[17]

In 1992, two teams of clinical medical ethicists conflicted over this point. In Chicago, physicians Alvin Moss and Mark Seigler argued that as ARESLD principally causes liver failure, as not enough livers are available for transplant, and as recidivism is likely among alcoholics, patients who develop liver failure "through no fault of their own" should have a higher priority for donor livers than patients with ARESLD, whose condition "results from failure to obtain treatment for alcoholism."[18]

Two medical ethicists at the University of Michigan, Carl Cohen and Martin Benjamin, disagreed. They maintained that alcoholics are not morally blameworthy and, after liver transplants, survive as long as nonalcoholics, and so should not be penalized.[19]

Kant and Rescher

Kantian ethics pulls in two directions on the question of penalizing alcoholics for liver transplants. On the one hand, Kant believes that people choose to drink and should be held responsible. For him, to say the alcoholic's actions are caused by a disease is to treat the person as a "mere means," as if he were the passive vehicle of causal forces over which he has no control. Herbert Fingarette's research shows that most so-called alcoholics are really voluntary heavy drinkers who can moderate their behavior, given proper incentives and contexts. Fingarette also emphasizes that Alcoholics Anonymous assumes that drinkers can choose not to drink.

As said, all other things being equal, Kantian ethics also pulls for a lottery in distributing a scarce liver, to treat each person equally and as having equal moral worth. Can these two strains of Kantian ethics be reconciled?

Perhaps. In 1969, philosopher Nicholas Rescher argued that the God Committee had been correct to use criteria that included social worth.[20] Rescher favored considering life expectancy, number of dependents, potential for future contributions to society, and past achievements. Less controversially, he supported screening candidates for medical problems that were likely to make them do poorly on dialysis and waste machines. He suggested that such a system might be based on points, with ties broken by a lottery.

Kant would be sympathetic to Rescher's two-tiered approach. Those who had injured themselves through voluntary behavior do not deserve the same chance as those who lost kidneys through a genetic disease. Once such people are screened out, however, everyone should be considered equally by lottery.

Distribution Systems and Waiting Lists

In the 1970s, no system existed for distributing donated organs, and surgeons with organs in one medical center did not always share them with surgeons elsewhere. This was wasteful. Some hoarded organs soon were lost.

The National Transplantation Act (1984) and the federal Task Force on Organ Transplantation (1986) were combined in 1987 to create the United Network for Organ Sharing (UNOS). UNOS alleviated some regional competition and established national standards about which patient would get the next available organ. UNOS continually grapples with the ethical question: *what is the most fair, just way to allocate organs?*

UNOS deals only with candidates who are already in the system. Thus how and when applicants get onto waiting lists for donor organs remains a pressing issue. Specifically, if you don't have medical insurance or a hospital willing to take you as a charity case, you won't get on the UNOS list.

An especially vexing problem is the practice of *multiple listing*.[21] Some patients get appointments with surgeons at more than one transplant center and have themselves worked up at each; but only people who can take time off from work, can afford to travel, and have generous medical plans can arrange for multiple listings.

For a patient who needs a kidney, being on several lists may not be necessary to get one, but for a patient who needs a heart or a liver, a multiple listing may be a matter of life and death. One criterion for receiving a heart or liver is locality: a candidate must be within the area of the transplant center. A patient who registers at half a dozen such centers in southern California could significantly increase his chances of being selected.

Imagine that you are going to die if you don't get an organ, but you know that a hundred other patients want the same organ for the same reason. Suppose you hear that someone in, say, Pittsburgh or Houston has received an organ because he or she knew the right surgeon and therefore got onto the right list. It's one thing to feel unlucky because you're in a life-threatening condition, but quite another to feel that you are going to die of organ failure because someone else managed to get into line in front of you.

Two well-known crises occurred about listing for organ transplants. When former baseball star Mickey Mantle came to Baylor University Medical Center in Dallas on May 28, 1995, decades of alcoholism, as well as his Hepatitis C, had destroyed his liver. Physicians also diagnosed him with end-stage liver disease.[22] A CT scan found a large tumor on the center of his liver compressing his common bile duct.[23]

Mantle went on the UNOS waiting list for a liver transplant, classified as a Stage 2, the second most urgent.[24] Two days later, he received a liver.[25]

Many felt that Mantle's celebrity had vaulted him to the top. The transplant team was also criticized for giving a transplant to a person with first, liver cancer and second, a lifelong alcoholism. Many felt that Mantle had destroyed his liver on his own and that someone more deserving should have received the transplant. Three months after his transplant, Mantle died from cancer.[26] His case rocked the public's trust in UNOS and its methods of selecting candidates.

Similarly in 1993, the governor of Pennsylvania from 1987 to 1995, Robert Casey, was diagnosed with Appalachian familiar amyloidosis, a rare genetic disease. Seemingly within 10 hours of entering the waiting list, Casey got a combined liver-heart transplant, even though many other candidates were ahead of him.

It was later claimed he had been on the list for a year, but did not want his disease known for political reasons. Pittsburgh's famous transplant program in Pennsylvania also defended Casey's selection, saying he was the only person on a list of people needing both a liver and a heart. After the outcry, UNOS revised its criteria to say that a successful candidate must be atop one of the lists for single organs (which Casey had not been).

Multiple listing is generally permitted, but in July 1990, New York became the first state to ban it (New York is still the only state with such a ban). In 1992, some patients who were multiple listed argued in a hearing before UNOS that forbidding the practice denied them autonomy. They maintained that they had a right as individuals to choose their own physicians; that is, a ban on multiple listing would curtail their "liberty right" to contract for medical care.[27]

There are two powerful arguments against multiple listing. First, a primary attribute of a just medical system is equality of access, and the use of wealth to jump the line violates this norm. Second, multiple listing compromises the entire

UNOS system because some people are getting listed above others arbitrarily. UNOS should be impartial not only in dealing with candidates who are already listed, but also in the actual process of deciding who gets listed.

A similar problem surfaced in the early 1990s, when it was revealed that candidates for neonatal heart transplants were being identified prenatally and then being placed on waiting lists immediately, while they were still fetuses.[28] Because time accumulated on a waiting list gives a candidate extra points, such a practice would offer a significant advantage. In this case, prenatal listing was made possible by the ability to diagnose hypoplastic left heart syndrome (HLHS) in utero; but such early diagnosis is not uniformly distributed in the United States, and early listing of babies diagnosed in utero seemed unfair to babies who were not diagnosed until birth. Moreover, fetuses with HLHS remain relatively safe while they are in the womb, whereas at birth HLHS babies are almost always at great risk and are in NICUs. For these reasons, UNOS changed its policy in June 1992 and put fetuses on a separate list from babies. UNOS also decided to allocate a heart to a fetus only when no baby could use it.

Retransplants

Retransplantation of the same patient raises other issues about justice. Since patients often reject transplanted organs, a second or third transplant can be done. But is it fair to give a particular patient a second heart or kidney when thousands of others never get one? Shouldn't patients only get a second organ when everyone has had a chance at one?

UNOS treats patients waiting for retransplants as first-time patients. This does not lead to the best outcomes. Nearly 82 percent of first-time transplants survive one year, but only 57 percent of retransplants do. Retransplanted patients fare worse than first-transplant patients because they usually are sicker.

Utilitarians see justice as creating the greatest years of life per donated organ. Under such constraints, UNOS should give first-time patients priority over retransplant patients.

But maximal years per organ is not the only value in play. Shouldn't medicine save those who are about to die? Shouldn't others, who are less sick, wait?

Transplant teams bond with patients and find it difficult not to save them. Consider a hypothetical 41-year-old Judy Rogers, a former bank teller now on dialysis and disability who suffers severe depression. This is understandable: the medical team has worked very hard—over many years—to save Judy's life, and when she rejects an organ, the team does not want to be forced by UNOS to watch her die. Medical staffs would see this as *patient abandonment*. More simply, Judy is personally known to nurses, medical students, and the surgeon, whereas new patients are abstractions.

But it is reasonable to ask why identified patients should take priority over new patients: a new patient may benefit more and be more meritorious. Moreover, if the medical teams are allowed to select who gets a new organ, "patients who are better at forming relationships with transplant teams" will be favored.[29]

Although transplant teams identify with retransplanted patients, others may identify with the patients who are waiting. Consider a hypothetical Max Loftin, a 53-year-old accountant with severe depression and dialysis patient waiting for a kidney transplant. A new kidney might cure his depression. But if present patients in hospitals get all next month's available kidneys as second or third retransplants, Max goes on to miss his appointments and hence to die, a nameless victim.

An actual patient named Ronnie DeSillers in Miami, who received *three* liver transplants, caused bitter feelings among patients waiting for a liver. Because his father knew how to work the system, Danny Canal of Wheaton, MD in 1998 received *three quadruple* organ transplants (the first due to multiple-listing). Did eleven other people deserve never to get an organ so Danny could get 12?

The Rule of Rescue

The rule of rescue, named by bioethicist Albert Jonsen, refers to giving scarce medical resources to an identified patient, rather than to equally deserving and equally endangered anonymous people.[30] We can cite countless examples of this rule.

Frequently, the media identify the person. If television follows the plight of a small girl trapped in a deep well, thousands will send dollars for her rescue; meanwhile television doesn't cover the plight of another young boy in peril, he is not rescued, and he dies. Is this just?

In 1982, hospital administrator Charles Fiske interrupted a televised news conference to successfully plead for a liver donation for his daughter, Jamie. For over 25 years since, desperate parents have used such methods to save their children in organ failure.

From the perspective of distributive justice, why is the rule of rescue problematic? Why is it an unjust way to distribute organs?

First, television often identifies the rescued person, but who gets to live shouldn't be decided by who gets on television. Television favors people who look good on television, which means cute, articulate people and families who know how to work reporters. But who gets to live shouldn't be decided by who is most photogenic.

The rule of rescue makes journalists and their editors the gatekeepers of life and death. The rule of rescue replaces the God Committee with the assignment editor ("Oh, we just did a child transplant story. Let's wait a month before we do another.")

And for every identifiable person who is saved, there are a dozen anonymous patients who are lost. If one life is worth the same as another, why is identification by a newspaper important?

When a physician admits a hypothetical Karen Smith to a hospital, Karen becomes identified as a candidate for rescue. Once she is inside, the medical team bonds to the smart, gregarious Karen. Once she is inside, physicians bestow a million dollars worth of publicly funded resources on her. Again, if there are many worthy candidates for a scarce medical resource, who gets to live shouldn't be decided by the likes of hospital staff or the whims of physicians in admitting patients.

Hospitals frequently set up rules and committees to prevent just this sort of thing. Left-ventricle assist devices (LVADs) can be bridges to heart transplants, but if hearts don't materialize, how long can a hospital keep patients on LVADs, especially if the patients have no coverage? The physician who initially admits his patient for an LVAD may feel like he's saved a life and is a hero, but he may be a villain to the hospital's administration, which must pay for the resulting care.

The rule of rescue is really a particular instance of the general conflict between impartial ethical theories and partial ones. On one side, we have Kantian ethics and utilitarianism, which treat everyone the same and which oppose the rule of rescue. On the other side, we have the ethics of care that values particular relationships. Our moral intuitions stem from both kinds of theories, which explains why they pull us in different directions.

It is precisely the pull of partialist theories that attracts us to rescuing the patient before us in the hospital bed. It is precisely such pull that impartial theories urge us to resist in seeking a more impartial way of deciding who gets into the hospital bed in the first place. Partial theories implicitly discount the value of unidentified people not in the circle of concern of the medical team.

Sickest First, UNOS, and the Rule of Rescue

As we have seen, utilitarianism clashes with the ethics of care over retransplants and the same clash looms larger in how UNOS allocates organs.

A utilitarian wanting to maximize human life in the lifeboat for the long row to Africa selects the strongest rowers, tosses the weak, sick, and elderly overboard, and eats the dog. Similarly, utilitarians wanting maximal years per organ only allocate organs to first-timers and allow no retransplants. For impartial ethical theories such as utilitarianism or Kantian ethics, one human life counts as much as another, regardless of whether that life is my father, my neighbor, my patient, my fellow citizen, or a complete stranger.

Piggybacking this logic on some facts leads to a surprising conclusion: giving organs to the sickest patients does not maximize the most years per life per organ. Why? Because some patients are too near death. When they die, the organs have been wasted.

Therefore, the best way to get the most organs per life is to give the organ to moderately sick people just experiencing organ failure. In that way, with a limited supply, more people live longer.

Congress, many surgeons, and the families of many patients reject such an impartial system. As their loved one grows closer to death, they grasp for life. Even if it wastes an organ, they feel that after waiting for years on the list for an organ, they deserve their one chance to live.

So strong is this feeling that in the fall of 2000, Congress *mandated* that the UNOS allocate organs on the basis of *sickest first*. As the Fact Sheet on the UNOS website states: "For heart, liver and intestinal organs, patients whose medical status is most urgent receive priority over those whose medical status is not as urgent."[31]

Howard Eisen, head of Temple University Hospital's heart transplant program, disapproves, "What you're doing is giving hearts to people who will do less well with them. People are waiting longer, so they get sicker, and end up getting two operations when they would otherwise need one."[32]

Sickest first equates the rule of rescue to a standard of distributive justice. Is this fair to the others down the line who took better care of their bodies and therefore who are not now as sick?

Living Donors

For many decades, an ethical bright line existed in transplant surgery of, "First, do no harm," which in part meant "Do not harm one person to benefit another." In 1954, Dr. Joseph Murray successfully transplanted a kidney from Ronald Herrick, a 23-year-old man, into his identical twin Richard, who was dying of kidney disease. Since the transplantation involved identical twins, immunological rejection posed no problem, and Richard accepted the transplanted kidney. Since no compatibility barriers existed, and since a brother's life was saved, the benefits of this surgery appeared to outweigh possible harms to the donor, and consequently ethical concerns were overridden. This precedent demonstrated the viability of live organ transplantation and paved the way for alternatives to cadaveric transplantation.[33]

As noted, half a century later a remarkable change occurred: in 2003, *the number of live donors has surpassed the number of cadaver donors* (brain-dead patients whose relatives consented to harvesting their organs).[34] In 50 years, transplant surgery had leapt from making one exception—an exception from a traditional rule in order to save a life—to a norm where the majority of organs today come from letting people volunteer to have surgeons risk harm to them to benefit another.

In 1989, the first transplant occurred from a healthy parent (a mother) to a daughter—from Teri Smith to Alyssa Smith. While he was removing the lobe of Teri's liver, surgeon Christopher Broelsch of the University of Chicago nicked Teri's spleen and had to excise it. Broelsch called the loss of Teri's spleen a "major complication," saying it gave him "the sickest feeling to have trouble with the first patient."[35]

Also in 1989, Marissa Ayala was conceived to provide stem cells for her sister Anissa, who had leukemia.[36] Preimplantation genetic diagnosis (PGD), the practice of analyzing artificially fertilized embryos, allowed Anissa's parents to choose an embryo that could serve as a compatible bone marrow donor for Anissa. Should Marissa have been conceived as a resource for Anissa? Marissa's bone marrow was taken and given to Anissa, which saved Anissa's life, but does one happy result justify creating a thousand more children to serve as resources for dying siblings?

In 1993, transplant centers accepted and recruited adult relatives of children for organ transplants, and Nilda Rodrìguez gave one-quarter of her liver to her sick granddaughter. In the same year, James and Barbara Sewell each donated part of a lung to their 22-year-old daughter, whose own lungs had been damaged by cystic fibrosis, a genetic disease that is typically fatal by age 30 (the patient usually dies from infection and collapse of the lungs). By 1997, as the practice became more accepted, California surgeon Vaughn Starnes had taken lung lobes from 76 donors for 37 recipients. One commentator in the same year noted that the practice was "ethically problematic," implying that a norm had not yet been established.

From 1990 to 2002, surgeons in St. Louis performed 207 lung transplants on 190 children.[37] All 190 children were under age 18, 121 were ages 10–18, and the most common reason for transplantation was cystic fibrosis. This means that surgeons took lung lobes from 207 healthy adults for these children. Italian surgeons reported similar results for 1996 to 2002, giving 55 people of mean age 25 years a lung transplant.[38]

Something similar happened with liver transplantation among relatives. From a few isolated cases in 1993–1994, such requests eventually became the norm: "There now exists an ethical imperative to develop this [live-donor donation of livers]," said Jean Edmond, MD, director of liver transplantation at New York Presbyterian Hospital in 1999.[39] Between 1996 and 1999, surgeons performed over 70 transplants among adult relatives, with 45 in the first half of 1999, showing exponential growth.

In 1999, officials confirmed the first death from adult-to-adult liver donation and they estimated that two to three other adults had died from donating parts of organs to their children.[40] By 2003, at least five people had died.[41] Exact figures are unknown.

The surgical journal *Transplantation* reported in late 2002 that 56 people who had previously been living organ donors later required a kidney transplant.[42] Of the 56 people, only 43 received transplants, and of these, 36 took. Of these 56 candidates, two died while waiting for an organ and one died after the operation.

Consider the sad case of Walter Wood, 45, who donated to his brother under the impression that kidney transplants were relatively safe and done only to save a life. Wood experienced an unexpected outcome during surgery: his abdominal muscles ruptured. He has since been in constant pain and has been unable to perform the simplest of tasks. As a result of his severe disability, Walter lost his job, had to sell his house, and approached bankruptcy. "I'm in constant pain from the surgeries I've had. I can't even move around in bed," Wood says.

Protecting patients such as Walter Wood is a problem in the system because the transplant team understandably focuses on the sick recipient of the organ, not the donor. Not only that, transplants occur only on people who have medical coverage, so the transplant team and its hospital get paid for medical services to the recipient. In contrast, they receive nothing for caring for donors and give such care at a financial loss. In sum, transplant teams have asymmetrical relationships to donors and to recipients.

After he donated part of his liver to this brother in 2002, newspaper reporter Mike Hurewitz of Albany, NY died a gruesome death at Mount Sinai Hospital in New York City. Also, 69-year-old Barbara Tarrant from North Carolina disastrously donated a kidney to her mentally retarded son and wound up paralyzed on her left side and without coherent speech.[43]

Widely regarded as heroic in the popular media, living donor transplantation carries real dangers. Surprisingly, no one knows how many donors have ended up like Mike Hurewitz, Barbara Tarrant, or Walter Wood. Why? Because living-donor transplant centers have no obligation to report deaths or injuries to the UNOS, nor does UNOS have any legal obligation to monitor such deaths and injuries.

Amazingly, no hospital, transplant center, or medical department tracks deaths and injuries from live donors such as Walter Wood. Once donors leave the hospital, they are on their own—for medical care, for insurance, for follow-up—and no one has done a long-term study on their problems.

Given the lack of such studies, an obvious question arises: without such data, how can donors really give *informed* consent about the risks of donation? If there is no long-term follow-up of the medical problems of past adult donors, how can new donors be really informed of the real risks of organ donation?

Costs and the Medical Commons

The cost of a liver transplant for a child is on average about $146,000 for the operation and $6,000 a year thereafter; a kidney transplant costs $60,000 for the first year and $6,000 a year thereafter; dialysis costs $32,000 a year; an average heart transplant costs $91,000 the first year and $6,000 a year thereafter; a bone-marrow transplant costs $100,000. Figures like these give many people pause.

During the 1970s, the biologist Garrett Hardin discussed the *tragedy of the commons*, a situation in which no one reduces his or her consumption of some public resource, until the resource becomes so ravaged that it disappears. The concept originated centuries ago in England, when pastures held in common were overgrazed: in each town, each shepherd increased his own flock until there were so many animals that the common could no longer support them. Point: unregulated pursuit of self-interest leads to destruction of public resources.

Former Colorado governor Richard Lamm agrees. He has emphasized that Americans cannot continue such extravagant policies and do well. In particular, as a matter of intergenerational justice, America cannot fund extravagant care for the elderly on the backs of the working young: "When a society faces fiscal reality and seeks to optimize its dollars, it not only starts on the road to financial sanity, but it also brings dramatic change to existing medical practices. Dialysis and transplantation will undoubtedly undergo major change."[44]

Lamm continues, "Dr. Thomas Starzl recently gave a liver transplant to a 76-year-old woman. It cost $240,000. Dr. Starzl should understand that with the average U.S. family making $24,000 a year, he has sentenced 10 U.S. families to work all year so that he could transplant a 76 year-old woman."

This topic will be explored much more in the last chapter of this book, where questions of fairness are raised about the 46 million working Americans without medical insurance and their subsidies of those who have insurance. Most of these Americans work and have FICA and Medicare taxes taken from their paychecks—Medicare taxes that pay for dialysis and kidney transplants. Ironically, the only medical care they are entitled to is to be stabilized in emergency rooms and to dialysis, should their kidneys fail.

Non-Heart-Beating Organ Transplantation: The Pittsburgh Protocol

The issue of exactly how a patient, whose body is a potential source of organs, gets declared dead, has simmered in the background of organ transplantation for nearly half a century. Between 1954 and 1967, organs for transplantation either came from living, related donors (e.g., a kidney from one twin to another) or by patients who were dead ("cadavers"). Patients who were declared dead were so declared by cardiopulmonary criteria, that is, their hearts stopped beating and they stopped breathing. This criterion was not ideal because when tissue no longer receives blood, damage occurs very fast, and such damage often occurs while the heart is stopping.

With the Harvard definition of braindeath in 1967, declaration of death in cadavers switched to neocortical criteria, allowing retrieval of organs from cadavers who had their breathing and circulation maintained artificially by respirators. Because the organs procured from patients declared dead this way were not injured, and because all states passed neocortical braindeath laws, procurement of organs for transplantation switched almost entirely to use of the neocortical standard because now organs could be transplanted in better shape for the receiving patient.

In recent years, improvements in automobile safety have reduced the pool of such bodies while burgeoning numbers of transplant programs have learned to transplant sicker people. Supply has dropped while demand has soared.

The University of Pittsburgh Medical Center has perhaps the most aggressive and voluminous transplant program on the globe. In 1993, it developed a protocol to start obtaining organs from patients who were declared dead by the old cardiopulmonary criteria. The novel idea of the Pittsburgh protocol was to manage death in the small class of patients where the cause of death has not damaged the organ already and where the patient or the family has already signed a "do not resuscitate" order. For example, a patient on a respirator is moved to the operating room where his respirator is removed, breathing stops, the surgical team waits two minutes for breathing to resume, the patient is declared dead, and then his organs are removed.

The official name of this protocol is "Non-Heart-Beating Donor" (NHBD). This phrase is not felicitous, for it seems to be an oxymoron (can a cadaver be a "donor"?).

The Pittsburgh protocol declares death after two minutes during which no pulse is detected and ventricular fibrillation, asystole, or electromechanical dissociation occurs. It allows drugs to be administered, such as vasodilators and anticoagulants, that are given solely to maximize health of organs to be transplanted. It declares that death occurs when there is irreversible loss of *cardiac function*, as opposed to the neocortical standard, which declares that death occurs when there is irreversible loss of *all brain activity*, including brain stem activity.

A 1997 study requested of the Institute of Medicine by the Secretary of Health and Human Services distinguished between *controlled* and *uncontrolled* NHBDs. Before the Harvard, neocortical definition of death was adopted, patients died in uncontrolled ways as their hearts stopped beating and injured their other organs. In the Pittsburgh protocol, the IOM said, "the (deaths of) donors are controlled because the timing and thus the process of donation are controlled through the timing of (withdrawal of) life support." These patients generally suffer from severe head injuries or progressive neurological illness.

One aspect of the new protocol that some people have trouble accepting is that the judgment of irreversibility differs from the judgment about lack of neocortical activity. The only way to know if such changes truly are irreversible is to start cardiopulmonary resuscitation (CPR), but in the Pittsburgh protocol, of course, the family and/or competent patient must explicitly decline CPR.

This point must be stressed. Consent of the patient distinguishes physician-assisted dying from murder. If the family has not consented to the Pittsburgh protocol, staff might be charged with accelerating death to harvest organs.

Another point to stress here is that CPR on a dying or elderly patient is a brutal way to die and often involves breaking chest bones. It is a peculiar form of torture practiced in our "advanced" and "modern" society. Fewer than 15 percent of hospital patients who receive CPR ever leave the hospital.[45] If a family understands these facts, it might elect to forgo CPR and allow the Pittsburgh protocol.

Hence the essential idea of the Pittsburgh protocol: Because the family, the patient, and the physicians believe the patient is going to die soon, why not manage the death to create life for others? For the family, something good may come out of the death: the gift of life to another person.

A 1993 conference explored the ethical issues of the Pittsburgh protocol, but did not achieve a consensus. Although all agreed that the dead-donor rule should continue—that is, that organs should only be taken from dead patients—they could not agree on whether families should be allowed to consent to organ procurement under the new protocol. "The Pittsburgh protocol gives an interpretation of irreversible that comes down to a low probability of auto-resuscitation and excludes the possibility of interventions that could restart the heart."

But what about the ethical issue where families consented but did not understand the issues? Critics object on Kantian grounds that the patient is not being treated as "an end in himself." Alan Weisbard argued that the Pittsburgh protocol indirectly brings about the death of some people to benefit others. Medical sociologist Renée Fox thinks it "morally offensive" to ask families, nurses, and residents to be involved in this effort, and criticizes the "macabre" public policy of championing maximal organ transplantation.[46]

In April 1997, the controversy made national news in the worst way when a bioethics professor in Cleveland went to a district attorney, charging that transplant surgeons at the famous Cleveland Clinic were about to violate the law. The headline of the *Cleveland Plain Dealer* was "'Murder, She Said" and a few days later, *60 Minutes* interviewed Mary Ellen Waithe and broke the story nationally. Other bioethicists criticized Waithe's elevation of a dispute in public policy to charges of illegal activities with overtones of criminal mischief.

The *60 Minutes* story on the Cleveland Clinic revealed that the University of Wisconsin Medical Center had been using a NHBD controlled-death protocol to harvest organs for over 20 years. During this show, a point of contention was whether the administration of heparin and regitine accelerated the death of donors. Heparin, a blood thinner, prevents clot formation, and regitine dilates blood vessels, keeping organs perfused with blood.

The claim that administration of heparin and regitine hastens death is hotly denied by surgeons at centers using the new protocols. The Institute of Medicine study vindicated such surgeons, noting the NHBD protocols across the country divided evenly between allowing the use at some stage in the donation process of one or both of these agents and expressly prohibiting or not mentioning them.

In most cases, it allowed careful administration. Nevertheless, because under certain circumstances in certain patients, there is a concern that these agents might be harmful, this report recommends case-by-case decisions on the use of anticoagulants and vasodilators and consideration of additional safeguards such as involvement of the patients' attending physician in prescribing decisions. The Institute of Medicine also recommended waiting five minutes, rather than two, after life-support was removed, before declaring death.[47]

The God Committee, Again

It's easy to criticize. Critics of the God Committee probably couldn't do a better job. Problem drinkers like Ernie Crowfeather, immature people, and people with poor personal hygiene fare poorly on dialysis and dialysis nurses often hate them.

Life on dialysis is not great. It has a high symptom burden, meaning that quality of life is low. As one nephrologist reports about the unpleasant daily life of his patients on dialysis,

> Insomnia is extraordinarily common and many [patients] experience severe muscle cramping and pains of different sorts. Itching is an equally common phenomenon, along with nausea, vomiting, and poor spirits. Our data indicates that among the roughly 300,000 patients undergoing dialysis in any given year, about 65,000 (or 23%) will die.[48]

So the God Committee was not so arbitrary after all to think about which people had the strength of character to endure these procedures. Today, when everyone is entitled to dialysis, many patients indirectly commit suicide by failing to comply with regimens or by missing appointments. The life-expectancy for dialysis patients is between one-eighth and one-third of the rest of the population, in part because many patients who are old and sick with other diseases get dialyzed in America.[49]

In 2006, a new form of home dialysis became available called *Rogosin dialysis* or *nocturnal dialysis*.[50] It requires a $13,000 dialysis machine at home and a $5,000 water purifier, but it can be done at home, six nights a week for eight hours each night. Complying with nocturnal dialysis means not needing to go to dialysis clinics three times a week for out-patient dialysis under nursing supervision.

But, as in the early days of home dialysis, nocturnal dialysis requires strict attention to cleanliness and personal hygiene. Even hair of dogs and cats may clog the machine, so they exclude patients. At present, patients with poor hygiene or unwilling to part with pets cannot use Rogosin dialysis. So history, and its ethical issues, repeat.

FURTHER READING AND RESOURCES

Renée Fox and Judith Swazey, *The Courage to Fail: A Social View of Organ Transplants and Dialysis*, 2d ed. rev., University of Chicago Press, Ill., 1974, 1978.

Institute of Medicine, *Non-Heart-Beating Organ Transplantation—Medical and Ethical Issues in Procurement*, National Academy Press, Washington, D.C., 1997.

René Fox and Judith Swazey, *Spare Parts: Organ Replacement in American Society*, Oxford University Press, New York, 1992.

Thomas Starzl, *The Puzzle People: Memoirs of a Transplant Surgeon*, University of Pittsburgh Press, Pa., 1992.

CHAPTER 14

Using One Baby for Another

Babies Fae, Gabriel, and Theresa, Plus Separating Conjoined Twins

This chapter discusses the 1984 case of Baby Fae, who briefly lived with a baboon's heart, the 1987 case of Baby Gabriel, an anencephalic baby whose heart went to another infant, Paul Holc, the 1992 case of the anencephalic Baby Theresa, whose parents wanted to donate her heart to another baby, and a series of cases about separating conjoined twins. All these cases raise issues about how dying babies are used in experimental medicine and about how one dying baby is used to help another.

The Case of Baby Fae, 1984

The infant known as Baby Fae was born at a hospital in Barstow, California, on October 14, 1984. Three weeks premature, she weighed five pounds. Noticing her pallor, the pediatrician transferred her to Loma Linda Hospital, a Seventh-Day Adventist facility near Riverside, California, about 60 miles from Los Angeles. Physicians there diagnosed her with hypoplastic left heart syndrome (HLHS).

Affecting one in 10,000 babies, HLHS leaves the normally powerful left side of the heart and aorta underdeveloped and thus too weak to pump blood. HLHS almost always kills infants within two weeks.

Fae's mother was 23-years-old, a Roman Catholic, unmarried, unemployed, and had no medical insurance; Fae's father was a 35-year-old laborer. The two had a son and had lived together for five years, but at Fae's birth, they were separated.

At Loma Linda, doctors told the mother that Fae would soon die; she was kept overnight in the hospital and then released. The mother had Fae baptized and took her to a motel to wait for her to die.

Transplantation of an organ from one species to another is a *xenograft*. Before this case, xenografts were rare and unpromising. In 1964, James Hardy implanted a chimpanzee heart into a 68-year-old man, who lived 90 minutes.[1] In 1977, Christiaan Barnard piggybacked a baboon heart next to the heart of a 25-year-old Italian woman, who lived 300 minutes; he later used the same technique to implant a chimpanzee heart in a 59-year-old man who lived less than four days. During the 1960s, Thomas Starzl and Keith Reemtsma performed six transplants each with simian (primate) kidneys and had better luck, but eventually abandoned the projects.[2] Baboon kidneys worked at best only two months. In 1975, a

British cardiologist connected veins and arteries of a dying one-year-old boy to a live baboon, neither of whom lived through the operation.

Leonard Bailey, the 41-year-old chief of pediatric surgery at Loma Linda, had been aggressively pursuing animal-to-human heart transplants for seven years. According to physician and critic Kenneth Stoller, during this period Bailey had performed "about 160 cross-species transplants, mostly on sheep and goats, none of whom survived more than six months."[3] For the previous 14 months, Loma Linda's Institutional Review Board had been considering xenografts by Bailey, and it had recently granted him permission for five operations.

When Baby Fae first came to the hospital and options were discussed with her mother, Bailey was away at a convention. When he returned on October 16, he called Baby Fae's mother to discuss a xenograft.

On October 19, Baby Fae was readmitted to Loma Linda and placed on a respirator. The surgeon discussed the operation for several hours with Fae's mother, father, and grandmother. Fae's mother watched a slide show about the operation. Both parents then signed a consent form, which had been reviewed in great detail by the IRB; they later signed a second form.

Bailey's immunologist, Sandra Nehlsen-Cannarella, began antigen-typing tests to find the best match for Fae among potential baboon donors; these tests would take six days. Using Fae's reaction to her own blood and tissue as a control, Nehlsen-Cannarella tested the following beings for compatibility: Baby Fae's mother (finding a weak immune reaction), some lab workers (strong reaction), herself (strong reaction), three baboons (strong reaction), and three additional baboons (weak reaction). A baboon named Goobers had a "very, very weak" reaction, so she became the source of the xenograft.[4]

The fact that a baboon heart might be used at all indicates a common ancestor of humans and primates. There is considerable similarity between human blood and the blood of primates, thus we might expect to find some close matches between humans and primates. Moreover, one-third of humans have a preformed antibody against tissue from other humans. About 70 percent of humans also have a preformed antibody against baboon tissue; Baby Fae was among the 30 percent who did not. Bailey gave this fact considerable weight, arguing that ignorance about human-baboon matching explained Hardy's earlier failures with xenografts.

Yet other primates are closer to humans in evolution, so Bailey was once asked on a radio show why, in view of these facts about evolution, he had picked a baboon rather than a chimpanzee. He surprisingly replied, "Er, I find that difficult to answer. You see, I don't believe in evolution."[5]

On October 26, the tissue-typing tests arrived, and Baby Fae's heart was said to have started dying and her lungs to be swelling with fluid. Whether Fae was dying at this point is important: According to the hospital's spokesperson, a baboon heart was used because there was no time to find a compatible human heart, so the transplant had to take place right away.

The source, Goobers, was a nine-month-old female baboon, purchased from the Foundation for Biomedical Research in Texas. According to standard procedure, Bailey placed Fae on a heart-lung machine that lowered her blood temperature to 68 degrees. Meanwhile, Goobers was sedated, and Bailey excised her walnut-sized heart. He then removed Fae's defective heart and replaced it with Goobers's healthy one.

Over the next four hours, he connected the transplanted heart and transplanted arteries. Then the heart-lung machine raised Fae's temperature to 98 degrees, and Goobers's heart began to beat spontaneously inside Fae.

On October 29, nurses weaned Fae from her respirator. On November 5, Bailey predicted that the animal heart would grow with Fae, and that she might celebrate her 20th birthday.

At the time, Christiaan Barnard predicted that soon medicine would have baboon farms for simian xenografts. Barney Clark's surgeon, William DeVries, said, "I really have sympathy for what [Bailey and his colleagues] are going through."[6]

Two weeks after surgery, Fae showed the first signs of rejection of the donor heart. Soon she deteriorated and went back on a respirator.

On November 15, Fae developed a heart blockage and renal failure; her physicians started closed-heart massage and dialysis. She then died, having lived 21 days with her baboon heart.

Bailey attempted no more xenografts, but other surgeons did. In 1992, Thomas Starzl at the University of Pittsburgh transplanted a baboon liver into a 35-year-old man with hepatitis B. He lived 70 days. The same year, a woman waiting for a human liver at Cedars Sinai Medical Center in Los Angeles received a pig liver as a bridge to a transplant, but died 32 hours later. In 1993, a man with hepatitis B received a baboon liver at the University of Pittsburgh; he was 62-years-old and near death at the time, and he died during the operation. Since 1905, baboon organs were transplanted to humans in 33 operations, but none succeeded.

Surgeons hope that transferring human genes into pigs will allow porcine xenografts, but none have worked to date. Even when drugs suppress immunorejection, a more lethal *hyperacute rejection* soon occurs in all xenografts.

ETHICAL ISSUES

Animal Donors and Animal Rights

Animal activists criticized Bailey: "This is medical sensationalism at the expense of Baby Fae, her family, and the baboon," said Lucy Shelton of People for the Ethical Treatment of Animals.[7] Activists protested outside Loma Linda Hospital, claiming that Fae's life was not intrinsically worth more than Goobers's. The philosopher Tom Regan claimed the operation had "two victims:" Fae and Goobers.

Regan argues that beings who "have a life" have a *right* to life. He held that Goobers had a biographical life in that it mattered to her whether she would live or have her heart cut out: "Like us, Goobers was somebody, a distinct individual." Regan argued that all primates have equal moral value, so Goobers did not exist as Fae's resource:

> Those people who seized [Goobers's] heart, even if they were motivated by their concern for Baby Fae, grievously violated Goobers's right to be treated with

respect. That she could do nothing to protest, and that many of us failed to recognize the transplant for the injustice that it was, does not diminish the wrong, a wrong settled before Baby Fae's sad death.[8]

Regan argued that even if human beings had obtained benefits in the past from using animals, such use was intrinsically wrong.

Other animal-rights philosophers emphasized that the difference between Baby Fae and Goobers, considering how young both were and what their individual potential might be, was not as great as the difference between Baby Fae and an anencephalic baby.[9] Anencephalic babies lack potential cognitive ability, whereas Goobers has more cognition, agency, and consciousness than either such a baby or a healthy newborn.

Some philosophers contemplated the large breeding facility from which Goobers had been bought and offered the image of a similar facility supplying anencephalic babies as sources of organs. If this image is repugnant, they asked, why do we tolerate such a facility for primates, especially when such primates are *more like us* than severely retarded humans? Are we just in denial?

So why not use an anencephalic newborn as a donor? As we shall see, this logic prevailed in the later cases of Baby Gabriel and Baby Theresa.

Bailey retorted that animal lovers picketing his campus were "born of a luxurious society" and implied that only in California would surgeons have to confront such activists: "People in southern California have it so good that they can afford to worry about this type of issue."[10] Moreover, "When it gets down to a human living or dying, there shouldn't be a question" of using an animal to save that human.

The director of Loma Linda's Center for Christian Bioethics agreed:

> On an ethical scale, we will always place human beings ahead of subhumans, especially in a situation where people can be genuinely saved by animals. That is the story of mankind from the very beginning. Animals, for example, have always been used for food and clothing.[11]

Of animal-rights activists, Fae's mother said, "They don't know what they're talking about."[12]

Alternative Treatment?

Was alternative treatment possible? One alternative to a xenograft for Fae was a human donor heart. Loma Linda claimed that the xenograft was necessary because Baby Fae was dying and no human heart was available. Bailey argued that it would be impossible to find a heart because the donor would have to be less than seven weeks old, and criteria for neonatal brain death were problematical ("You can have a flat EEG on a newborn, and yet the baby will survive").[13]

Most neonatal transplants come from anencephalic babies; and Bailey maintained that most parents of such infants would refuse to accept the fact that their baby was brain-dead, and would not agree to donate the baby's organs in time. He described the baboon heart as Baby Fae's "only chance to live."

An associate surgeon at Loma Linda defended Bailey:

> It would have to be the sort of case where an infant fell out of a crib and was declared brain dead but the heart was okay. Then all these tests would have to be done to insure a proper matching. With Baby Fae, we had five days to do those tests, getting the best possible [animal] donor. With a human heart, we might not have been able to keep the recipient alive.[14]

In his memoirs, surgeon Thomas Starzl describes Paul Teraski as a "symbol of integrity" in the transplant community.[15] Teraski, director of the Southern California Regional Organ Procurement Agency, said that an infant heart had been available *on the day* of Baby Fae's xenograft. Teraski added, "I think that they [the Loma Linda team] did not make any effort to get a human infant heart because they were set on doing a baboon."[16]

Bailey agreed that he didn't look for a human heart:

> We were not searching for a human heart. We were out to enter the whole new area of transplanting tissue-matched baboon hearts into newborns who are supported with antisuppressive drugs. I suppose that we could have used a human heart that was outsized and that was not tissue-matched, and that would have pacified some people, but it would have been very poor science. On the other hand, I suppose my belief that there are no newborn hearts available for transplantation was more opinion than data or science, but it is scientific to acknowledge that the whole area of determining brain death of newborns is very problematical.[17]

Another alternative existed. Pediatric surgeon William Norwood had developed surgery for HLHS that attempted to repair the left ventricle. He had performed his operation many times at Children's Hospitals in Philadelphia, with a success rate of 40 percent. Bailey claimed that children did not do well enough after the Norwood procedure to justify this operation for Baby Fae. But given Bailey's interest in xenografts, was he an impartial judge? Also, can you use the "poor science" retest and not believe in evolution?

Babies as Subjects of Research

For critics, what was objectionable about Bailey's surgery was not that it was risky or experimental—after all, surgery can discover what is possible only by trying. What was objectionable was that Bailey used a baby, who could not consent. In the decades since the earlier attempts at xenografts, the only new developments had been cyclosporin and better tissue matching, and both could have been used in a consulting adult.

In addition to questions about whether using Fae made sense medically, a more general question is whether parents should volunteer children as research subjects in any circumstances. Protestant theologian Paul Ramsey argued that it is always wrong for parents to volunteer their children as subjects of *nontherapeutic* research:

> If today we mean to give such weight to the research imperative, then we should not seek to give a principled justification of what we are doing with children. It is better to leave the research imperative in incorrigible conflict with the principle that protects the individual human person from being used for research purposes without

either his expressed or correctly construed consent. Some sorts of human experimentation should, in this alternative, be acknowledged to be "borderline situations" in which moral agents are under the necessity of doing wrong for the sake of the public good. Either way they do wrong. It is immoral not to do the research. It is also immoral to use children who cannot themselves consent and who ought not to be presumed to consent to research unrelated to their treatment. On this supposition research medicine, like politics, is a realm in which men have to "sin bravely."[18]

Catholic theologian Richard McCormick demurred, holding that parents can volunteer children for "low-risk" nontherapeutic research.[19] Based on the Roman Catholic tradition of natural law, he argued that just as adults should volunteer for low-risk, nontherapeutic research, infants should be volunteered for the same kind of research.

Interestingly, neither Ramsey nor McCormick uses the utilitarian justification of the greatest good for the greatest number. To many people, though, utilitarianism offers the most natural justification. If no one volunteered for such research, progress would halt, so for the general good, both adults and babies should participate. Because HLHS is a congenital defect of babies, how can treatment for it advance unless some HLHS babies participate in research?

Informed Consent

Many people wondered whether Bailey had carefully described the Norwood procedure to Fae's mother. Was she informed that a human donor was available on the day of Fae's surgery?

The crucial fact here is that Fae's mother had no medical insurance. The xenograft was offered for free. Fae's mother had no money for the Norwood procedure or for a human heart transplant. Costs for such a transplant can be $250,000 with immunosuppressive drugs costing $20,000 a year for life thereafter.

Bioethicist and University of Southern California law professor Alexander Capron summed up this criticism:

> Doubts linger, not only about the adequacy of the information supplied to Baby Fae's parents, but about whether their personal difficulties made it possible for them to choose freely, and whether the realization that their child was dying may have left them with the erroneous conclusion that consenting to the transplant was the only "right" thing to do.[20]

In most respects, the mother's poverty and lack of insurance rendered her consent meaningless. Faced with the death of her baby and no other realistic options, what else could she choose?

And was the mother informed about the probable outcome of the xenograft? Did Baby Fae's mother understand that Bailey's xenograft was a shot in the dark, unlikely to work, and a procedure that might merely extend her baby's dying?

Historically, lack of informed consent was always a problem with xenografts. Boston University law professor George Annas emphasized that in previous attempts to implant animal hearts in humans, patients were poor, vulnerable, and rarely consented.

In 1963, Keith Reemtsma at Columbia University implanted chimpanzee kidneys in a 43-year-old African-American man who was dying of glomerulonephritis. In 1964, James Hardy at the University of Mississippi implanted a chimpanzee heart into a poor, deaf, mute man who was dying, was carried to the hospital unconscious, never consented to the operation, and survived for only two hours. These operations were experimental, not therapeutic, and were characterized by exploitation and lack of consent. Annas saw Baby Fae's case as a continuation of such practices. Calling Bailey the champion of the "anything goes" school of experimentation, he concluded:

> This inadequately reviewed, inappropriately consented to, premature experiment on an impoverished, terminally ill newborn was unjustified. It differs from the xenograft experiments of the early 1960s only in the fact that there was prior review of the proposal by an IRB. But this distinction did not protect Baby Fae. She remained unprotected from ruthless experimentation in which her only role was that of victim.[21]

The Media

This case drew an enormous amount of attention from the media. True, Loma Linda tried to protect the family's privacy and confidentiality, but it and Bailey withheld more than identifying details. Their account of events leading up to the surgery was confusing; hospital spokespersons gave occasional misstatements of fact; and Loma Linda refused to release a copy of the consent form which Fae's parents had signed. Journalists complained about secrecy and the public's right to know.

This situation formed an interesting contrast to the case two years earlier of Barney Clark's artificial heart. Just as many reporters came to Loma Linda as to Utah, but they got much less information. William DeVries had held daily press briefings; Bailey held fewer. Reporters accused Loma Linda of ineptitude and said that aspects of the case begged for clarification.

While Bailey and Loma Linda were accused of reticence, they were also accused of publicity seeking, self-promotion, grandstanding, and adventurism.[22] In contrast, Keith Reemtsma at Columbia University gave no news conferences until his patient had been discharged from the hospital and until he had prepared and submitted a scientific paper. Reemtsma argued:

> Science and news are, in a sense, asymmetrical and sometimes antagonistic. News emphasizes uniqueness, the immediacy, the human interest, in a case such as [Baby Fae's]. Science emphasizes verification, controls, comparisons, and patterns.[23]

Law professor Alex Capron argued similarly:

> There was a time when the public learned of biomedical developments after they had been reviewed by, and generally reported to, the researchers' scientific and medical peers [a procedure that protected everyone's dignity and meant that the public would learn only of genuine advances] rather than merely being titillated by bizarre cases of as yet unproven import.[24]

As we shall see below, this criticism also applies to separation of conjoined twins, which has almost never been done as part of a scientific protocol where results are carefully studied over decades.

Therapy or Research?

Was Fae's xenograft therapy or research? Was alternative treatment available? Did the xenograft have a chance to help Fae, or was she just one sacrifice among thousands on the altar of medical research?

A *therapeutic* procedure offers a patient a reasonable chance of benefit; a procedure which offers little chance is *research* and *experimental*. This medical distinction can be expressed in Kantian ethics as the difference between treating people as "ends in themselves" and using them as "mere means." Essayist Charles Krauthammer wrote:

> Civilization hangs on the Kantian principle that human beings are to be treated as ends and not means. So much depends on that principle because there is no crime that cannot be, that has not been, committed in the name of the future against those who inhabit the present. Medical experimentation, which invokes the claims of the future, necessarily turns people into means.[25]

Was Bailey's best scenario possible? Was there a probability that Fae could have lived to 20 with a baboon heart? At one point, Bailey phrased his claim differently, saying that Fae had a chance to "celebrate more than one birthday with her new heart."[26] Was this modest scenario possible?

Bailey claimed his operation had *therapeutic intent*:

> I have always believed it would work, or I would not have attempted it. . . . There was always therapeutic intent. My dilemma has been educating the university and the medical profession.[27]

He made these comments nine days after the operation, when Baby Fae was still alive and seemed to be doing well. He also said that xenografts might soon be preferable to human transplants.

Immunologist Nehlsen-Cannarella argued that, if a perfect match had been found with the best-matched lymphocytes, the operation could have been therapeutic. With such a perfect match, Fae could have accepted the heart.

Other surgeons castigated Bailey, rejecting the idea of *therapeutic intent* and saying that Bailey needed *therapeutic probability*. Almost any experimental surgery has a remote chance of being therapeutic, but that's not enough.

These surgeons also rejected Bailey's and Nehlsen-Cannarella's claim about tissue typing. In 1970, Paul Teraski had discovered that while tissue typing can improve transplants within families, it couldn't outside of families. Surgeons resisted Teraski's findings, but accepted the limitations his results suggested. Thomas Starzl wrote in 1992:

> Twenty years later the only controversy is whether matching under all circumstances means enough to be given any consideration in the distribution of cadaver kidneys. By exposing the truth, Teraski had made it clear that the field of clinical transplantation could advance significantly only by the development of better

drugs and other treatment strategies, not by vainly hoping that the solution would be through tissue matching.[28]

Most transplant surgeons agreed. The American expert on pediatric transplants, John Najarian at the University of Minnesota, said of the Baby Fae case: "There has never been a successful cross-species transplant. To try it now is merely to prolong the dying process."[29] He also said that Fae's death on November 15 was "reasonably close to what could be expected," because three weeks was about how long it usually takes for rejection to do its damage.

In a review of this case, the editor of *Journal of Heart Transplantation* concluded:

> These clinical attempts demonstrated that the human body could acutely tolerate primate hearts, at least for a few days, but no evidence was found to suggest that these grafts could be accepted for prolonged periods of time with the available methods of immunosuppression. . . . Using presently available means of immunosuppression and immunomanipulation, there is no evidence that a vital organ can be transplanted from one species to another and result in prolonged survival of the recipient . . . .
>
> From the experimental data and past clinical attempts, there is nothing to indicate that a human infant will tolerate a primate heart for months or years using today's means to induce and control tolerance. The Loma Linda surgical team has not informed the medical community, as yet, of any new evidence that might suggest the contrary.[30]

The case against Baby Fae's transplant as therapy may be summed up as follows:

First, it had been known since 1970 that better antigen matches between donor and recipient would not improve transplants.

Second, even the best matches required long-term maintenance on cyclosporin. Bailey claimed that infants can be given larger dosages of cyclosporin than adults, but cyclosporin eventually produces toxic side effects.[31] The autopsy on Baby Fae indicated that her kidneys were probably poisoned by the massive dosages of cyclosporin she received.

Third, Bailey argued that since an infant's immune system is not fully developed, babies might initially tolerate xenografts. But this is not certain; and even if it were true, an initial success would be followed by failure as the baby's immune system developed and rejected the xenograft.

Fourth, only one heart xenograft had been tried previously, and this had a disastrous result.

Fifth, Loma Linda was a small medical institution. In their zeal to perform a xenograft and be famous, the staff was blind to their own limitations.

Sixth, Bailey himself was an amateur: He had never performed a human heart transplant, and he had never published about xenografts.

Taking all this into account, Baby Fae had no chance of surviving one year, let alone reaching her 20th birthday. Thus the surgery was not therapeutic but experimental. *Nature* concluded that "the serious difficulty over [Bailey's] operation . . . is that it may have catered to the researchers' needs first and to the patient's only second."[32] In his essay in *Time*, Krauthammer said that Baby Fae had lived and died in the realm of experimentation:

> Only the bravery was missing: no one would admit the violation. Bravery was instead fatuously ascribed to Baby Fae, a creature as incapable of bravery as she was of circulating her own blood. Whether this case was an advance in medical science awaits the examination of the record by the scientific community. That it was an adventure in medical ethics is already clear.[33]

In a review of the case, the American Medical Association and top medical journals criticized Bailey, concluding that xenografts should be undertaken only as part of a systematic research program with controls in randomized clinical trials.[34]

Baby Gabriel and Paul Holc, 1987

Like the Terri Schiavo case two decades later, the Baby Fae case received saturation coverage in the media, making Bailey and Loma Linda household names. When his xenograft program failed, Bailey tried to use his new fame to create a center for heart failure on infants with HLHS with donated hearts from anencephalic babies.

In 1987, surgeons and medical ethicists at a conference in Ontario, Canada, who were sympathetic to Bailey's goal (Bailey had been a resident in cardiac surgery in Ontario in 1974), created guidelines for using anencephalics as organ donors, guidelines called the *Ontario Protocol*.

The most important of its guidelines was that an anencephalic baby could become a donor only after being pronounced dead by the classical criteria of brain death. Another guideline was that the potential donor could not be expected to live more than one week; this standard was meant to ensure that the donor was born dying. At birth, an anencephalic was to be put on a respirator to preserve its organs, then taken off every six hours to see if it could breathe on its own. If a baby failed to breathe for three minutes, it could be declared brain-dead by three physicians independent of the transplant team.

It should be noted that the respirator is necessary in this protocol because the normal course of anencephaly is for the heart gradually to stop beating: this diminishes blood flow, so the organs become anoxic and start to deteriorate; by the time the brain stem is dead, the heart and kidneys are no longer useful for transplantation.

Because maintaining the brain stem may prevent a potential donor from becoming brain dead, the Ontario protocol was ill-conceived.

UCLA pediatric neurologist Allan Shewmon severely criticized the Ontario Protocol (he also criticized the idea of "minimally conscious state" in the Schiavo case). The leading authority on anencephaly, Shewmon held that anencephalic babies should not be used as donors at all because there was no consensus in neurology about determining brain death in them.[35]

The Ontario protocol was not applied to a case until February 1988, though it had been in the news for some time before that.

In October 1987, a Canadian couple, Karen and Fred Schouten, learned after eight months of pregnancy that their fetus was anencephalic. They decided to bring it to term and to donate its organs. When her heart began to fail after birth, the baby, a girl named Gabriel, was ventilated. The United Network for Organ Sharing (UNOS) was alerted, but no potential recipients were found in Canada or the northeastern United States.

Meanwhile, at Loma Linda Hospital, Bailey was working with another couple, Gordon and Paul Holc, also Canadian, whose eight-month fetus had HLHS and needed a heart transplant and who had come to Loma Linda because of the publicity it was receiving. The Schoutens and Gabriel flew to Loma Linda. There, the Holcs' baby, Paul, was prematurely delivered by cesarean section to get the donor heart. Three hours later, Gabriel Schouten's heart was excised and transplanted into Paul Holc's chest.

This was the first time a transplant from an anencephalic baby to another infant resulted in a baby who could grow up and lead a normal life. In gratitude to the Schoutens and to Bailey, the Holcs named their baby Paul Gabriel Bailey Holc. Karen Schouten later said that she felt good about her decision and how it had benefited Paul Holc: "Paul is very special to me because he has a part of our baby inside him. One day maybe I'll see him. I hope he comes to me when he's 30 years old and says, 'Hi. Guess what? I made it.'"[36]

In 1994, NBC aired a TV movie about the case, which ended by showing the real Paul playing in first grade and hugging the real Karen Schouten. Paul Holc, aka "The Incredible Holc," turned 13 in 2000 and was healthy and doing well.

Perhaps waiting too long for a consensus, Bailey never applied the Ontario Protocol in the Schouten-Holc case. Its first application came at Loma Linda in 1988 with Michael and Brenda Winners and their anencephalic baby. That case had a sad result: No recipients were found.

This was the first of 12 unsuccessful attempts by Bailey to transplant organs from anencephalic babies to other babies.[37] Of these 12 potential donors, 10 lived beyond the one-week limit, one could not be matched to a recipient, and in the remaining case the physicians decided against a transplant. In 1988, Bailey suspended his transplant program. There was a de facto moratorium on transplants from anencephalics until the 1992 case of Baby Theresa raised the issue again.

Baby Theresa, 1992

In 1991 in Fort Lauderdale, Florida, Laura Campo and Justin Pearson—who were not married—conceived a child. Like Fae's mother, Laura had no medical insurance and did not see a physician until her 24th week of pregnancy. During her eighth month of pregnancy, she learned that her fetus was anencephalic.

Anencephaly is a congenital neurological disorder characterized by absence of the cerebrum and cerebellum, as well as the top of the skull, resulting in exposure of the brain stem.[38] However, anencephaly "does not mean the complete absence of the head or brain."[39] Because there is a brain stem, an electroencephalogram can be taken, and autonomic functions such as breathing and heartbeat may be present. Anencephalics do not meet Harvard criteria of brain death.

Because the diagnosis of anencephaly was made so late in Laura Campo's pregnancy, and because Laura's health was not in danger from the fetus, no legal abortion could be performed. Like most mothers of anencephalic fetuses, Laura said that if she had known the diagnosis earlier, she would have aborted.

After hearing a talk show about organ donation from anencephalic babies, Laura decided to bring the fetus to term to serve as a source of organs.

Anencephaly occurs in one in 500 pregnancies. Over 95 percent identified pre-natally are aborted. Of those carried to term, 60 percent are stillborn. Since an anencephalic is likely to have a swollen head (hydrocephalus), vaginal delivery may kill it, and Laura had a cesarean delivery to keep the organs healthy for transplantation.

Anencephaly is perhaps the most serious of all birth defects, because the baby essentially lacks the higher brain necessary for personhood. Anencephalics are born dying. There is no hope of growth into childhood or adulthood. The open skull is vulnerable to infection, and most anencephalics die within one week, though in rare cases some have lived for one year.[40]

Anencephalics are the major potential source of donor organs for other babies born with congenital defects. When the recipient is an infant, a donor organ must be very small, and so an infant donor is needed. However, few infants are involved in accidents that leave them brain dead but with healthy organs. Babies who die as a result of abuse or from sudden infant death syndrome usually have damaged organs that are unsuitable for transplantation.

In the United States, 2,000 babies a year need organ transplants; this number includes 600 babies with HLHS, about 500 with liver failure, and another 500 with kidney failure. About 300 anencephalic babies are born alive each year.

Using anencephalics as organ donors has been possible since 1967. A few days after Christiaan Barnard's transplant, Adrian Kantrowitz transplanted a heart from an anencephalic baby into another infant, who died six hours later.[41] Kantrowitz had almost performed a similar operation 18 months earlier, but he had to wait for the anencephalic donor's heart to stop beating, and then restart it, which proved impossible.

Laura Campo's baby girl was born on March 21, 1992, and named Theresa Ann Campo Pearson. Some physicians expected her to die within minutes, but she did not. Pictures of Theresa showed a beautiful baby wearing a pink knitted cap that covered the top half of her head. Underneath the cap were no skin, no skull, and no cerebrum. Removing the cap revealed the brain stem inside a partial skull.

Under Florida law, before Theresa's organs could be donated, she had to be declared brain dead. Like most states, Florida used the Harvard standard of brain death. The neonatologist said that unless Baby Theresa was declared brain dead, he would not remove the organs.

Laura Campo and Justin Pearson then asked Judge Estella Moriarty of the cir-cuit court to rule Theresa brain dead so her organs could be donated. But Judge Moriarty correctly ruled against the couple: "[I am] unable to authorize someone to take your baby's life, however short—however unsatisfactory—to save another child. Death is a fact, not an opinion."[42]

The couple appealed to Florida's District Court of Appeals, which affirmed Judge Moriarty's decision and which ended the case medically. On March 29, Theresa began to experience organ failure. At this point, the neonatologist said, "We had to tell the parents [that] all they were doing was prolonging the baby's death."[43] The respirator was removed and Theresa died the next day. By that time, her organs were useless for transplantation.

On the day of their baby's death, Laura Campo and Justin Pearson appeared on television to plead for a change in Florida's laws regarding brain death. Laura Campo was upset and depressed, and it was questionable whether she should have been allowed to undergo the strain of being on the show (but that is a question of media ethics, isn't it, not medical ethics?). A calm, eloquent surgeon joined them and discussed the need for donor organs.

Even though Baby Theresa was dead, in September the Florida Supreme Court heard arguments in the case for purposes of public policy. It decided not to change the law and that anencephalic newborns should *not be* considered dead for organ donation.[44]

ETHICAL ISSUES

Infants as Donors

The cases of Baby Theresa and Baby Gabriel raised basic questions about using such infants as sources of organs. Should any baby be used for the good of another baby? If so, what are the criteria?

One argument against using infants as organ donors is their vulnerability. In general, the more vulnerable people are, the less defensible it is to do something to them without their consent, and babies are considered the most vulnerable of all.

In this regard, a question of terminology arises. When an infant's organ is used as a transplant, who is giving what as a "gift"? Terms like donation and "the gift of life" seem to be inappropriate in this situation; since no baby ever consents to donate his or her organs, a baby cannot really be described as providing a gift.

More accurate terms are: "organ salvage," "organ transfer," "organ recovery," "organ reassignment," and so on. Such terms seem cold, and this connotation suggests why people resist using infants' organs as sources for other infants and why organ procurement agents prefer phrases such as "gift of life."

On the other hand, one possible argument in favor of using infants' organs for transplants would be analogous to McCormick's argument: Parents should choose for a child as the child ought to choose in adulthood. Another possible argument is utilitarian: Infants' organs should be used for transplant if that resulted in the greatest good for the greatest number.

Anencephalics and Brain Death

One vital question in the debate over anencephalics as donors has to do with brain death. Some critics have argued that there are no good criteria for brain death in infants, and whether or not this is true, brain death in anencephalic infants is unclear.

Anencephaly is a medical term describing a range of gross congenital brain deficits, all of which entail no chance of normal brain function but some of which do not entail immediate brain death.[45] The fact that most babies do not die the first week—and thus could not be donors under the Ontario guidelines—illustrates this problem, because some kinds of anencephaly are something like persistent vegetative state (PVS); therefore, with maximal supportive care, some anencephalic infants could survive indefinitely. One critic said, "I have an uneasy feeling that what lurks behind the anencephalic issue is the vegetative state issue."[46]

Some commentators have suggested creating a new category of legal brain death, or an exemption from the usual legal criteria of brain death, to allow for transfers of organs from anencephalic babies. Such a new category or exemption is needed for organ donation because anencephalic infants are neither dead nor about to die quickly enough, and allowing them to die naturally could destroy their organs.

So the question boils down to this: Should we change our criteria of brain death for infants to get more organs from other dying infants?

The parents of Baby Theresa hoped that their case would help create pressure for such an exemption in Florida. Disability advocates opposed changing the Florida law: "Treating anencephalics as dead equates them with 'nonpersons,' presenting a 'slippery slope' problem with regard to all other persons who lack cognition for whatever reason."[47]

Two physicians considered a proposal to adopt a system used in Germany, where anencephalics are considered "brain-absent" and therefore brain-dead. They rejected this proposal for America:

> Not only are the brains of such infants not completely absent, but there is also a remarkable heterogeneity of morphologic and functional features in the infants considered anencephalic. . . .The causes of the neural-tube defects, including anencephaly, are complex and multiple—a fact that confounds the issue and supports the concept that the condition is quite variable. It is worrisome, but not surprising, that the diagnosis of anencephaly is occasionally made in error. Indeed, too many errors have been made for the diagnosis to be considered reliable as a legal definition of death. We conclude that anencephalic infants are not brain-absent and that the condition is sufficiently variable that the establishment of a special category is not justified.[48]

Another problem is that diagnosis of anencephaly, even as a range, is often problematic. Diagnosing brain size or brain function at birth is controversial (see Baby Jane Doe case). Will overzealous physicians and parents, wanting to bring some good out of a tragedy, declare babies anencephalic when they have some lesser defect—say, microcephaly? The media sometimes report cases of retarded children allegedly diagnosed as anencephalic who now function well.

A slippery slope might occur here: If borderline anencephalics can become a source of organs, there might be a tendency to use infants with closely related disorders such as atelencephaly (incomplete development of the brain) and lissencephaly (unusually small brain parts). It has been argued that "the slippery slope is real," because some physicians have proposed transplants from infants with defects less severe than anencephaly."[49] Judge Moriarty wrote in her medical review for her decision, "There has been a tendency by some parties and *amici* to confuse lethal anencephaly with these less serious conditions, even to the point of describing children as 'anencephalic' who have abnormal but otherwise intact skulls and who are several years of age."[50]

Some critics have asked whether less was being done for anencephalic babies when these babies were seen as potential organ donors. Alex Capron described the situation as follows: "By far the most fundamental problem . . . was trying to sustain an anencephalic's liver, heart, and kidneys without temporarily giving life to its brain stem, the one organ that needed to die for transplant to begin."[51]

According to the Ontario Protocol, a potential anencephalic donor is to be maintained on a respirator, but periodically removed from the respirator to see if independent breathing will occur. Is this removal in the best interest of the infant? Is the anencephalic infant really being seen as a patient? Or as an organ source? (The Pittsburgh Protocol raises the same questions.)

A counterargument here is that with anencephaly, birth is not morally relevant. That is, most fetuses diagnosed as anencephalic are aborted (indeed, anencephaly is one of the best reasons for aborting a fetus during the second term), and the birth of an anencephalic does not make a moral difference. If abortion is appropriate in anencephaly, why should it be considered immoral to do less to prolong the life of an anencephalic who is a potential organ donor? It might be argued, along these lines, that since anencephalics almost always die a few days after birth, why not allow physicians to kill anencephalics painlessly and transplant their organs at the optimal time?

Another question concerns keeping an anencephalic fetus alive to be a later source of organs. There seems to be a real distinction between keeping a fetus alive for this purpose and simply using the organs of a baby who has accidentally become brain dead or who has unexpectedly been born anencephalic. Some critics say we shouldn't cross this line.

So how many anencephalic organ sources are we talking about? Most anencephalics are identified in utero and most are aborted. Of the approximately 650 anencephalics brought to term each year in the United States, about 60 percent will be stillborn. Of the approximately 300 anencephalics who are born alive and survive immediately after birth, about half will be possible donors of hearts, kidneys, and livers; the others will be unacceptable for various reasons, including organ malformation, low birth weight, and lack of consent by family. The number of possible donors would be further reduced after blood and tissue matching. Taking all this into account, one study estimates that *only about 30 recipients a year* would benefit from using anencephalics as sources of organs.[52]

Given that serious problems exist about using anencephalics as organ sources, is this figure—30 babies a year—large enough? Would it justify changing our criteria of brain death? Most ethicists and doctors decided negatively: The numbers were too small for so big a change.

Costs and Opportunity Costs

In the Baby Fae case, many critics questioned whether so much money should be spent on a single case when the same amount of money could have done so much good for so many others. Although Loma Linda never revealed the cost of Fae's surgery and the associated treatment, it was probably at least $500,000. Would it make sense to perform, say, 500 to a 1,000 such operations a year, at a cost of maybe

$1 billion, while thousands of babies are born deformed because their mothers could not afford prenatal tests like amniocentesis and sonograms?

In the case of Baby Gabriel and Paul Holc, the surgery alone cost $140,000; in addition, there were costs of flying everyone to Loma Linda and, for the Schoutens and the Ontario hospital, the cost of keeping Gabriel Schouten alive for a week. Consider that thousands of pregnant women in the United States get no prenatal care and that as a result, many babies are born with preventable defects. Isn't the system biased in favor of dramatic surgical cases and against these anonymous women and their children?

What about costs of separating conjoined twins in 14-hour operations with dozens of surgeons? Millions of dollars can easily be spent on one case. Why is so much free care given on these dramatic cases, while other babies are ignored? How many poor women with babies with HLHS go to motels to wait for their babies to die?

Criteria of Success in Surgery: Conjoined Twins

Separation of conjoined twins also raises issues about use of babies in risky surgery and about surgeons seeking fame. On any given day in any major children's hospital, surgeons operate on two desperately ill infants and no one notices. Spectacular surgery occurs, teams spend weeks nurturing each child back to health, but the public is indifferent.

Now make one change and have the two infants enter the hospital as conjoined twins, connected at the head, sternum, or pelvis, and everyone takes notice. Why is that?

Philosopher Alice Dregger argues that it's a modern freak show, the kind of thing that people once paid to see in exhibits.[53] In the 18th century, physicians paid such people to exhibit themselves. But as this philosopher and historian of science argues, at least back then such people got paid and were allowed to exhibit their bodies with dignity. Today, the only message they get is: "You're abnormal. We can surgically normalize you, even at risk of killing you. Be grateful."[54]

Separating conjoined twins, especially adults, may often be a reach for fame by the hospital and by the surgical team, saying, "Hey. We can do this and nobody else can! We're the top dogs!" More charitably, it may be just another version of the rule of rescue: We can separate these two conjoined babies, give them separate lives, and feel good about doing so.

In lionizing these cases and their surgeons, the media often describe twins undergoing separation as "brave little fighters," the surgeons as "heroes," and the hospital as performing operations that are "medically necessary." But is this really so?

Johns Hopkins's Ben Carson became famous in 1987 for successfully separating seven-month-old German craniopagus twins (joined at the head and sharing part of the same brain). Since then, he has written several best-selling books about his surgeries on conjoined twins and his life.[55] In 1994, he and his team tried to separate seven-month-old South African craniopagus twins, who both died during the operation. In 1997, he traveled with a 50-member team to successfully separate two Zambian craniopagus twins facing in opposite directions, who did not share any organs.[56]

In 2003, he joined the team of surgeons separating Ladan and Laleh Bijani, the adult Iranian women who both died during the operation. Dregger criticizes what Carson said he told the twins in obtaining consent, that a 50 percent chance existed that one of them would die or be disabled from the surgery:

> But as a leading expert in the field, Carson surely knew of the most comprehensive study of craniopagus separations, which had concluded that 'mortality and morbidity after surgical separation of craniopagus twins is horrendous: of the 60 infants operated on, 30 died, 17 were impaired, 6 were alive but ultimate status unknown, and only 7 were apparently normal.'"[57]

As Dregger points out, at their advanced age, experts agreed that their skulls had thickened and hardened, their brains had matured and were less resilient, thus making their chances of success even worse than the above dismal statistics.[58] Dregger wonders whether these women were given true information about the dismal prospects of the surgery.

In 2004, Carson attempted to separate the German craniopagus twins Lee and Tabea Block. His surgery was only partially successful, as Tabea died during the surgery.[59]

Conjoined children can live and grow into late adulthood while conjoined. Eng and Chang lived into their 70s, each married and fathered several normal children.

But don't conjoined twins do better when separated to live separate, independent lives? "The problem with this question is that conjoined twins almost invariably state that, from their point of view, they don't need to be separated to be individuals, because they are *not* trapped or confined by their conjoinment."[60]

Perhaps the most spectacular issue here is *how little is known about long-term survival for conjoined twins who were separated and about their subsequent quality of life.* As Dregger notes, the one extant study merely asked whether separated twins were later alive or dead, with no other questions asked. How can surgeons get informed consent without real data? The assumption always is: anything is better than living like this.

But is it? What is the resulting quality of life for survivors? In retrospect, what do the separated twins think of the operation? Would they do it for their own children, if they were conjoined? How many mourn the loss of a twin killed in the operation?

Some adult conjoined twins claim surgeons and parents are prejudiced against life as conjoined adults, thinking that their quality of life is so low that likelihood of death for one during surgery to free the other is preferable.[61] Dregger calls these *sacrifice surgeries* and argues that they pose the most challenging ethical questions. Surely they raise the most controversial assumption of all: that a chance of normalcy for one is worth the death of the other.

In discussing separation of the conjoined twins Angela and Amy Lakeberg in 1993, Dregger writes, "Yet no matter how justified the ends, it is troubling to see surgeons actively cause the death of a child like Amy—who was obviously conscious and as entitled to the conjoined heart as her sister."[62]

In August 2002, UCLA surgeons separated one-year-old Guatemalan craniopagus twins in a 22-hour operation. The story received saturation coverage nationwide, illustrating the rule of rescue. In July 2006, Dr. Carson announced he would separate 10-year-old craniopagus twins from Delhi, India.

Conclusion

There is an old saying in medicine: "Beware the surgeon with one case." That sums up many of the cases in this chapter and sums up a continuing ethical problem in surgery. As Alice Dregger states the problem, "Unlike drugs and many non-surgical medical procedures, surgeries, at least in the United States, are largely exempt from systematic review. There is little tradition or regulation in support of rigorous systematic review."[63]

When experimental surgery is done, it should be in a well-conceived research design. One surgeon grandstanding for fame should not be allowed. Loma Linda's website still features the Baby Fae and Paul Holc cases. Should it be proud of Leonard Bailey and what happened there? Should Hopkins boast of separating conjoined twins? What's the opportunity cost of all this surgery?

FURTHER READING AND RESOURCES

George Annas, "Baby Fae: The 'Anything Goes' School of Human Experimentation," *Hastings Center Report*, 15, no. 1, February 1985, p. 15–17.

"Baby Fae: Ethical Issues Surround Cross-Species Organ Transplantation," *Scope Note* 5, Kennedy Institute of Ethics, Georgetown University, Washington, D. C.

Denise Breo, "Interview with 'Baby Fae's' Surgeon," *American Medical News*, November 16, 1984.

Alice Dregger, *One of Us: Conjoined Twins and the Future of the Normal*, Harvard University Press, Cambridge, MA, 2004.

Charles Krauthammer, "The Using of Baby Fae," *Time*, December 3, 1984.

Thomasine Kushner and Raymond Belotti, "Baby Fae: A Beastly Business," *Journal of Medical Ethics*, 11, 1985.

CHAPTER 15

Involuntary Psychiatric Commitment

The Case of Joyce Brown

This chapter describes a homeless woman living on the Upper East Side of Manhattan who was committed against her will for treatment for schizophrenia. Defended by the ACLU, her cases raised ethical issues about paternalism, political uses of psychiatry, rights of mental patients, and compassion.

THE CASE OF JOYCE BROWN

In the 1980s, mentally unstable, homeless people overwhelmed Manhattan; mental health professionals and the public wanted something done. In 1987, New York City started Project Help, but the people it tried to help resisted. Could insane homeless people just be left to "die with their rights on?" Or could Project Help seize them for psychiatric evaluation and involuntary commitment?

Controversially, Project Help broadened its standards for involuntary commitment beyond the legal requirements of mental illness and dangerousness. It added two new criteria: "self-neglect" and a "need to be treated for mental illness."

The first person picked up was Joyce Brown, a 40-year-old African-American woman. For 18 months, she slept outside a Swensen's ice cream parlor on Second Avenue and 65th Street, not too far from Gracie Mansion, where Mayor Ed Koch lived. During the day, she panhandled for money to buy food, cigarettes, and toilet paper. Brown was chosen as a test case by Project Help and Mayor Koch, who saw her sometimes and spoke to her on the street.

Her physical appearance suggested mental illness. Her teeth were unclean; her hair was matted underneath a bulky white knit cap. She had a glazed look, muttered as she panhandled, and often talked to herself. She sometimes sang "How Much Is That Doggie in the Window?" Once, when a resident of the block gave her money, she tossed it back while screaming angrily at an invisible man. One neighbor described her in a letter to the *New York Times* as "full of rage." She cursed at black men she encountered, although she liked babies. She sometimes defecated and urinated in the gutter. On bitterly cold nights, the police tried to take her to a shelter, but she resisted.

When Project Help forcibly brought her to the emergency room of Bellevue Hospital, she was injected against her will with five mg. of Haldol, an antipsychotic drug and two mg. of Ativan, a fast-acting short-term tranquilizer, and then taken to a new 28-bed, locked psychiatric unit on the 19th floor.

The Legal Conflict

After Joyce Brown was evaluated at Bellevue, Mayor Koch was informed that she was neither sufficiently insane nor sufficiently dangerous for involuntary commitment. Although diagnosed as schizophrenic, Brown was not dangerous to herself or others. Bellevue psychiatrists did agree however that Brown was "in need of treatment for mental illness," so Joyce met one of the new criteria for commitment.

Once a person is brought to a psychiatric facility, release is unlikely until a commitment hearing occurs before a judge. New York state law allowed involuntary injections only in emergency rooms; and in the psychiatric unit at Bellevue, Joyce Brown exercised her right to refuse further drugs.

Prior to her hearing before Judge Robert Lippman, she called the American Civil Liberties Union (ACLU). It agreed to represent her if she would waive confidentiality and would agree to publicity about her case to help other homeless people, which she did.

At the hearing, her three sisters from New Jersey arrived. Married, working, and middle class, they said they had been searching for Joyce for the last 18 months. They said their family was from Elizabeth, New Jersey, and their father was a Methodist minister; all the children had gone to church.

Brown had been a "bright, attractive, and happy-go-lucky child." She had graduated from both high school and business school, and had held several jobs at Bell Laboratories. During these years, her sisters said, she had been a "big, healthy girl" who wore nice clothes and jewelry and "always drove around in a new Cadillac."

They said that Brown had started taking heroin in her 20s, and later cocaine. She worked for 10 years as a secretary for the New Jersey Human Rights Commission. In 1982, her mental health and her job performance plummeted. In 1985, at age 38, she was fired because of absenteeism and use of drugs. She was living with her sisters and her parents, but she left them and went to a shelter in Newark. There, she was expelled for assaulting someone.

Her sisters admit that they then tricked her into a voluntary commitment in the psychiatric ward of East Orange General Hospital in New Jersey. There she was diagnosed as psychotic and given antipsychotic drugs. She resisted these injections. She was locked up for two weeks, during which attendants restrained her in an isolation room. After these two weeks, she was released.

She then fled New Jersey and starting living under various aliases on East 62nd Street. She avoided shelters for the homeless, considering them dangerous for unattached women. She did not contact her sisters, fearing they would commit her.

At her hearing, Brown was articulate, called herself a "professional street person," and answered probing questions:

Q: Why had she torn up paper money given to her? A: "I only need $7 a day to live on. I tore up additional money given to me to prevent being robbed of it at night."[1]

Q: Why did she defecate on herself? "I never did," she replied, although she had used the streets because no local restaurant would let her use its restroom. "I offered to buy something and they still refused."

Four psychiatrists testified for the city that Brown suffered from schizophrenia, should be treated in an institution, and, if left on the street, would deteriorate. They denied that this was "political psychiatry" and stated that Joyce Brown's "self-neglect" was "so severe" that she should be helped against her will. They noted that schizophrenics are often bright and have periods of rationality.

Three psychiatrists testified for ACLU that she was not psychotic, not dangerous, not unreasonable in her answers, and not incapable of caring for herself on the streets. In his summation, an ACLU attorney said the city had not proved that Brown was dangerous to herself or others: "The only evidence the city had is that she goes to the bathroom in the streets. I see that in New York City every day, because there's a lack of public restroom facilities."

In her rebuttal, the attorney for the city replied: "Decency and the law and common sense do not require us to wait until something happens to her. It is our duty to act before it is too late."[2]

In November, Judge Lippman ordered Joyce Brown freed. He had found her "rational, logical, and coherent" throughout her testimony;[3] he said that she "displayed a sense of humor, pride, a fierce independence of spirit, [and] quick mental reflexes"; and he noted that she met none of the conditions set forth in *O'Connor v. Donaldson.*

He stressed that even if all the psychiatrists had diagnosed her as psychotic, the city had still not proved Brown was dangerous to others or herself:

> I am aware that her mode of existence does not conform to conventional standards, that it is an offense to aesthetic sense. [Nevertheless] she copes, she is fit, she survives. . . . [s]he refuses to be housed in a shelter. That may reveal more about conditions in shelters than about Joyce Brown's mental state. It might, in fact, prove she's quite sane. [Also] there must be some civilized alternatives other than involuntary hospitalization or the street.[4]

After the hearing, Brown's sisters called the judge's decision "racist" and "sexist." They argued that if his own wife or mother were sleeping on the streets, "he would not stand for it." They insisted that she needed treatment.

The sisters then revealed that after Brown had been hospitalized, they had gotten her declared mentally disabled and she had accordingly received $500 a month in social security disability payments, which they had been holding for her. Brown had refused the money, rejecting the "lie" that she was mentally disabled.

After her victory, Brown and her ACLU lawyers held a press conference, where she said, "I didn't want to play the game before, but now I am. . . . I am going to get an apartment, go back to work, and get my life together." She criticized the city for spending $600 a day on her care: "I could be living at Trump Tower."[5]

Why did Brown appear so different at her hearing than on the streets? Her psychiatrists claimed she had improved rapidly in the hospital. She dismissed their claim, asserting she had never been crazy. She resented being taken into Bellevue like "cattle" and affirmed that living on the street was a rational choice. Her sisters dismissed this assertion: "You might be able to survive one winter, or even two, but you can't survive that way forever."

Mayor Koch blasted Judge Lippman's decision: "If anything happens to that woman, God forbid, the blood of that woman is on that judge's hands." Reminded by a reporter that Lippman had found Brown lucid, Koch replied, "This woman is at risk. When she lay on the ground in the rain, in the snow, uncovered—was that lucid?"[6] When asked if Brown's commitment was "political psychiatry," Koch asked, "*Who* would claim that?" When told that it had been Brown herself, he replied, "That alone proves she's crazy."[7]

The city and Koch appealed to a five-member New York State Appellate Court, before which the ACLU argued that Brown would not return to the streets but would live in a supportive residence for the homeless. The city argued that where she would live was irrelevant: "She was not hospitalized because she was living on the streets [but because] three psychiatrists said she needed medical and psychiatric help."

The appellate court reviewed the testimony of a social worker who said she had observed "fecal matter" on the sheets in which Brown wrapped herself. The appellate court also reviewed the testimony of one psychiatrist who said that Brown had told him she often defecated and urinated on herself. It found that "the evidence presented in this case clearly and convincingly demonstrated her past history of assaultive and aggressive behavior."[8]

The appellate court overruled Judge Lippman, saying he had placed too much emphasis on Brown's testimony instead of the testimony of the psychiatrists who believed she would harm herself. Surprisingly, the majority noted that this case required the high standard of proof of "clear and convincing evidence" rather than the weaker "preponderance of evidence" standard, and that the city had met the higher standard.

After the appellate decision, Koch said, "Up until this moment, the only treatment has been a loving safe environment. Now we will seek to treat her medically." But New York state law required the city to get a court order to medicate her against her will. In 1988, a state judge ruled against forced medication. Bellevue Hospital then released her, saying there was no point in holding her there.

After being held for 84 days and then released, Brown said:

I was incarcerated against my will. . . . [I was] a political prisoner. The only thing wrong with me was that I was homeless, not insane. You just can't go around picking everyone up and automatically label them schizophrenic. I'm angry at Mayor Koch, the city and Bellevue. They held me down and injected me . . . They took my blood against my will. . . .

I need a place to live; I don't need an institution. . . .

People are treated differently just because of your economic status, [because of] what you look like and where you live. . . .

I was mistreated, mentally abused, and I will never, ever, forget this.[9]

The Aftermath

Joyce Brown was released to live in a hotel for women run by a nonprofit agency. She received several job offers and worked temporarily as a secretary in the ACLU office. In early 1988, she became a celebrity. She received half a dozen movie and book offers and dined at Windows on the World, a restaurant atop the World Trade Center. She appeared on *The Donahue Show* and *60 Minutes*. She loved the attention.

She lectured to law students at Harvard on "The Homeless Crisis: A Street View." She observed, "It looks like I have been appointed the homeless spokesperson."

Then things worsened. Her roommate at the hotel said that Joyce had "a lot of anger inside" and frequently talked to herself. One day, while walking to work, she was heard muttering racial slurs and obscenities. In March 1988, Joyce was begging on a street in Times Square shouting obscenities at passersby. Asked how she was doing, she insisted, "I'm not insane."[10]

In September, she was charged with possession of a small amount of heroin and two hypodermic needles in a Harlem housing project.[11]

During 1989, Joyce lived in a supervised residence for formerly homeless women in Manhattan. Unconfirmed reports indicated that she was in and out of psychiatric hospitals between 1989 and 1994. After a decade of interventions, her physicians discovered that that her primary problem was addiction to drugs, not schizophrenia. At last report, she was drug-free and living on her own, and attended a daily support group for former drug-users.

Thus she never was a true schizophrenic, and hence did not meet the commitment standards of *O'Conner v. Donaldson.*

BACKGROUND TO THE CASE

Ideology and Insanity

Early humans believed that the voices characteristically heard by schizophrenics came from the gods. Julian Jaynes claims that the first humans to have identifiable thoughts experienced them as terrifying internal voices, and thinks the human brain evolved as bicameral to control them.[12]

Hippocrates held that mental disorders had natural causes. Plato thought insanity was an imbalance between parts of the mind. Roman physician Galen accepted Hippocrates' naturalistic concept.

The Middle Ages abandoned this naturalistic approach, substituting demonic possession and exorcism. The insane sometimes lived on a *ship of fools*, which sailed from port to port to take on food and water, but which never disembarked its human cargo.

From the 15th to the 18th century, the insane were seen as possessed by demons or as witches, and often killed.

Yet the 16th century saw the founding of Bethlehem Royal Hospital in London, based on naturalistic principles. It had more patients than it could handle. Its name is the origin of "bedlam."

The French physician Philippe Pinel (1745–1826), head of the Bicàtre Hospital for the Insane in Paris, unchained his patients, used compassion, and looked for natural causes, all with therapeutic results.

In the 19th century, Quaker institutions practiced "moral treatment," allowing patients to roam the grounds, work in gardens, and to live in a homelike atmosphere.

In the 20th century, psychiatry embraced pharmacological treatments. Its two major ethical issues then were political diagnoses and patient rights against involuntary treatment.

Patients' Rights

If one accepts that the insane need therapeutic help rather than criminal justice, then they need no trial to commit them for treatment. In a benevolent system, committing psychiatrists act in the best interests of patients.

In the 1960s and 1970s, movies such as *King of Hearts* (1966) and the Oscar-winning *One Flew over the Cuckoo's Nest* (1975) attacked such commitment as unjust. Lawyers who defended patients' autonomy argued that psychiatric diagnoses were subjective, that large public mental institutions were coercive, and that checks and balances were needed. These lawyers would eventually batter down the locked doors of psychiatric wards.

On the other side, psychiatry saw itself as benevolent and held that the insane needed treatment. It emphasized that schizophrenia is biochemical and can be objectively identified and treated pharmacologically, but that schizophrenics must be made to take their medications.

Thomas Szasz, a famous gadfly to psychiatry, saw no problem with patients who voluntarily sought help, for the proper role of psychiatrists was to help them. He criticized situations where people like Joyce Brown had psychiatrists forced on them—people who did not see themselves as mentally ill and who resisted intervention. Szasz held that involuntary commitment rarely benefited patients and existed to rid society of strange people.

Szasz's basic position was this: A physical disease, such as AIDS or cancer, has a physical cause. Some mental illnesses have a physical cause in the brain, and these mental illnesses are real. But some so-called mental illnesses have no physical cause; they result from mere problems in living. A mental illness with no physical cause, Szasz famously held, is a *myth*, not a disease. (Note that Szasz did not claim that most mental illness is a myth.)

Szasz concluded that psychiatry could not be objective, or value-free in nonbiological cases. He held that it was "much more intimately related to problems of ethics than is medicine in general."[13] Consider that interpersonal relations—relationships between wife and husband, between the individual and the community, among colleagues, among neighbors—inevitably involve stress, conflict of interests, and strain. Much of this disharmony has to do with incompatible values, and to pretend that psychiatrists can offer value-free approaches is ludicrous: "Much of psychotherapy revolves around nothing other than the elucidation and weighing of goals and values—many of which may be mutually contradictory—and the means whereby they might best be harmonized, realized, or relinquished."

Szasz wonders who truly defines norms of "correct" and "psychotic" behavior. He opposed classification of personality disorders as mental illness. According to Szasz, psychiatry presumes that love, continued life, stable marriage, kindness, and meekness indicate mental health; and that hatred, homicide, suicide, repeated divorce, chronic hostility, and vengefulness indicate mental illness. These presumptions are evaluative, not factual.

A famous study by D. Rosenhan, "On Being Sane in Insane Places," figured in the patients' rights movement. In this study, several sociologists, psychiatrists, and others voluntarily entered mental hospitals, saying that they were "hearing voices"—a major symptom of schizophrenia.[14] Once committed, they acted normally and no longer mentioned "voices." Because of the label "schizophrenic" in their medical charts, the staff continued to treat them as schizophrenic. Ironically, although the staff did not see through the sham, several of the genuine mental patients did.

Legal Victories for Psychiatric Patients

In 1972, in *Wyatt* v. *Stickney*, Alabama federal judge Frank Johnson ruled that a committed mental patient must either receive treatment or be released. Johnson's decision specified the institutional conditions necessary to ensure minimal treatment: at least two psychiatrists, 12 registered nurses, and 10 aides for every 250 patients. For years, most states had not met this minimal standard.

Johnson required state mental institutions to provide individualized treatment plans, to allow patients to refuse invasive electroconvulsive therapy and lobotomies, and to establish the least restrictive conditions necessary for treatment.

Johnson's ruling prefigured the *O'Conner* v. *Donaldson* decision by the United States Supreme Court in 1975.[15] In 1943, at age 34, Kenneth Donaldson got into a fight with coworkers over politics and was knocked out. His parents considered him crazy and petitioned a Florida judge to commit him. Committed, he underwent 11 weeks of electroshock treatment, and was then released.

In 1956, while he was visiting his parents in Florida, his father asked for a sanity hearing, saying that his son had a persecution complex. Donaldson was then committed to Florida State Mental Hospital, where he was held against his will for 15 years. During those years, he constantly petitioned the courts for a new hearing. All the while, he rarely saw a physician and never received treatment. Inside the institution, he was presumed insane and—like Rosenhan's impostors—could not prove otherwise. Finally, in 1971, when his case was about to be heard, he was released.

A lawyer then helped Donaldson sue for damages against the superintendent of the institution, J. B. O'Connor, and the case eventually reached the Supreme Court. The Supreme Court decided for Donaldson, ruling that he should not have been held against his will, even if he was mentally ill, unless he had been dangerous to himself or to others and had no means of existing outside the institution.

The *O'Connor* decision established two necessary conditions for involuntary commitment:

1. Suffering from mental illness (being "insane").
2. Being dangerous to others or being dangerous to oneself.

Note that both conditions, (1) insanity and (2) danger to oneself or others, must be met for involuntary commitment. Judges later interpreted dangerousness as imminent risk to life or imminent risk of bodily harm; "imminent" means within days or hours. The arbiters are two psychiatrists. Evidence of dangerousness to oneself would consist of:

(a) Threats of suicide.

(b) Gross neglect of basic needs.

With these legal changes, the courts moved from a medical model of civil commitment, which had been used in the early 1960s, to a patient's rights model in the 1970s.

In the 1990s, many states added a third requirement for involuntary commitment:

3. Provision of the least restrictive environment by the institution.

Conditions 1 (mental illness) and 2 (dangerousness) applied in all states, since the Supreme Court had established them; two-thirds of the states also applied condition 3 (least restrictive environment).[16]

In some states, the *O'Connor* criteria have been interpreted to mean that a person must commit an *overt act* in order to warrant a hearing for involuntary commitment. This interpretation is controversial and has been opposed by relatives, who can often perceive a pattern of threats and hostility and do not want to wait until someone is injured or killed before a hearing takes place. At present, courts and legislatures are struggling with the implications of this "overt act" requirement.

Deinstitutionalization

These legal decisions entailed the release of many mental patients from large state institutions, because such institutions often could not provide individualized treatment (as required by *Wyatt*) and were not the least restrictive environment.

Other factors also contributed to deinstitutionalization. New psychotropic medications allowed more outpatient treatment. The Kennedy administration had advocated small, community-integrated facilities rather than large, impersonal state institutions. In the words of President Kennedy, "Reliance on the cold mercy of custodial isolation will be supplanted by the open warmth of community concern."[17] Other factors included tight budgets, psychiatrists who sought lighter workloads, and a general distrust of authority in the early 1970s.

All these factors emptied American mental institutions. During the 1970s, 50 to 75 percent of the patients in state institutions were released. In 1955, nearly 560,000 patients lived in state mental institutions; in 1988, there were only 130,000, so over 30 years, nearly a half million mental patients were deinstitutionalized. All levels of government saved money, the ACLU was appeased, and mental patients flooded into communities.

But the "warmth of community concern" envisioned by John Kennedy did not appear. Communities rejected halfway houses, and few facilities were created. Mental patients "living in the community" scraped by on warm-air grates more

often than in group homes. More bag ladies appeared on city streets. Local charities set up soup kitchens for hungry street people. In the 1980s, Reaganites hailed
soup kitchens as proof that government intervention was unneeded.

Deinstitutionalization failed to help people with mental illness. It failed
because government funds were never allocated for community homes; because
communities rejected such homes; because mental health services were fragment-
ed between county, state, and federal agencies; because housing was scarce; and
because the legal pendulum had swung toward patients' rights.[18]

During the month Joyce Brown was released from Bellevue, under the
expanded criteria, Project Help helped 466 homeless mentally ill people. It estimated that 800 to 1,000 such people were still out on the city streets.

When New York City officials planned Project Help, they assumed that people such as Joyce Brown would stay for a few weeks in psychiatric hospitals and
would then be moved into community facilities, where they could live under
supervised conditions. When Project Help picked up these people, however, they
were far sicker than had been expected. Many more places were needed in psychiatric hospitals than had been planned for.

Violence and the Mentally Ill Homeless in the Cities

In 1977, Juan Gonzalez, a homeless man suffering from symptoms like Joyce
Brown's, went berserk on the Staten Island Ferry and killed two people with a
sword. As a result, the public clamored for incarceration of *potentially dangerous*
mentally ill people. The concept of potential danger soon came to be used to justify holding someone temporarily for a "cool-down" observational period.
Gonzalez had been picked up for just such a period and diagnosed as a paranoid
schizophrenic just before the killings, but he had not been considered imminently
dangerous to others, so he had been discharged.

In 1991, Keven McKiever, a homeless man who had gone to Bellevue Hospital
seeking care and had been turned away, stabbed to death Alexis Walsh, a former
Radio City Rockette. In 1993, Christopher Battiste, a homeless mentally ill drug
abuser, allegedly murdered an elderly woman in the Bronx on a Sunday morning
as she came home from church.

Larry Hogue, a homeless, mentally ill, African-American, Vietnam veteran,
sometimes lived peacefully on a street corner in the upper west side of Manhattan,
but when he took illegal drugs, he became hostile, violent, and what *60 Minutes*
called the "wild man of 96th Street." A state judge ruled that he could be involuntarily committed against his will for detoxification, but that he would have to be
released "as soon as he decides to seek outpatient care."[19] In 1994, shortly before
he was due to be released from Creedmore Hospital, he escaped, committed a
robbery for small change, and was soon picked up. He was then returned to
Creedmore.

In 1999, two schizophrenic men not taking their prescribed medications
pushed innocent people in front of oncoming subway trains in New York City,
killing a young woman named Kendra Webdale and leaving the other victim
without legs. Both men had a history of violence. In previous years, similar events
had occurred:

Reuben Harris, who suffered from paranoid schizophrenia, had 12 hospitalizations and a history of violent behavior, pushed Song Sin to her death in the same manner in 1995. Jaheem Grayton, who also had a history of violence and severe mental illness, pushed Naeeham Lee to her death after struggling to steal her earrings in 1996. Mary Ventura pushed Catherine Costello into the path of a subway train in 1985, three weeks after being discharged from a psychiatric hospital.[20]

These cases resulted in passage in New York in 1999 of *Kendra's law*, where a psychiatrist or relative can force hospitalization for a mentally ill person who has been hospitalized within the last three years, who has a history of violence, and who will not take his medication. At least 41 states passed laws implementing such Assisted Outpatient Treatment programs, where outpatients can be forced to take medications and remain under supervision (California, Maine, Maryland, Massachusetts, New Jersey, Pennsylvania, and Rhode Island have not).[21]

The courts and the general public have come to expect psychiatrists to be able to predict dangerousness among the mentally ill, but can they? To assess the potential for violent behavior, emergency-room psychiatrists simply ask patients about their own tendencies toward violence and their own past acts of violence.[22] This is not a sophisticated tool, although in practice it seems to work better than anything else.

The famous legal decision *Tarasoff* should be noted here.[23] In this case, Prosenjit Poddarin 1969 confided to his psychotherapist at the University of California that he planned to kill Tatiana Tarasoff, which he did. Tarasoff's parents sued the therapist and university saying they should have broken confidentiality and warned the girl and parents of Poddarin's threat. The actual decision has been misinterpreted to say that therapists must breach confidentiality and warn potential victims when life is at stake. In fact the 1976 decision merely said that, in such situations, therapists have a duty to take "reasonable steps" to protect potential victims, such as notifying police or seeking involuntary commitment.

ETHICAL ISSUES

Paternalism, Autonomy, and Diminished Competence

Paternalism in medicine is treatment of adult patients as incompetents who do not know their own best interests. Under which conditions might paternalism be justified? One condition is *temporary incompetence*, followed by a return of competence. In these situations, paternalism would be justified if patients later agreed with it (for example, people prevented from committing suicide who later agree that they are glad to be alive).

Questions about patients' competence are important in any discussion of paternalism. In this regard, one question has to do with the basic concept of competence. The American legal system tends to treat mental patients as if they were either totally competent and autonomous, or totally dysfunctional and subject to mandatory treatment. Many observers argue that this is a false dichotomy that harms patients. Competence is not an either-or capacity, but a matter of degrees on a gradient.

Another question has to do with what constitutes proof of competence and incompetence. This issue is not necessarily clear-cut: the psychiatrist Virginia Abernethy argues, for instance, that "disorientation, mental illness, irrationality, [and] commitment to a mental institution are not conclusive proof of incompetence."[24]

Abernethy describes the case of "Ms. A," a highly intelligent, independent woman who lived alone in a large house with six cats, in an unheated garbage-strewn room.[25] After a fire in her house, Ms. A was hospitalized but found competent and released. As winter came, a concerned social worker investigated; he found her with her feet black, ulcerated, and bleeding. When he tried to get her to go with him to a hospital, she chased him away with a shotgun. The police later came and forcibly hospitalized her. At the hospital, her feet were diagnosed as gangrenous, and surgeons wanted to amputate; when she refused, psychiatrists began to evaluate her.

It turned out that Ms. A's feet had blackened once before, a few years earlier, and she had recovered. She now hoped for another recovery, but the psychiatrists interpreted this as "psychotic denial" and tried to get her to say that she wanted to live, so that they could amputate. She refused, avoiding their questions. Ms. A was faced with a dilemma: either she had to let the surgeons amputate, or she had to let the psychiatrists conclude that she was in denial and therefore psychotic. It might seem unfair to present a patient with such a choice, and trying to avoid the choice would seem to be reasonable. Amazingly, according to Abernethy, "Her rejection of the two-choice model became the grounds, finally, for concluding that Ms. A was not competent to refuse amputation."

Abernethy analyzed the psychodynamics of this process. First, a false aura of medical emergency "pervaded the psychiatric consultations and judicial process." Second, "Ms. A herself was quick to anger and regarded most interactions with medical personnel as adversarial." Third, Ms. A's anger created anger in those evaluating her competence: "Professionals who think of themselves as altruistic, or at least benevolently motivated, may be particularly sensitive to hostility because they feel deserving of gratitude." Abernethy says that psychiatrists are outcome-oriented and cannot tolerate a patient's self-destructiveness, even in the name of autonomy and even when self-destruction results from an underlying disease that they ultimately cannot stop. Abernethy notes, moreover, that "hope is not a criterion of psychotic denial."

In some ways, Joyce Brown resembled Ms. A. Like Ms. A, she rejected her diagnosis, hoped that she was sane, and thought she could take care of herself. Like Ms. A, she saw psychiatrists as enemies. Acknowledged to be generally competent, both women were claimed to have a *focal incompetence,* a specific incompetence to make decisions about their own treatment. Abernethy notes, "The criterion of a focal delusion is dangerously liable to error because a patient can easily be seen as delusional in an emotionally charged interchange, when in other circumstances he addresses the same issue appropriately." Abernethy sums up: "Competence is presumed and does not have to proved. Incompetence has to be proved."

Homelessness and Commitment

What was the issue in the Joyce Brown case—insanity or homelessness? Mayor Koch and New York City were accused of wanting Brown committed because she was a public nuisance and homeless. Her neighbors were accused of wanting her out of their sight because she offended their affluent sensibilities.

The ACLU, noting that Joyce Brown did not want to leave the street and had never been proven dangerous, argued that her presence embarrassed the rich people in the neighborhood. New York City had thousands of people like her, so why was there no outcry about others? Why did no one write letters to the *New York Times* about the Joyce Browns in the Bronx? Once Brown was gone, how many of her former neighbors on the upper east side inquired about her?

Norman Siegel, executive director of ACLU, extended this argument to Koch and the city as well: "In sweeping up the homeless, the Mayor is attempting to place these people out of sight and out of mind and hide the crisis from the public consciousness." Siegel claimed that Project Help targeted areas seen by tourists and inhabited by the rich.

Even though Koch and the city cared about quality of life in public places, they emphasized that homeless people were picked up for treatment, not to remove them from public places. Homeless people gravitated to rich areas because they were safer there and such places offered them better opportunities for begging.

City officials claimed that Brown's insanity was the true issue and her homelessness merely a side issue. Her ACLU lawyers disagreed: "The Joyce Brown story has captured the issue of the homeless that a lot of people have been trying to deal with for years."[26] The city's goal, the ACLU implied, was how to get homeless people off the streets, not how to treat the mentally ill; city officials didn't seem worried about schizophrenics who camped out in bad neighborhoods.

The ACLU suggested reinstituting public baths (which had been widely available in the city during the depression and earlier) and using condemned housing as temporary shelters. Incarcerating the homeless "for their own good" was a cheap solution; building homes for street people was much more expensive.

No one could deny that the housing situation in New York City was bad: affordable housing was rare. The problem of creating permanent housing for the city's homeless had frustrated many good minds. The city maintained thousands of families in squalid welfare hotels at exorbitant rates. Critics feared that providing rented housing would encourage more people to depend on government handouts; they also pointed out that the city was one of the most expensive places in the United States in which to subsidize public housing.

Psychiatry and Commitment

During this case, ACLU lawyer Robert Levy and psychiatrist Robert Gould, who testified for Brown, emphasized the political dangers of involuntary roundups, handcuffing, forcible injections of medication, and confinement in locked wards. Levy and Gould said that Brown had been examined at least five times previously and had been found "not to require involuntary hospitalization." They claimed that nearly half of the 215 people brought to emergency rooms by Project Help did "not require involuntary hospitalization." Gould and Levy argued that to allow "preventive detention based solely on nebulous predictions of 'future self-destructive behavior'" would invite abuse. They warned of "totalitarian regimes" using psychiatry for control of dissidents.[27]

When confronted with arguments like this, Mayor Koch replied, "This is not political psychiatry! This is not Russia! We're trying to help this woman!"

On the other hand, how broadly should standards of commitment sweep? In cases like Brown's, how many people might be forced into mental hospitals by uncaring or even malevolent relatives? (Isn't this what Barbara Streisand portrayed in *Nuts*?) How many psychiatrists might use medication, time-out rooms, restraints, and continued commitment not as treatment but as punishment for patients who thwart their will?

Part of the debate about Brown's case concerned the ability of psychiatry to help schizophrenics. Judge Lippman noted that the four city and three ACLU psychiatrists had disagreed dramatically, and concluded, "It is evident that psychiatry is not a science amenable to the exactness of mathematics or the predictability of physical laws."

Most psychiatrists objected to this view. They point to schizophrenics who were dysfunctional but who gained years of ability after being forced to take medication. They say that such patients stabilize and become free from delusions and that many patients, if they take their medication regularly, can even return to life outside institutions. The psychiatrist Paul Chodoff defended limited involuntary commitment as follows:

> Is freedom defined only by absence of external constraints? Internal physiological or psychological processes can contribute to a throttling of the spirit that is as painful as any applied from the outside. The "wild" manic individual without his lithium, the panicky hallucinator without his injection of fluphenazine hydrochloride and the understanding support of a concerned staff, the sodden alcoholic—are they free? Sometimes, as Woody Guthrie said, "Freedom means no place to go."[28]

In fact, many people suffering from paranoid schizophrenia can be improved by treatment. All psychiatrists today believe that schizophrenia is a biological disease caused by chemical imbalance, so it makes sense that chemical treatments can help such people.

Suffering and Commitment: Benefit and Harm

Columnist Ellen Goodman argued that the ethical questions in this case boiled down not to whether people like Joyce Brown were likely to harm themselves, but whether they were suffering. Brown should be taken off the streets before she dies there "with her rights on."[29]

But was the matter really so straightforward? To say that commitment is justified to end suffering assumes first that a person is really suffering, and second that involuntary psychiatric commitment can ease his or her suffering.

Consider the first assumption, that the person is suffering. When someone like Joyce Brown protests that she does not need or want help, it can be asked—as Thomas Szasz asked—who can determine that she is "suffering" enough to be locked inside a psychiatric ward? Who bears the onus of proof, the patient or the psychiatrist?

With regard to the second assumption, that involuntary commitment can help, it is important to consider the nature of involuntary commitment. What Brown feared most was another commitment to an inpatient unit like the one at East Orange Hospital. Would she really be helped by involuntary psychiatry, involuntary medication, and involuntary therapy in a locked unit within a large public institution?

Brown's court-appointed psychiatrist had found that she suffered from "serious mental illness" and would benefit from medication—but that she would suffer more from forced treatment than from the mental illness itself. In such a situation, she might harm herself while trying to resist the administration of antipsychotic medications and tranquilizers. Also, commitment might destroy her fierce independence; and if it did not—if she continued to resist—she might end up a zombie, like McMurphy in *One Flew over the Cuckoo's Nest*.

Moreover, the long-term side effects of antipsychotics and tranquilizers can be as bad as the original disorder: antipsychotic drugs, such as neuroleptics, administered over years create tardive dyskinesia in 10–25 percent of patients. This condition impairs voluntary movement, is untreatable, and persists in two-thirds of affected patients when medication is stopped.

It can also be argued that the potential benefits of involuntary treatment cannot be defined objectively. Most psychiatrists, of course, tend to think that people such as Brown benefit from living on medication and thereby losing their inner voices and delusions. But aren't benefit and harm, above the level of basic needs, defined by each person's own self-concept and life plans? As three lawyers write,

> When faced with an obviously aberrant person, we know, or we think we know, that he would be "happier" if he were as we are. We believe that no one would want to be a misfit in society. From the very best of motives, then, we wish to fix him. It is difficult to deal with this feeling since it rests on the unverifiable assumption that the aberrant person, if he saw himself as we see him, would choose to be different than he is. But since he cannot be as we, and we cannot be as he, there is simply no way to judge the predicate for the assertion.[30]

Isn't it a rather shaky application of paternalism to say that Joyce Brown had to be treated so that she could obtain someone else's idea of a benefit? Psychiatrists imply that mentally ill patients suffer internal pain; but if that is so, why don't all patients want to get rid of it? Isn't it illogical—isn't it begging the question—for psychiatrists to explain that patients don't want to get rid of this pain "because they're crazy"?

Housing for the Mentally Ill as an Ethical Issue

Recently, the term "homeless" has been attacked by a new wave of critics as inappropriate for the wandering mentally ill; instead, these critics emphasize substance abuse. They have challenged the ACLU's view that people like Joyce Brown are primarily victims of a greedy or indifferent society which failed to provide affordable housing; they say there is evidence that as many as 85 percent of panhandlers are alcoholics, substance abusers, or mentally ill—and that all of these need treatment.[31] These new critics advocate mandatory treatment and police intervention to prevent panhandling. They urge people not to give money to beggars, saying that those who do give money are "enablers of addiction."

The sheltered or supervised group home remains an elusive ideal. Whether we are discussing severely physically disabled people like Larry McAfee, welfare reform, or the mentally ill homeless, the best living facility for many people is a supervised group home. Living in such a home is much better than being warehoused in a large institution or being left to fend for oneself. Supervised group homes in safe neighborhoods are the perfect compromise between institutionalization and independence.

Urban revitalization made new residents in old neighborhoods intolerant of homeless beggars. No one denied that lack of affordable housing caused homelessness, but few citizens felt government should raise taxes to build such housing. The problem, then, is not with group homes as a concept but with the practical matter of getting group homes for those who need them.

Funding has been one difficulty. In New York, for example, because of AIDS and years of limited funding to balance its gigantic medical budget, places in group homes are scarce; in fact, the shortage of homes has caused a crisis in the city since 1988. Budgets were cut for existing homes, so that some staff members had to be fired and some patients released. The funds saved by cutting group homes were used by legislators for other projects; and now no one seems to know how to get the funding—or the patients—back.

Meanwhile, deinstitutionalization has continued. In 1993, in New York, 2,400 new group home beds had been planned in preparation for the release of 1,000 more people with mental illness from large institutions in 1994, but the number of new beds was later cut to 800. When New York's highest court ruled in 1993 that the City must provide housing for homeless mentally ill patients discharged from city hospitals, the city estimated that it would cost $300 million to do so and disputed the ruling. Nine years later, a study by the *New York Times* exposed widespread failings in the city's adult homes for mentally ill people, "allowing some of its most vulnerable citizens to be exploited in a system plagued by inept, wasteful and fraudulent services."[32]

Many cities emulated New York City's mayor Rudolph Giuliani, who forced homeless people off the streets in the 1990s and into city-funded shelters away from tourists and the affluent. Cities such as Sacramento, Seattle, and Atlanta forced homeless people to move out and did not build new shelters.

When cities tried to build group homes, fights ensued. Residents on Earle Street in Greenville, SC, one of its oldest neighborhoods, sued in 1994 when charities tried to open a sixth group home there. In Alabama, Birmingham's Southside, Forest Park, and Avondale neighborhoods had too many group homes, while surrounding, affluent suburbs had none. All around the country, certain neighborhoods in each city became categorized as "the" area for group homes, where too many were built. Such identification made other neighborhoods passionately resist having even one such home, lest more such homes follow.

In the first decade of the 21st century, lack of housing remains a problem for mentally ill homeless people plagued by drugs, dysfunctional families, poverty, and often, all three.

FURTHER READING AND RESOURCES

Alice Baum and Donald Burnes, *A Nation in Denial: The Truth about Homelessness*, Westview, Boulder, Colo., 1993.

Paul Chodoff, "The Case for Involuntary Hospitalization of the Mentally Ill," *American Journal of Psychiatry*, vol. 133, no. 5, May 1976.

Saul Feldman, "Out of the Hospitals, onto the Streets: The Overselling of Benevolence," *Hastings Center Report*, 13, no. 3, June 1983.

Charles Krauthammer, "How to Save the Homeless Mentally Ill," *New Republic*, February 8, 1988.

J. Livermore, C. Malmquist, and P. Meehl, "On the Justification for Civil Commitment," *University of Pennsylvania Law Review*, 117, November 1968.

The video "Brown vs. Koch" from *60 Minutes* may be available for purchase for a reasonable fee.

CHAPTER 16

Testing Adults for Genetic Disease

Diabetes, Breast Cancer, and Huntington's Disease

This chapter discusses ethical issues in testing for genetic diseases using cases of three adults whose symptoms may not appear for many years. Perhaps the most important case involves Maria, a 30-year-old mother struggling with type 2 diabetes who represents 25 million people in North America with diabetes and 50 million who are prediabetic. The most famous case is that of Nancy Wexler, whose mother died of Huntington's disease and who has a 50 percent chance of inheriting her mother's disease. Finally, we discuss Joan, a 50-year-old mother and survivor of breast cancer, who, like Maria, has several daughters. Ethical issues in these cases of testing arise about families, personal responsibility, and money.

CASE 1: TESTING FOR DIABETES

Maria Lopez, a 30-year-old woman, has type 2 diabetes and struggles to control it.[1] Her extended family in East Harlem in New York City includes many older diabetic relatives. At 5 feet, 6 inches, Maria weighs 267 pounds and considers herself overweight. She has always fought to control her weight, finding it hard to exercise, and loves French fries and soft drinks. Diagnosed with diabetes at age 15 after she was hospitalized for spells of fainting, she once lost 100 pounds, but has since gained it back.

Diabetes mellitus is a disease of high blood sugar levels (hyperglycemia) caused by insufficient secretion or function of insulin, a hormone produced by the pancreas. *Type 1 diabetes*, once called juvenile onset diabetes or insulin-dependent diabetes mellitus, has low or no secretion of insulin. *Type 2 diabetes*, once called adult-onset diabetes, obesity-related diabetes, or noninsulin dependent diabetes mellitus, has resistance by the body's cells to insulin.

Diabetes may soon reach epidemic proportions: The Centers for Disease Control estimates that 21 million Americans suffer from diabetes and another 41 million are prediabetic.[2] At some point during their lives, one of three American children will become diabetic. Worldwide, more and more people who previously avoided diabetes will succumb to it as they adopt Western diets high in fats and processed corn sugars. Americans of Chinese, Korean, and Japanese ancestry develop type 2 diabetes at a rate 60 percent higher than whites.[3]

Worldwide, 171 million people suffer from diabetes. That number is expected to double by 2030.[4]

In 2006, epidemiologists discovered an epidemic of type 2 diabetes in New York City. Over 800,000 of its citizens, more than one in eight, have diabetes.[5] This incidence in this city is a third higher than in the nation. In East Harlem, as many as one in five people has diabetes.[6]

Maria Lopez says her diabetes makes her miserable. "I have never wanted this disease to control my life." Since she was first diagnosed, she has denied that she has a disease and that it could lead to her early death. "I'm a traditionally-built woman from a culture of strong, big women," she says. "I eat what I like. To hell with needles and machines."

Diabetics must monitor their blood sugar several times a day. In the past, they had to do so by drawing blood with needles, but new technology now avoids that. Nevertheless, Maria and others find it socially embarrassing to constantly take out monitors to check their blood sugars, so they frequently omit doing so and fake numbers on their daily sheets.

Diabetics are told to give up beer, cokes, French fries, potato chips, pies, cakes, and "everything else that tastes good," Maria says. But many diabetics in East Harlem are poor with high levels of stress, are trying to keep families and jobs together, live around people whose lives have been affected by drugs, violence, divorce and unemployment, and hence find it difficult to eat right.

Public health educators urge Maria to exercise daily and to eat a low-fat diet high in fresh fruits and vegetables. "That's not so easy to do," she says. "And my two daughters (aged 10 and 8) like to go to McDonald's." Blood sugar monitoring is time-consuming and requires effort, and many patients dislike it.

Uncontrolled diabetes leads to very bad results: kidney failure, retinal damage that leads to blindness, gangrene (especially in legs, leading to amputation), damage to nerves, and heart failure.

In public health and primary care, diabetes is a stealth epidemic. "It's the Rodney Dangerfield of diseases," says the director of a diabetes center.[7] Compared with cancer and AIDS, less money is allocated to find cures for diabetics. Most medical care is oriented to managing crises rather than preventing diabetes.

In 2006, scientists at DeCode Genetics discovered a gene for type 2 diabetes. People who get two copies of the gene from their parents have twice the likelihood of developing diabetes as those who don't carry any copies. Being born with one copy raises the risk above average by 40 percent, and about 38 percent of Northern Europeans carry one copy of the gene, as well as many African-Americans. The head of DeCode explained:

> "If you have one copy of this variant, which 38 percent of people do, your risk of developing type 2 diabetes is increased by 40 percent," Stefansson, who is chief executive officer of DeCode, says. "Seven percent have two copies and have a 140 percent increase in risk."[8]

He also noted that he saw variants of this gene in other populations around the world not present in Iceland, where DeCode has a license to test the country's population for genetic diseases. Presumably, Far Eastern Asians carry a similar gene, explaining the incidence of diabetes in this population when they migrate to developed countries.

One philosophical question we want to consider in this chapter is this: Is Maria *responsible* for her diabetes? Normally, we recoil at this question because we realize that if we hold her responsible, she can be blamed for her disease. It's bad enough to have diabetes, why add to that by being moralistic?

Moreover, using the Golden Rule, we imagine what it would be like to get a diagnosis of diabetes ourselves: Do we want a moralistic physician or nurse condemning us, saying, "You should have eaten better! Now you have nobody to blame but yourself."

And if type 2 diabetes is genetic, then isn't such blame incorrect? Wouldn't Maria have gotten diabetes anyway, no matter how she ate? In the words of the debate over free will, isn't it false that she "could have done otherwise"? Even if her disease is partly environmental and due to poor diet, didn't something cause her to *crave* bad foods? Prediabetic people crave sweets, but some people with different genes have no sweet tooth and do not. So isn't blame about diabetes just stupid? Later in this chapter, we return to this question and provide some answers.

BACKGROUND: BASIC GENETICS

The gene is the basic unit of heredity. It consists of DNA, an organic molecule. Packed inside each of the 46 chromosomes in humans is a complicated strand of interwoven DNA, the famous double helix. The number of genes varies on each chromosome.

The pattern of the four nucleotide bases (A, C, T, and G) in the 46 double helices makes up a person's genetic code. Between 30,000 and 40,000 sequences of these 138 billion pairs of bases are genes.

The Human Genome Project, one of the greatest projects in the history of science, began in October 1993 with the goal of mapping which parts of human DNA were genes. Costing $3 billion, it finished in 2003, having mapped all the human genes.

Francis Collins headed this project. According to a biography about him, he

> developed innovative methods of crossing large stretches of DNA to identify disease genes. . . . That gene-hunting approach, which he named 'positional cloning,' has developed into a powerful component of modern molecular genetics. In contrast to previous methods for finding genes, positional cloning enabled scientists to identify disease genes without knowing in advance what the functional abnormality underlying the disease might be.[9]

Collins's lab also identified the first known gene for cystic fibrosis.

If we think of the 46 strands of human DNA (each with billions of base pairs) as, say, North America, the Human Genome Project showed the territory and its major highways; on this map, the 30,000 to 40,000 genes are the towns and cities. The largest gene, comparable in size to Los Angeles, is the gene for muscular dystrophy, composed of 2 million base pairs. The genes for globulin and insulin are like towns, with only about 1,000 base pairs each.

Knowing which parts of DNA are genes, and where they are, begins genetic knowledge. In the next steps, scientists must identify what genes do, with what other genes, and through which mediating proteins (proteinomics). In addition, some genetic diseases stem from variants in standard genes, or from nonfunctioning genes, so the causes of disease are complex. Finally, varying environmental inputs determine how many genes express themselves. Exposure of the fetus to drugs, nutrition in childhood, and use of tobacco affects how genes control bodily characteristics. In genetics, this is called the *norm of reaction*.[10]

Genetic diseases are inherited disorders. Some genetic diseases are caused by a dominant gene, as in Huntington's disease, where just one copy of the bad gene is needed to get the disease. However, most of us carry genes for recessive genetic diseases, but are not affected by them. We are *heterozygous*, having a dissimilar pair of genes for an inherited recessive disease. Heterozygotes of recessive traits will not experience a disease, but can pass the gene for it to their offspring. If two parents who are heterozygous for a disease both bequeath the gene for the disorder to an offspring, that person will be *homozygous* for the disorder—will have an identical pair of genes. Homozygotes always express the disease.

As many as 15 million Americans suffer from genetic disease. Over 3,500 established and 2,500 suspected disorders are hereditary. These are large figures; in fact, every family may include someone who is a potential victim of genetic disease or is susceptible to a disorder that may be linked to genetic causes, such as diabetes, cancer, or coronary artery disease. Genetic diseases account for over one-third of acute-care hospitalization of children under 18.

CASE 2: NANCY WEXLER AND TESTING FOR HUNTINGTON'S DISEASE

Clinical psychologist Nancy Wexler, born in 1945, graduated from Radcliff College in 1967. After a 10-year deterioration and catatonia, her mother died of Huntington's disease, a devastating, fatal neurological disease lacking cure or treatment. Because the Huntington's gene is dominant, Nancy and her sister Alice each had a 50 percent risk of inheriting the disease. Because the average age of onset is 36, victims usually have children before learning they are affected.

A severe, progressive neurological disease, Huntington's causes neurons in the caudate nuclei region of the brain to rapidly shed. Although age of onset varies, Huntington's is completely *penetrant* by age 65: the gene affects everyone with the disease.

Huntington's progresses through several stages (about five years each). First comes loss of muscular coordination and changes in personality, making victims angry, hostile, depressed, and sexually promiscuous. Next comes slurred speech, distorted facial expressions, constant muscular jerkiness, and staggering and falling. The third stage brings incontinence, dementia, and dependence on others, usually in an institution. In the last stage, victims are vegetative.

At present, 25,000 Americans have Huntington's, and about 100,000 Americans have an afflicted parent. Most victims are white. People at risk of Huntington's constantly wonder if each stumble augurs onset of the disease.

Unlike others at risk for genetic disease, Wexler helped both to discover the gene for Huntington's and to develop a predictive test for it. Around 1800, a European sailor with Huntington's jumped ship around Lake Maracaibo in Venezuela. He had 14 children, and because families there were large, by 1981 he had 3,000 descendants. Of these, 100 had Huntington's and another 1,100 were at risk. In 1981, Nancy led an expedition there to obtain blood samples from these descendants and to test them to find a genetic marker for Huntington's. Co-researcher James Gusella found such a marker in 1983.

In 1987, though the gene had not been discovered, Gusella developed a linkage test for Huntington's, meaning he could test for a batch of genes that included the Huntington's gene which tended to be inherited (or "linked") together. The linkage test allowed people such as Nancy to know odds about their risk, for example, 5 percent versus 80 percent. In this way, it prefigured today's genetic tests where people can know that they have an 80 percent risk of hereditary breast cancer or little risk, but do not get a simple yes-or-no answer.

In 1986, before the linkage tests, Nancy Wexler taught as a professor of clinical neuropsychology at Columbia University. She then said she would like to take the test when it became available. However, famously, she later changed her mind, deciding *not* to take the test.

The implications of her decision stunned people in medical genetics because a leading advocate for testing, who carried a 50 percent risk, had decided at the last minute to not know her risk. And she had spent a decade helping to develop this very test. Moreover, she was a clinical psychologist who should have known her own values.

Indeed, not only did Nancy not take the test, but over the next decades, she became an advocate for others not to take it. What was going on?

To people who want to be tested so that they could decide to go to law school, she said: "Go to law school! Develop your mind! What are you going to do if you're positive? Spend the rest of your life waiting to be a patient?"

In 1983, when James Gusella discovered the marker for Huntington's, he thought that finding the gene would take three to five years. In fact, it took *ten* years. Over the next decade, geneticists followed many false trails. Meanwhile, other researchers discovered single genes for muscular dystrophy, cystic fibrosis, neurofibromatosis ("elephant man" disease), colon cancer, ataxia, and sickle-cell anemia.

In 1993, an international team of six genetic laboratories discovered the exact molecular location of the Huntington's gene.[11] Now people could test directly for the gene, opening a new era in genetic testing. By 2007, Nancy Wexler had still not taken the test but frequently commented on genetic issues. Presumably, at age 62, she does not have the gene.

THE EUGENICS MOVEMENT

Before genetics became a science, a number of ill-founded ideas about heredity abounded. American pragmatist philosopher George Santayana famously said, "Those who cannot learn from history are doomed to repeat it." Knowing the mistakes of the eugenics movement helps us to spot mistakes in public policy about today's genetics.

One mistake, *phrenology*, claimed that the inherited size and shape of the head determined intelligence and character. Although it seems ludicrous now, physicians then palpated the skull to assess character and IQ.

Other misconceptions stemmed from crackpot versions of Charles Darwin's theory of evolution by natural selection, especially his concept of "survival of the fittest." Darwin used fittest simply to mean "best adapted," so "fit" referred to the adaptation between an organism and its environment. Unfortunately, many people misunderstood "fit" to apply to social positions.

This misconception, *social Darwinism*, saw evolution in terms of group competition in human societies. Elitist, white social Darwinists held that social advantages implied biological superiority; therefore upper classes would prevail in any competition. They claimed that the fittest races would prevail in struggles for existence, so they predicted that blacks (whom they saw as biologically unfit) would not survive into the 20th century.

Social Darwinism can most charitably be described as unsophisticated. Not based on any understanding of evolution, it failed to take into account the vast numbers of organisms involved in attempts to survive, the enormous length of time over which these attempts evolve, or the ongoing role of adaptive mutations.

The *eugenics movement* flourished from 1905 to 1935 and hoped to improve hereditary characteristics through voluntary, selective breeding. Charles Darwin's cousin, Francis Galton, coined the term "eugenics" in the late 1880s.

Eugenics popped up worldwide: in Germany, Austria, Scandinavia, Italy, Japan, and South America, but as historian Daniel Kevles writes, "the center of this trend was the American eugenics movement. Its headquarters was at Cold Springs Harbor on Long Island, New York . . . ."[12] This point bears emphasizing: although many people identify modern eugenics with German Nazis, Americans—with their heterogeneous population—most passionately championed eugenics. American politicians, popular media, and scientists espoused it, advocated "eugenic marriages" and sterilization of the unfit, and declared that the American gene pool had declined through interbreeding with unfit races.

At the beginning of the 20th century in the United States, a few prominent families—largely of English, Swiss, German, and Dutch ancestry—exercised enormous wealth and power; they controlled many newspapers, magazines, and even universities, so they controlled many ideas of the time. These families obsessed about "breeding" and feared that the "purity" of Americans would be "contaminated" if their children bred with Irish, Italians, Turks, Jews, Asians, African-Americans, or anybody else whose origin differed from their own.

Wealthy and powerful families desired not only to preserve the purity of their own stock but also to control the growth of other groups. Watching the many progeny of Irish, Italian, and Greek immigrants, they saw Malthusian doom approaching. They thought the "unfit" had no right to bear children. A prominent New York urologist, William Robinson, proclaimed about people with mental retardation, "It is the acme of stupidity to talk in such cases of individual liberty, of the rights of the individual. Such individuals have no rights. They have no right in the first instance to be born, but having been born, they have no right to propagate their kind."[13]

Even on their own terms and in their own time, these ideas made little sense. Social Darwinism and eugenics contradicted each other: if the white race would emerge triumphant, why worry about excessive breeding among other races? If the lower classes were so "unfit" as to be destined to die out, why prevent them from breeding?

Eugenics enjoyed popularity because of a pervasive climate of bigotry (the same climate in Germany led to the rise of Hitler, anti-Semitism, and the Holocaust). The newspaper magnate William Hearst and Theodore Roosevelt thundered against "yellow niggers" who had invaded America from Asia. When Henry Ford ran for president in the 1920s, he promised to rid the country of the "Jew bankers," whom he accused of having caused America to enter World War I; later, he would accuse Jewish bankers of causing the Depression.[14]

The eugenics movement affected critical legislation in the United States. One kind of legislation permitted mandatory sterilization. While the Nazis famously sterilized 225,000 "mental defectives," the United States also practiced large-scale involuntary sterilization. In 1907, Indiana first required sterilization of the retarded and criminally insane; 30 other states soon followed. California led the nation in sterilizations, accounting for nearly a third of the national total; Virginia was second and Indiana third.[15] By 1941, physicians had sterilized over 36,000 Americans against their will, often for the vague condition of "feeblemindedness" or because victims had been born into large families on welfare. Some states did not reverse their sterilization laws until the 1960s.

The eugenics movement lay behind the famous (1927) *Buck* v. *Bell* decision by the United States Supreme Court. Supposedly retarded like her mother, Carrie Buck had been committed at age 18 to a state mental institution in Virginia. Pregnant when committed, Carrie gave birth to a daughter inside the institution.

Harry Laughlin, an influential geneticist who worked at Cold Springs Harbor, concluded that Carrie Buck's retardation was hereditary. He based this conclusion not on his own examination but upon reading a written report of a social worker, who said Carrie had a "feeble look" about her. Laughlin then declared that Carrie Buck "lived a life of immorality and prostitution," and that all the Bucks belonged to the "shiftless, ignorant, worthless class of anti-social whites of the South."

The U.S. Supreme Court upheld the legality of the Virginia law permitting Carrie Buck's sterilization. Justice Oliver Wendell Holmes wrote the majority (8 to 1) opinion:

> We have seen more than once that the public welfare may call upon the best citizens for their lives. It would be strange if it could not call upon those who already sap the strength of the State for these lesser sacrifices, often not felt to be such by those concerned, in order to prevent our being swamped with incompetence. It is better for all the world, if instead of waiting to execute degenerate offspring for crime, or to let them starve for their imbecility, society can prevent those who are manifestly unfit from continuing their kind. The principle that sustains compulsory vaccination is broad enough to cover cutting the Fallopian tubes.

He concluded, "Three generations of imbeciles are enough."

The legal legacy of eugenics also included the *Immigration Restriction Act of 1924*. Hailed by eugenicists as their greatest triumph, it assumed the inferior genes of Asians, Africans, Greeks, Irish, Poles, and Italians, and the superior genes of the English, Dutch, Scotch, Scandinavians, and Germans. President Calvin Coolidge enthusiastically signed the Act into law. As Vice President he said, "America must be kept American. Biological laws show . . . that Nordics deteriorate when mixed with other races.[16]

This Immigration Act established quotas according to countries of origin. Based on how many people from a given country were already in America, such quotas denied entry to people from "inferior" countries.

Indeed, America as a "melting pot" originally poured scorn on immigration. Similarly, the Statue of Liberty today symbolizes freedom, but after 1924, thousands of the world's "huddled masses" had only a glimpse of it before their boats were sent back.

In sum, eugenicists incorrectly assumed many things, among them:

1. *The reductionist assumption* that each trait identified by morality or social distinctions was caused by a gene in a one-to-one relation. Prostitution, retardation, poverty, and criminality were each supposedly caused by a single gene.

2. *The reductionist assumption* that genes cause diseases in a simplistic, one-gene-to-one-disease way. A few genetic diseases, such as Huntington's and sickle-cell, do work this way, but most do not.

3. *Ignorance about recessive inheritance.* Two unaffected carriers can each pass a gene for a recessive trait to a child, who will then be homozygous for the trait.

4. *Ignorance of environmental effects on expression of genes.* How a gene, or a combination of genes, is expressed depends in part on what happens during gestation, in early childhood, and in the overall environment. Genes have a fan-like range of expression (their norm of reaction), and which point on the fan manifests in a particular person depends on what happened in his or her environment.

5. *Naiveté as to the ease of controlling reproduction* in couples. Humans are driven to have sex, and if they aren't careful, children result. When informed of risk of a child with genetic disease, few humans can or will prevent birth of children, especially without access to contraception!

6. *Ignorance of mutations and chromosomal breakage.* Not knowing about these aspects of genetics, eugenicists mistakenly believed that if all retarded people could be prevented from reproducing, retardation could be eliminated from the gene pool.

7. *Ignorance of population genetics.* Eugenicists hoped to perfect humanity through selective breeding, but population genetics have since shown that there will be a regression to the mean. *Regression to the mean* is the inherent tendency in stable populations to return to an average value over time; in population genetics, the underlying causes creating a mean value in a population will eventually normalize any deviant values.

After 1935, the eugenics movement declined in the United States. Geneticist Hermann J. Muller said that eugenics was "hopelessly perverted," a cult for "advocates for race and class prejudice, defenders of vested interests of church and State, Fascists, Hitlerites, and reactionaries generally."[17] Another leading geneticist, J. B. S. Haldane, said at the time of the sterilization programs that "many of the deeds done in America in the name of eugenics are about as much justified by science as were the proceedings of the Inquisition by the Gospels."[18] Advances in population genetics prompted Haldane to remark, "An ounce of algebra is worth a ton of verbal argument."[19]

The overall lesson of the eugenics movement is that politicians, educators, clergy, and some scientists hastily promoted laws and moral attitudes that had little to do with complex scientific facts. Paradoxically, the appeal of the solidity and inevitability of real, scientific facts gave plausibility to these nonfactual laws and attitudes. Unfortunately, many of the assumptions made were falsely reductionistic, based on ideology, or just plain wrong. If we call such laws and moral attitudes "public policy," then the eugenics movement showed that public policy can leap past verified facts in creating dangerous laws that harm people, all in the name of the very facts that are lacking.

CASE 3: GENES FOR BREAST CANCER

Like diabetes, breast cancer is more complicated than Huntington's. Most breast cancer is not caused by a single gene, has both preventive and curative treatments, and is not uniformly fatal.

Joan is a 50-year-old woman who had breast cancer at age 45 and had the affected breast removed, followed by radiation and chemotherapy and a maintenance course of tamoxifen. In high school and college, she smoked one to two packs of cigarettes a day, and for a decade in college and graduate school, used oral contraceptives. Cancer in females is associated with smoking and the pill, especially both together.

Joan blames herself for her cancer, but because her mother and aunt had breast cancer at the same age, wonders if she might have hereditary breast cancer. If she did, her daughters might take precautions. Moreover, if she did have the gene, her smoking and use of contraceptives might not have given her breast cancer.

Is most breast cancer caused by a gene? Despite the conventional wisdom, it is not. In fact, 95 percent of breast cancer is not caused by a gene. But the 5 percent that is caused by a gene is the center of controversy here.

In 1990, Mary Claire-King discovered a single gene, BRCA1 (BReast CAncer1) causing one form of breast cancer and ovarian cancer; its exact location was identified in 1994. Alan Ashworth in 1995 discovered another gene, BRCA2. In 2002, researchers discovered a third gene, CHEK2. Mutations in any of these genes cause breast cancer. Women in families expressing mutations in these BRCA1 or BRCA2 run an 80 percent risk of developing breast cancer in their lives, compared with a 9 percent risk for other women. Both BRCA1 and BRCA2 are autosomal dominant genes.

The science of presymptomatic testing for these genes is complex. Many mutations of BRCA1 and BRCA2 carry varying degrees of risk, which must be interpreted correctly for each family. The same mutation may act differently in different families or in twins with different lifestyles.

ETHICAL ISSUES

Testing as Self-Interest

Testing for genes for breast cancer may benefit the woman affected. Even with surgery, radiation, and chemotherapy for breast cancer, about 20 percent of women will still die from it. For this reason, significant percentages of women testing positive for breast cancer or for the genes BRCA1 or BRCA2 decided to remove both breasts in hopes of living to old age.

This is a significant ethical issue whose pedigree requires some explanation. In the 1960s, many women under 50 with breast cancer elected to have a bilateral mastectomy to remove both cancerous and precancerous tissue from their breasts.[20] In the 1970s and 1980s, studies showed that for most women with breast cancer, women getting a lumpectomy fared no worse than getting bilateral mastectomies. Because significant percentages of women experienced loss of femininity and self-esteem after their mastectomies, sparing them this surgery was thought to be a benefit.

However, the current views is that women with the breast cancer genes have an 80 percent chance of developing breast cancer during their lives, so for them bilateral mastectomy holds out a chance to prevent the cancer from starting at all.

Even before clinical trials finished, large numbers of women testing positive for BRCA1 and BRCA2 had preventive bilateral mastectomies. In 2002, a clinical trial proved that, five years after surgery, women with a BRCA1 or BRCA2 mutation undergoing prophylactic bilateral mastectomy have a statistically significant lower risk of breast cancer.

However, if there is any lesson in the ethics of genetic testing, it is that everything is complicated. Later studies suggested that the figure of 80 percent risk was exaggerated. Women with breast cancer initially recruited for studies of the two breast cancer genes came from families with breast cancer in grandmothers, mothers, daughters, and sisters, resulting in a selection bias.[21] So other women probably had their breasts removed based on data showing a much greater risk of breast cancer than they had.

Now add another twist. Besides the three mutations of BRCA1, BRCA2, and CHEK2 that cause breast cancer, hundreds of variant mutations now are known, each conferring a different degree of risk. Moreover, the risk of each variant may vary with the peculiarities of each family. Conveying all this information accurately requires sophistication by patient and genetic counselor.

But the history of genetics shows that sophistication and understanding of subtle, complex issues are not strengths of public policy or among the public. Women are likely to think "I have the breast cancer gene" and fear death in a few years from breast cancer.

If a woman has BRCA1, BRCA2 or CHEK2, the benefits of knowing early are that taking birth control pills reduces risk of ovarian cancer by 60 percent and taking the drug tamoxifen reduces risk of breast cancer by nearly half. More radically, prophylactic bilateral mastectomy increases longevity.

These same benefits apply to men, who account for about 2 percent of all cases of breast cancer.

Similarly, testing for the gene for type 2 diabetes could lead to benefits for Maria Lopez, especially if she could adopt a healthy lifestyle. For Maria and especially her daughters, it will be important to eat a low-fat, low-processed sugar diet and to exercise to keep their weight normal. In some cases, a positive test for the type 2 gene could be a wake-up call to adopt a healthy lifestyle.

Testing Only to Hear Good News

When people take genetic tests, do they really understand what they're doing? One Huntington's counselor says, "When people say they want this test to find out if they have the gene so they can make decisions, they really want to find out that they don't have it. The trouble is that fifty percent of them do. And there's no way to prepare them."[22]

In the first study of the linkage test for Huntington's, most people at risk (63–79 percent) originally said they would take the test, but some changed their minds later.[23] Some had expected to test negative and had intended to take the test to confirm this. This expectation indicated that they were in denial and were unprepared for a positive result; when they were well-counseled, counselors broke through their denial and they decided not to test.

The same study reported that "participants found to be probable gene carriers reported being surprised or shocked by the test result."[24] They had not expected to have the lethal gene.

Another consideration is that self-knowledge is seldom perfect. Many people simply cannot predict how they will react to testing positive—what they will feel or do if they learn the worst. Since Huntington's cannot be cured or ameliorated, a positive test will tell someone like Nancy Wexler that she is going to die an early, terrible death. Not everyone can deal with such knowledge. Moreover, isn't it inhumane to give people such a diagnosis when no treatment is possible? Perhaps people at risk of Huntington's should not be burdened with more truth than they can bear.[25]

On the positive side, testing for genes for breast cancer or diabetes allows intervention at an early stage. In one family, one of two sisters at hereditary risk worried about developing breast cancer and had planned to have her breasts removed as a preventive measure; she took the test for breast cancer genes, turned out to be negative and canceled her plan. Her sister did not think she was at risk and had refused mammograms but discovered she had the BRCA1 gene. A previous examination of her breasts had found nothing, but a reexamination found a minuscule node, and a biopsy determined that cancer had already begun, so a radical mastectomy was performed. Without the genetic test, this second sister might not have discovered her cancer until many years later.

Testing also allays fears of women who are "certain" they have such genes when they do not. Also, for some women, a mysterious, random turn of fate becomes testable and predictable. Although all women who test positive dislike the news, and although some who tested negative felt guilty, almost all think it's better to have a way to know.

Testing as a Duty to One's Family

Knowing one's likely genetic fate isn't just a concern of individuals. People are not atomistic; they come embedded in families, with children and parents, brothers and sisters.

The major argument favoring testing for serious genetic disease concerns childbearing. Nancy Wexler did not have children for fear that one might inherit Huntington's, yet perhaps her decision was misguided. If she had taken the test and been negative, she could have had children unaffected by Huntington's.

On the other hand, people who test positive should not have children or should test embryos and implant ones lacking the Huntington's gene. Why is that? Because parents should want the best lives for their children, and such lives start with freedom from genetic disease. No parent should willingly inflict a serious genetic disease on his or her child.

A second argument for testing concerns spouses and caretakers. Consider the following example. A man who was at risk for Huntington's but had decided not to take the test discussed his reasons before a large medical class. His reasons were greeted with respect; but as the class ended and the students started to file out, a woman cried out from the back of the room, "What about me and the kids? What about my view about testing him?" It was the man's wife.

She wanted to be able to plan for the future. If her husband were positive, she would be taking care of him. She might also have been thinking of money: if her husband were positive, he would eventually need custodial care, and they would have to start saving up for that or, if possible, arrange for life or health insurance. Moreover, when Huntington's strikes, the family as well as the victim will suffer emotionally; they should prepare themselves for this. Finally, they might try to make the most of whatever time remains before onset.

Besides a strict duty to one's family, compromises are possible. For instance, middle-aged people who do not want to know may feel that they have escaped the disease and that they can now take the test as a gift to their children. Another compromise is to have blood samples taken and stored at the International Research Roster for Huntington's in Indianapolis, Indiana, or at similar blood banks around North America. If someone dies before symptoms appear, his blood can be tested postmortem.

Testing One's Family by Testing Oneself

In any genetic testing, testing one family member has inevitable implications for other members of the family. In more ways than one, the results of testing affect the entire family.

Catherine Hayes gives an example:

> A case in point involves a pair of identical twins, only one of whom wanted to be tested. She swore that she would never reveal the results to anyone else in her family, in particular her twin. Once she was informed of the results—that there was a high probability that she would have Huntington's—the information spread quickly throughout the entire family. This meant that the twin who did not want to know her genetic status was now faced with the unwelcome knowledge that she too would probably have the disease.[26]

Hayes had five brothers and eight nieces and nephews. Though she tested negative, one of her brothers already has symptoms of Huntington's and another has tested positive; both already have children.

In one family where a woman tested for hereditary breast cancer, confidentiality was very difficult to maintain among the women of these extended families. It was hard for a woman to resist her family and not discover her status: in testing a middle-aged woman, one is also telling her mother and her daughters their risk of developing breast cancer.

It is important to keep in mind that in testing for dominant, single-gene diseases, such as Huntington's and the breast cancer genes, there is no such thing as testing only a fetus or testing only a parent: a positive fetus reveals a positive parent; a positive parent reveals that any children are at risk.

Helping families understand that genetic testing is difficult. Hayes notes, "Many medical professionals have difficulty viewing genetic issues in a family context. . . . Most researchers cannot possibly know what it is like to grow up in a family haunted by a genetic disease . . . ."

Testing may tear families apart. Consider the right to know. Even in a life-or-death situation, judges have ruled that relatives cannot be compelled to be tested for compatibility as bone-marrow or organ donors. Such decisions indicate that judges will not force genetic tests on relatives.

If a person tested positive for Huntington's and concealed it from a prospective spouse, could that be grounds for annulment? Does a prospective spouse have a right to know about such a test? Or does marrying "for better or worse" cover such questions?

Can one parent have a child tested in order to find out if the other parent is affected? Suppose that a father tests positive for Huntington's and refuses to tell his teenage daughter, Laura. Suppose that a genetic counselor is aware of the father's result. When Laura gets married, what should the counselor do? Recommend general genetic tests to her? Suppose she refuses. If she knew that her father was positive, would she agree to testing? If so, should the counselor violate the father's confidentiality? To many people, the good of preventing another child with Huntington's outweighs the harm of violating privacy, especially where there is a strong sense that the affected parent had an obligation to reveal his result in the first place.

One advocate for families afflicted with genetic disease believes that:

> first and foremost, genetic testing must be viewed as a family issue, not an individual one. The person who enrolls in a testing program should be strongly encouraged to involve other family members, within reason. Testing one member of a family will affect other members. Persons who refuse to involve their families may not have considered fully the consequences for other members or for themselves.[27]

Personal Responsibility for Disease

Let us return to the question of whether Joan and Maria are responsible for their diseases. The answer may be, "Yes and no." We can approach the question of responsibility in a less moralistic way by taking a different approach. Suppose

Joan and Maria each have three teenage daughters and that both Joan and Maria want to inoculate these daughters against a similar fate. The absolutely crucial question here is this: *Can these daughters avoid their mother's diseases?*

Put this way, we are not being moralistic or looking for a way to cast the first stone. Instead, we are doing preventive work, albeit in a conceptual way. "Conceptual" because we can assume ideal conditions: good education, maximal free will, good familial support for good eating, and so on. We can then ask, "Under ideal conditions, if they inherit their mother's genetic risk, can these daughters avoid breast cancer and diabetes?" Notice that this question has several dimensions: metaphysical (is there free will at all?), moral (are patients partly responsible for their diseases or good health?), and clinical (practically speaking, how much change can physicians expect of patients at-risk for breast cancer and diabetes?).

Type 2 diabetes is an especially good candidate for prevention because we know that many Asian people do not get diabetes until they adopt Western lifestyles. (Similarly, for Asian men immigrating to North American, incidence of prostate cancer jumps from 1 per 100,000 to 70 per 100,000.[28]) The prevailing view about preventing diabetes is this:

> What is especially disturbing about the rise of Type 2 [diabetes] is that it can be delayed and perhaps prevented with changes in diet and exercise. For although both types are believed to stem in part from genetic factors, Type 2 is also spurred by obesity and inactivity. This is particularly true in those prone to illness.[29]

So are 21 million Americans "failures" in personal responsibility because they have diabetes? Are another 10 million "successes" because they staved off genetic predisposition?

Let us take a larger perspective. Cancer occurs when tumor-suppressing genes or DNA repair mechanisms cease to work, resulting in wild, uncontrolled growth of cells. Diabetes occurs when the body fails to turn food into glucose, the body's chief source of energy.

Both diseases occur when environmental inputs trigger potential in an inherited genetic template. At the very least, avoidance of the inputs can delay onset of disease and perhaps avoid it altogether (people with genetic dispositions to alcoholism do not become alcoholics in countries where alcohol is banned). As a person ages, her immune system and organs deteriorate, and mutated cells in her body accumulate, making her more vulnerable to cancer and diabetes, so some people, despite healthy lifestyles, may eventually succumb to their genetic risk.[30]

Individuals and societies have some control over how many carcinogens are introduced to human bodies: tobacco sales can be banned in schools and hospitals, smoking can be forbidden in public, and people can avoid or quit tobacco. Similarly, junk foods and sodas can be banned from schools. Individuals at risk for cancer and diabetes can eat low-fat diets high in fiber, fresh fruits, and vegetables. In this way, both societies and individuals can reduce the likelihood of cancer and diabetes.

But what if a daughter gets cancer or diabetes anyway? Should she be blamed? Answer: probably not. To say that these diseases can be partially preventable by healthy living is not to say that some cases aren't, like Huntington's disease, genetically inevitable. Second, other factors in a person's life may have prevented healthy living such that a person truly could not have done otherwise. In these cases, blame would be wrong.

Testing and Sick Identities

Nancy Wexler rejects an attitude she found dominant among the medical community about testing, which might be expressed as: "Come on! Take your knowledge like a man and don't be a sissy!" So everybody is expected to find out his or her genetic fate as soon as possible. The problem with this attitude is that it seems to benefit the medical community and family more than the individual affected. If there is no cure or treatment, as with Huntington's, what's so good about knowing?

Nancy Wexler thinks that people who test positive may adopt a "sick identity" for any genetic disease long before they experience any symptoms. That is one of her primary arguments against genetic testing. If you're going to get the disease, she argues, you will in fact get it, so there's nothing you can do about it. Why burden yourself being identified as "sick" long before you are?

Moreover, some people are highly suggestible. People who are concerned about suicide often focus on the consequences of testing teenagers—a population that is already highly suicidal. Youngsters who are merely at risk for Huntington's, breast cancer, or diabetes already agonize about going to college and spending their parents' money, and those who learn for certain that they have these genes may be even more vulnerable.

Should girls under 18 years of age be tested for these genes if they run in their families? At first glance, the answer seems no, for a positive answer might take away the fun of childhood and adolescence. Moreover, great danger exists of developing a sick identity as a "woman with breast cancer" or a "woman who will get diabetes." On the other hand, eating junk food and smoking start early in many teenagers, so early testing might be beneficial.

Preventing Suicide by Not Knowing

Because 25 percent of people with Huntington's consider suicide and 10 percent carry it out,[31] scientists have debated whether the test for Huntington's should be made available at all. Nancy Wexler said, "We have to understand that the day you tell someone he has this gene, his life and view of himself change forever. We're worried about the potential for suicide."[32] This argument might also be a factor, although to a lesser extent, in testing people for breast cancer or diabetes.

Should suicide be prevented at all costs, such that people who say they might commit suicide should not be tested for Huntington's? As Wexler emphasizes, "Huntington's patients know their family and they know what's happening to them. So in a way, it's worse than Alzheimer's."[33]

Is suicide an adequate reason for not testing? Even if 10 percent commit suicide, 90 percent do not. Nancy Wexler says, "Suicide is not unreasonable. It's not so awful that we can't discuss it or consider it." She observes, "For some of my friends who have Huntington's, knowing that they can commit suicide gives them a certain sense of control. They want to feel that if it gets too bad, they can have a way out. They can do something."[34]

Some scientists argue against paternalism: "I think we can trust people to make these decisions. I'm not so convinced we researchers should be dictating how the technology gets used."[35]

Testing Only with Good Counseling

Many people who are not absolutely opposed to testing—and even people who generally favor testing—argue that testing should only be offered *with good counseling*, especially because the results will be probabilistic for most people (not "You don't have the gene," but "You have a 90 percent chance of not having the gene").

This is, of course, paternalistic. However, it is true that some of those who test positive will wish they hadn't taken the test and some may develop emotional problems, and that counseling can help such people.

As a matter of public policy, should people, through their private physicians, simply be allowed to "buy" their own test results, or should counseling be required?

The President's Commission on Bioethics (1983) emphasized that counseling should be guaranteed: "A full range of prescreening and follow-up services . . . should be available before a program [of genetic testing] is introduced."[36] Note, though, that the recommendation here is for making counseling available, not mandatory.

This is not a realistic policy. First, 44 million Americans lack medical insurance and would need to buy genetic counseling, an expensive proposition. Second, just finding a trained genetics counselor is not easy, and many people do not live near a major medical center that has such a skilled counselor. Even for people with good medical coverage for physical illnesses, most policies today do not provide good coverage for genetic counseling.

Genetic Testing and Insurance

Genetic testing raises financial issues. For example, when one woman who tested positive decided to have a preventive radical mastectomy, she didn't want to tell her insurance company the reason for her decision because she was afraid her company would cancel her policy or raise her premiums, and perhaps even do the same for her daughters. Because her insurer didn't know anything, it thought she was being irrational and wouldn't pay for her surgery.

An important issue about genetic testing and medical insurance concerns confidentiality. Several national companies (such as Medical Information Bureau of Boston) inform insurance companies about applicants who are risks.[37] For people who take presymptomatic genetic tests and test positive, insurers could raise premiums for families. Worse, they could consider the result evidence of a preexisting condition and exclude that disease from future coverage.

For this reason, it is crucial to control the distribution of test results: that is, to decide who should and should not receive them. Many large institutions, such as the military, universities, and large companies, "self-insure" themselves and pass their losses along to employees through increased premiums. Moreover, some employers may not keep test results confidential, especially if key employees are involved; consequently, a positive result may keep an executive off the fast track.

Violation of confidentiality might also keep a physician out of a medical group, a student out of a university or graduate school, and so on.

Congress has considered a proposal, the Human Genome Privacy Bill, to ban insurers from access to genetic tests. A task force of the Human Genome Project has recommended that " . . . all individual risk information be excluded from decisions about who gets insured, what they get insured for, and how much they get charged. We see no other practical, sustainable plan for health care coverage than community rating."[38]

Genetic testing reveals the gaps in our national, medical *nonsystem*. If everyone who tests positive for genetic disease can get expensive medical coverage, while those who test negative are allowed to opt out, insurance companies will quickly go bankrupt. As genetic testing stresses our stopgap system, inequities of future health that it reveals may force us to adopt a national, single-payer system (for more on this, see the last chapter).

Genetic testing for diabetes exposes similar problems. Almost no money is spent by medical centers for education and counseling to prevent diabetes because doing so generally loses money. In contrast, waiting until crises develop and then amputating gangrenous legs produces profits (because insurance reimburses physicians well for doing surgical procedures, not for talking to patients).[39] Similarly, insurance companies curtail benefits to diabetics to discourage them from enrolling in their plans: "In a 2003 survey, 87 percent of health insurance actuaries . . . said that if they were to improve coverage [for diabetics] with richer drug benefits or easier access to specialists, they would incur financial problems by attracting the sickest, most expensive patients."[40]

Caveat Emptor: Making Money from Genetic Testing

In 2002, Myriad Genetics of Salt Lake City expanded its sales force from 85 to 600 agents to market BRCA1 testing directly to doctors and their patients. The tests, which cost between $750 and $2,750, would only benefit the 5 to 10 percent of people with breast cancer caused by these genes.

Unfortunately, BRCA1's discovery offered hope of a screening test only for women with hereditary breast and ovarian cancer—not for the 90 to 95 percent of women who develop nonhereditary breast cancer.

In some ways, marketing such tests is a win-win situation for Myriad Genetics. For the people who test positive, they get their money's worth and advance news. For the people who test negative, they get relief and will not complain about the money spent. The ethical issue arises when thousands of people seek relief who are really not at risk: they waste their money in getting a negative result. But it would be patronizing to say they can't spend their money as they choose, even irrationally.

Note that similar tests could be offered for genes for prostate cancer or diabetes, only a small percentage of which is caused by a single gene. For most people, such testing would be a waste of money.

Premature Announcements and Oversimplifications

Almost every week, the mass media report the discovery of a genetic basis for a disease or a trait (such as humor). Yet almost all such reports mislead us into thinking that the genetic revolution has come. In fact, when we examine the practical aspects, in other words, when we look to see applications in ordinary medicine, we see the reality: progress is slow, hesitant, and results are usually complicated with many qualifications.

Recall that scientists created a linkage test in 1983 for Huntington's, predicted it would take 3 to 5 years to find the gene, and in fact, it took 10 years to find the gene. A good clinical test was not routinely offered until 1996. During the same decades, optimists predicted discovery of a gene for breast cancer, which finally came in 1994 and 1995, but practical tests for the three mutations took much longer. Scientists didn't discover a diabetes gene until 2000 and it took until 2006 to discover its exact location.

Just as the search for the these genes took longer and proved harder than expected, many early reports of discoveries of genetic causes of illnesses were premature. In 1987, researchers retracted an earlier claim that manic-depression was linked to a gene on the X chromosome.[41] By this time, earlier claims about genetic causes of schizophrenia and alcoholism had been retracted.

Today, geneticists believe that psychiatric disorders such as schizophrenia will not be found to be single-gene disorders. According to one leading researcher, common forms of mental illness may be caused by three to five genes acting together, probably with environmental co-factors.[42]

Like eugenics, much of the news about genetics in today's mass media is simplistic, alarmist, and premature. The movie *GATTACA* sums up these misconceptions, scaring us about imminent presymptomatic testing that may in fact be a century away.

Blame and Responsibility: Final Thoughts

Genetic testing may lead each of us to think more carefully about causes of gene-associated diseases. Presymptomatic testing may give some people a small window of preventive control. People at risk for cancers of the breast or prostate may be able to avoid smoking or being around second-hand smoke (exposure of children to the latter among smoking parents is strongly associated with later development of diabetes when children grow up[43]).

Previously, three standards of evidence were discussed that are used in the law: preponderance of evidence, clear and convincing evidence, and beyond a reasonable doubt. These standards can be used to make a point. We know beyond a reasonable doubt that no one with Huntington's disease can do anything to prevent this disease from destroying their brains and killing them. We also know that, for people with genes for breast cancer, unless they have double mastectomies, 80 percent of them will develop breast cancer.

This brings us to diabetes. Probably the best chance that prediabetics have to prevent diabetes is as children and adolescents, before they become overweight and have high levels of blood sugar. If they enter young adulthood overweight and accustomed to eating lots of processed sugars, the probability that they will develop diabetes is high.

Does that mean they should be blamed for their disease? No. To hand out blame, we would need to know, at least with clear and convincing evidence, that they could have acted otherwise and eaten/exercised differently. It may be true that they could have, just as it may be true that the presumption of innocence allows some of the guilty to go free. But people who do not have genes for type 2 diabetes cannot really know what it's like to crave fats and sugars and to be tormented by these cravings. Yes, everyone is tempted, but some are tempted so much more intensely and continually than others! Until we have evidence that prediabetics could have acted otherwise, we should not blame them as individuals or in public policy.

That is compatible with educating young people and acting as if they can transcend their genetic dispositions. We want to think the best of people and to give them hope, but at the same time, we don't want to condemn them when they turn out to be less than ideal.

Finally, the history of eugenics shows that we almost always make huge mistakes in public policy about genetics, especially in oversimplifying complex issues. Responsibility may exist on a gradient, corresponding to a gradient of free will, such that some people have more than others. Two people with the same genes, placed at birth in different families (like Twain's *The Prince and the Pauper*) might as adults have differing degrees of free will and responsibility for their health or disease. On this perspective, poor people from dysfunctional families with no medical insurance, with genes predisposing them to diabetes or cancer, and little education will have less free will than well-educated young adults from loving, well-off families with good medical coverage who are blessed to have inherited good genes.

FURTHER READING AND RESOURCES

Catherine Hayes, "Genetic Testing for Huntington's—A Family Issue," *New England Journal of Medicine*, 327, no. 20, 1993.

Daniel Kevles, *In the Name of Eugenics: Genetics and the Uses of Human Heredity*, Knopf, New York, 1985.

CHAPTER 17

Preventing the Global Spread of AIDS

This chapter emphasizes prevention of AIDS as a worldwide problem and as a challenge for bioethics. In a sense, such prevention is the ultimate classic case because already in human history, someone has become infected or died of HIV over 65 million times. Millions more new people become infected each year, raising the question of how we can slow this scourge.

The heart of the chapter discusses four approaches to stopping AIDS. As it explains, part of our problem stems from conflicts between these approaches, where each accuses the others of being part of the problem.

The chapter also discusses past epidemics, misunderstandings of AIDS, the transmission, clinical course, and treatment of AIDS, the scandal over HIV-infection of the blood supply, Kimberly Bergalis' case, homosexuality, contact tracing, mandatory screening, and preventive programs that exchange needles.

BACKGROUND: EPIDEMICS, PLAGUES, AND AIDS

Throughout human history, epidemics have always terrified humans. The deadly bacterial disease known as *the black death* or simply, the *plague,* had its great outbreak in 1348 in Europe.

It had two forms: *bubonic plague*, the most common and classic, is characterized by inflamed swellings of the lymphatic glands in the groin and armpits, and is transmitted by fleas. Rats and other small mammals carried fleas to humans, and the bites of fleas transmitted plague to humans.

The bacillus *Yersinia pestis* causes bubonic plague. Untreated bubonic plague killed 50 percent of its victims. Today, antibiotics treat its earliest stages.

A virulent complication of untreated bubonic plague, *pneumonic plague,* involves the lungs. Easily transmitted when one person coughs on another, the microbe kills almost universally. Because of it, many physicians of the 14th century decided their calling lay elsewhere.

In the same century, astrologers claimed that plague resulted from the conjunction of Saturn, Mars, and Jupiter; others claimed it resulted from sulfurous fumes released by earthquakes. Clergy taught that God had sent it to punish humans for great sins.

Historian Barbara Tuchman tells us that during medieval epidemics, "Organized groups of 200 to 300 . . . marched from city to city, stripped to the waist, scourging themselves with leather whips tipped with iron spikes until they bled. While they cried aloud to Christ and the Virgin for pity, . . . the watching townspeople sobbed in sympathy."[1] In so marching, they spread infected fleas.

The fearful ignorance of the times required *scapegoats* (in the Bible, goats were sacrificed to atone for bad things and to ward off worse things). So people accused Orthodox Jews, with their distinctive dress, of poisoning wells and spreading plague. When atonement processions reached cities, they often attacked the Jewish quarter, trapped Jews inside, and set the area on fire. When plague followed, Jews were blamed, not the procession.

Leprosy, cholera, and syphilis also terrified people. Leprosy, or Hansen's disease, creates lesions on the skin and kills slowly over years. Twentieth century medicine learned that people only get infected through exposure over many months through the skin or mucosa. Before then, society banished lepers and forced them to live in isolated places in lepers' colonies, and if they walked out, to ring cowbells to warn people off.

Great epidemics of cholera from infected water also created fear and loathing of its victims. During the epidemic of 1813, Americans blamed those who fell ill, especially wanton prostitutes, drunk Irish, lazy blacks, and the dirty poor who lived along creeks used for both drinking water and defecation. Ministers praised God for cholera for "cleansing the filth from society."

In 1854, physician John Snow realized that cholera only broke out in the district that received water from the Broad Street pump in London; he discovered that infected water spread cholera and that clean water could prevent it. Nevertheless, Americans preferred to believe that sin and being Irish caused cholera, so many more died in the third great cholera epidemic of 1862.

Not until acceptance of the germ theory of disease after 1900 did public health prevent epidemics of cholera. In other words, it took a half century for a medical insight to be translated into public policy to save millions of lives.

Victims of syphilis were also blamed for their disease. As discussed earlier, moralists blamed vice for the disease whereas scientists blamed spirochetes. (Ch. 10 on the Tuskegee Study discusses syphilis.)

A Brief History of AIDS

The first proven case of HIV came from a blood sample collected in 1959 from a man in Kinshasa, Democratic Republic of Congo. Genetic analysis of his blood suggests that HIV-1 may have stemmed from a virus that existed in the early 1940s or even the late 1930s.

Researcher Beatrice Hahn and her team at UAB proved in 1999 by DNA sequencing that the virus spread to humans from wild chimpanzees in southern Cameroon; HIV infected the blood of hunters there through catching, killing, and cutting up these chimps for bushmeat.[2]

Around 1978, gay men in the United States, Sweden, and Haiti begin to show signs of what would later be called AIDS. Between 1979 and 1981, Kaposi's sarcoma, and *Pneumocystis carinii* pneumonia (PCP) unexpectedly showed up in gay males in Los Angeles and New York.

On June 5, 1981, the Centers for Disease Control (CDC) announced the discovery of a mysterious "gay-related infectious disease" (GRID) that had killed 3 gay men; only a month later, 108 cases of GRID were reported and 46 gay men were dead.

Three months after the first report of GRID in the summer of 1981, CDC announced that babies of drug-dependent women in New York City also had the disease; GRID was changed to *acquired immune deficiency syndrome* or *AIDS*.

In 1982, when physicians in New York and California had already seen hundreds of cases of AIDS, they did not know its incubation or causative agent. CDC guessed that incubation could be many years and that many thousands of people could be infected. No one then diagnosed with AIDS had ever lived more than two years, so the disease frightened everyone.

In 1983, Luc Montagnier and the Institut Pasteur in France discovered that a virus, the *human immunodeficiency virus,* HIV, caused AIDS. Today his virus is called HIV-1. In 1986, scientists discovered a second form in West Africa, HIV-2, where it may have been infecting residents for decades. HIV-2 seems to develop more slowly and to be milder than HIV-1 but to be more easily transmitted heterosexually (the United States has reported few cases of HIV-2).[3]

As early as 1982, the CDC warned that donated blood could carry the agent causing AIDS. Blood then could have been screened for hepatitis, thereby indirectly screening for HIV, but officials deemed this too expensive and unfortunately did not do it.

In 1984, the FDA approved the ELISA test for antibodies to HIV. Now blood donated or otherwise obtained could be tested for HIV. However, authorities running blood banks did not immediately test blood using the ELISA test. Why?

First, at the time, each opposing group politicized every fact about HIV and AIDS. A little historical background shows how this occurred. This background may predict what would occur if SARS or a lethal bird flu became epidemic.

AIDS and Ideology

By the end of 1981, CDC epidemiologists realized that gay men were being killed by a new kind of infectious disease of unknown nature and transmission. CDC postulated that sex among gay men might be spreading the disease, especially sex with anonymous partners in bathhouses in cities such as New York and San Francisco.

These bathhouses constituted what epidemiologists call an *amplification system* for the spread of a disease. Because some of the men had many anonymous sexual partners, some of whom, in turn, traveled to other places for sex with numbers of partners, the virus could spread quickly. Another such system was cheap travel by jet around the world. Indeed, CDC identified a gay airline steward as Patient Zero, the first person to bring HIV from Africa to the United States and to introduce it to gay bathhouses.[4]

Sharing needles and syringes to inject drugs constitutes another amplification system. Blood withdrawn from a user's vein mixes both with a drug in the syringe and with viral particles from previous users.

Another amplification system is a community's blood supply. Because plasma is pooled from many sources and because clotting factor for hemophiliacs is similarly pooled, one infected donation can infect many recipients.

The CDC called upon federal and state governments to fund studies to see if a new lethal disease had appeared in the blood system, but none did anything. At the time, medical experts believed that all lethal infectious diseases had been discovered, so no one expected a new one to emerge.

Also in 1981, gay men and lesbians had won some freedom from historical prejudice against them: resistance against oppressive police round-ups began in June 1969 at a bar called the Stonewall Inn in Greenwich Village in New York City. The resistance to harassment shown by gay men in the *Stonewall Riots* fostered a new pride in being gay and encouraged gay men to come out of the closet (of shame and secrecy in which they had been hiding their sexual identity).

Also in North America and Europe during the 1970s, a new sexual freedom ruled among heterosexuals, fueled by birth control, permissive attitudes towards nonmarital sex, Woodstock, mind-altering drugs, and social rebellion against authority. So gay men and lesbians rode the crest of a larger fire of sexual change burning through the forest of traditional society. In medicine, psychiatrists removed homosexuality from their list of psychiatric illnesses.

But many people still feared and ridiculed gay men. Reverend Jerry Falwell, who founded Moral Majority, a religious political organization, blamed gays for AIDS. In 1982, the Secretary of Moral Majority, Greg Dixon, wrote, "If homosexuals are not stopped, they will in time infect the entire nation, and America will be destroyed—as entire civilizations have fallen in the past."[5] This attitude persists, as seen in 2001 when the World Trade Center was destroyed: ministers Falwell and Pat Robertson blamed gays and atheists for the event, saying it was God's punishment on America, echoing earlier clergy who had scapegoated Jews for plague and the Irish for cholera.[6]

The head of the Southern Baptist Convention said that God had created AIDS to "indicate His displeasure with the homosexual lifestyle."[7] Monsignor Edward Clark of St. John's University in Queens, New York, claimed that, "If gay men would stop promiscuous sodomy, the AIDS virus would disappear from America."[8] Politician and media commentator Patrick Buchanan decried, " The poor homosexuals—they have declared war on nature and now nature is exacting an awful retribution."[9]

Reverend Falwell advocated shutting down bathhouses where gay men engaged in anonymous sex. Owners of such bathhouses countered with ads in gay newspapers extolling freedom and lambasting Falwell as a bigot. When gay activist Larry Kramer argued that shutting down bathhouses would save gay men's lives, gay men ridiculed him as a bigot.

Between 1983 and 1987, conservative politicians and clergy sparred verbally about AIDS with liberals and gay people. French philosopher Michel Foucault asserted that HIV did not cause AIDS and that HIV was not spread sexually. Foucault himself patronized bathhouses in the 1970s and died of AIDS in 1984, becoming perhaps the only philosopher in history to have his views empirically refuted by the manner of his own death.

In the *New York Review of Books*, contributing editor Jonathan Lieberson, a graduate student in philosophy at Columbia University, wrote several influential articles about AIDS in the mid-1980s. In one long article in 1986, he claimed that irrationality about AIDS was running wild, that only 10 percent of HIV-infected people would ever get AIDS, and that contact tracing should never be used to track down sex partners of HIV-infected men, even to save lives, because the newly won freedom of gay men and their sex lives was too important to sacrifice.[10] Around 1989, Lieberson himself died of AIDS (this periodical never apologized for these inaccurate pieces).

Transmission of HIV

Despite many rumors to the contrary, HIV is transmitted in only three ways: through blood, through semen, or to babies during birth or breast-feeding.

Without treatment, HIV causes a progressive weakening of the immune system, resulting in the body's inability to ward off normal infections. Without antiretroviral drugs, the average time between HIV-infection and full-blown AIDS in 2005 was 9.5 years, and 9.2 months between AIDS and death.

Cells called T4 lymphocytes (or simply T4 cells) indicate the health of the immune system: the lower the number of cells, the worse it is doing. When the count of T4 cells drops below 200, a person with AIDS usually gets *opportunistic infections* such as Kaposi's sarcoma, PCP, a fungal infection called oral thrush, or cervical cancer.

Testing Blood, Again

In the midst of the above controversies, authorities in 1984 weighed whether to test America's blood for hepatitis as an indirect test for HIV. Those *against* testing won.

Encouraged by people such as Foucault and the *New York Review of Books*, some vocal gay men argued that their donations of blood should not be "quarantined" and that HIV had not really been proven to cause AIDS. Blood banks worried that, if they screened blood, they might lose income (although they do not technically charge for blood, they make money classifying, transferring, and storing blood).

In May 1984, Stanford University started screening blood for HIV. Two months later, defending a national decision *not* to screen, Health and Human Services Secretary Margaret Heckler said, "I want to assure the American people that the blood supply is 100 percent safe . . . ."[11]

Joseph Bove, MD, who chaired the FDA's committee overseeing the safety of the nation's blood, said the "overreacting press" was causing hysteria about blood.[12] When the CDC counted 73 cases of deaths from AIDS caused by transfusion in March, 1984, Bove dismissed this danger: "More people are killed by bee stings."[13] Six months later, 269 people had died of AIDS from tainted blood.

In so assuring Americans, Bove and Heckler either lied, were incompetent, or both. In March 1985, most American blood banks began using the ELISA test to screen blood, a full year after they should have. Because of this lag, thousands of Americans and most hemophiliacs became infected with HIV. One of them was Ryan White, a hemophiliac who died at age 18 in 1990.

In 1985, a woman who was a prostitute and intravenous drug-user tested positive for HIV. Now that Ryan White and she had the disease, it seemed to be no longer just a gay disease. Now it had infiltrated heterosexuals and the blood supply.

Until 1986, people had hoped that most HIV-infected people would not die. Then that changed dramatically when researchers predicted that, without treatment, almost all the HIV-infected would get AIDS and die.

The same year, a few gutsy people founded ACT-UP to help people with AIDS. Its demonstrations forced the FDA to shorten by two years its process for approving new drugs and in 1987, AZT (zidovudine) became the first anti-HIV drug.

A decade later in 1996, scientists discovered protease inhibitors. These drugs block the protease enzyme, needed to create new, mature particles of HIV. These drugs allowed people with AIDS to live somewhat normal lives.

At the start of AIDS, 25 percent of women born of infected mothers became infected. AZT blocks such *vertical transmission* to less than 1 percent.

Protease inhibitors plus AZT can cost $10,000 a year and cause severe complications. Because they require an obsessive attention to daily regimens, few people taking them work regular jobs. In short, they do not cure AIDS, but provide a way to survive it.

Kimberly Bergalis's Case

In December 1987, David Acer, a dentist in Jensen Beach, Fla., extracted two molars from 21 year-old Kimberly Bergalis, a junior at the University of Florida in Gainesville. After graduating in 1990, Kimberly tested positive for HIV.

A young white male in his early 30s, Dr. Acer admitted to having had sexual relations over the previous decade with 100 to 150 men. In September 1987, he developed Kaposi's sarcoma. In July 1989, he sold his practice, sold his tools and destroyed his records. In September 1990, he died of AIDS.

When his former patients tested themselves for HIV, six others tested positive. By using DNA sequencing, CDC proved that Dr. Acer was the source of infection in all his infected patients.

All the patients felt betrayed by the health professions. Kimberly Bergalis died publicly and painfully. In 1991, with little hair and weighing only 70 pounds, she testified before Congress, urging it to pass a law making it a felony for HIV-positive health professionals to interact with patients without revealing their HIV status. The law never passed and Kimberly died in December 1991 at age 25.

Exactly how or why Dr. Acer infected his patients remains a mystery. Some people believe that he deliberately infected heterosexuals so that Americans would no longer see AIDS as a disease of gay men. What he did will never be known for sure.

In some ways it is better if Dr. Acer deliberately infected Kimberly. Why is that? Because if he did, then she did not get infected through unsafe dental/medical practices, and hence, no reason exists to test dentists/physicians for HIV. Retrospective analysis of cases of HIV+ dentists, surgeons, and internists reveal virtually no cases of accidental infection of patients. In general, probability of infection varies with amount of blood injected, how deeply the injection goes, and how much virus the blood contains. Also, the same procedures (double-gloving, masking, and not reusing needles) that protect patients from infection also protect physicians and dentists from patients.

THREE ETHICAL ISSUES IN STOPPING THE SPREAD OF AIDS

Homosexuality

Some people believe that teaching gay men how to practice safe sex condones sex between men. Although similar objections can be made to teaching safe sex, many people feel that sex between men should not be tolerated. Homosexuality has existed for thousands of years. In ancient Greece, bisexuality among men was popular, and leading Greek men such as Socrates preferred male lovers. Gay figures include Roman emperor Hadrian, King Frederick the Great of Prussia, playwright Tennessee Williams, and novelist Gore Vidal. According to the late Yale historian John Boswell, Christianity tolerated homosexuality more before the 12th century than in later centuries.[14]

Although a minority of people see homosexuality as a choice, virtually all medical researchers believe that sexual orientation is biologically determined. In 1991, cancer researcher Simon LeVay published a paper in *Science* asserting that a specific region of the X chromosome in 40 pairs of gay men was associated with their sexual preference for men. The media dubbed this "the gay gene." Some people believe that if a person has one copy of this gene, he or she may or may not become gay, depending on the person's experiences. But if the person gets *two* copies of the gene, it is inevitable that the person will be gay.

The lived experience of gay men and lesbians testifies to the truth of this *biological view*. Virtually every gay man and lesbian reports as children and teenagers fighting against his or her inner sexual attraction and trying to fit the norm of heterosexuality in advertising and culture. Because teenagers want to fit in, most gay and lesbian teenagers resist being attracted to members of the same sex and date heterosexually. Their sexual orientation appears to be a resisted discovery rather than a choice.

Many people harbor the false belief that state or federal laws protect sexual orientation. Only if Congress, a state, a city, or a county passed such a law would it be illegal to evict or fire someone because of homosexuality. Currently, except for San Francisco and two cities in Colorado, it is legal to do so almost everywhere.

Indeed, in *Bowers* v. *Hardwick*, the U. S. Supreme Court in 1988 allowed Georgia to keep a law making forms of anal and oral intercourse illegal between members of the same sex. Ironically, a footnote to the decision did *not* allow the state to criminalize the same behavior among heterosexuals. Obviously, this decision violates Mill's harm principle and cries out for an explanation of why such sexual behavior between members of the same sex is a crime, but not a crime when between members of different sexes.

Five years later in 2003, the U.S. Supreme Court admitted in *Lawrence* v. *Texas* that it had made a mistake, that the issue was not (as the *Bowers* court said) whether the Constitution conferred upon "homosexuals a right to engage in sodomy," but whether the Constitution conferred a liberty interest to all Americans broad enough to allow consenting sex among adults.[15]

As we will see below, worldviews collide over homosexuality and stopping AIDS. Is conceptualizing homosexuality as an evil lifestyle *homophobia*? Part of the problem of stopping AIDS? Or is tolerance of homosexuality, drugs, and other "immorality" a root cause of the spread of AIDS?

Needle Exchange Programs

Needle exchange programs (NEPs) prevent the spread of HIV by giving drug users a clean needle and syringe each time they inject drugs, eliminating the need to share a possibly contaminated syringe. One study in New Haven, Connecticut achieved a 33 percent reduction in HIV transmission by giving out clean needles to at-risk persons. A 1992 study by the CDC of 23 NEPs seemed to show no increase in drug usage by giving out clean needles.

But do such NEPs encourage nonusers to try hard drugs? If using such drugs had no risk of disease, might not more people use them?

Public health officials worry about *the exposure rate*. What that means is, in most populations, a small percentage of people will always become addicted after exposure to an addictive drug, be that alcohol or heroin. If the same, say, 2 percent of people always become addicted, it matters a lot whether the population exposed is 20 thousand or 20 million.

Prohibition kept alcohol's exposure rate low. Similarly, keeping cocaine and heroin illegal keeps their exposure rate low.

HIV Exceptionalism

In the first decade of AIDS, authorities in public health bowed to pressure from AIDS activists and did not pursue contact tracing the way they had with other sexually transmissible diseases. Because of prejudice against gay men, they feared that tracing those exposed to HIV might lead to some people losing their medical insurance or jobs. Besides, until AZT arrived in 1986, authorities could offer no treatment, so the benefits of identification were scant. So authorities made an exception for contact tracing for HIV.

Today, with AZT and protease inhibitors, early notification can save lives by helping the infected get prompt treatment.

Now if a HIV+ person knowingly practices unsafe sex, he can be charged in many states with a crime. In 1997 in New York, Nushawn Williams knew he was HIV+ and infected 28 teenage girls; he went to jail for doing so. In this case, contact tracing prevented even more girls from becoming infected.

HIV exceptionalism is now generally regarded in public health as a mistake. It succumbed to pressure from gay activists, and may have cost some of them their lives.

In 2006, the CDC recommended routine testing of all patients by doctors for HIV. Of course this created controversy. Conservative religious groups retorted that no reason existed to test people in traditional marriages.

STOPPING THE WORLDWIDE SPREAD OF HIV: FIVE VIEWS

In the first edition of this book in 1990, it seemed shocking that by 1987, 60,000 Americans had died of AIDS, more people than had died in the Vietnam War, and researchers guessed that in 1990, 10 million people might be infected worldwide. In 1992, Larry Kramer wrote:

> When I first became aware of this disease, there were only 43 cases in the United States; now there are 12 million people infected with AIDS around the world; within the next eight years, this figure could rise to 40 million. From 43 [people] to 40 million should be enough not only to cause some level of panic, but also to make everyone ask: how is this plague spreading so quickly? Indeed, 1 million new people worldwide were infected with the AIDS virus last year alone.[16]

Fourteen years after Larry Kramer wrote this, and after a quarter century of AIDS, we have little more wisdom on how to stop AIDS. Meanwhile, the number of victims of AIDS in the world now ceases to shock people and even numbs them.

By 2001, AIDS had killed nearly a half a million Americans, but in America, HIV-infection had become a chronic infection that people could live with. American patients then could even morally think about getting married or becoming parents. But in the developing world where most people lived, AIDS seemed unstoppable.

In the summer of 2001, when the virus had killed 20 million people and infected another 40 million, Secretary-General Kofi Annan of the United Nations called for a special, new, concerted effort to arrest the disease. Rock stars such as Bono pressured America to give more aid, which it did.

Five years later in the summer of 2006, Kofi Annan offered a depressing assessment: despite great progress in human events, the spread of AIDS was "the single greatest reversal in the history of human development."

Why was he so gloomy? Answer: *exactly 25 years after Americans first heard of AIDS, the disease had killed 25 million people on the planet.* The small bit of progress was that "only" 40 million people worldwide were then infected, the same number as five years before (although five million of the previous 40 million had since died). The 2001 conference had aimed at universal access to treatment, costing $20 billion a year, but only $10 billion had actually been donated each year.[17]

Year	HIV+ People	Number Killed[18]
1981	600	200
1990	10,000,000	1,000,000
1999	30,000,000	10,000,000
2006	40,000,000	25,000,000

The most urgent issue now in medicine concerns stopping the spread of AIDS. Bad answers affect more people's lives than any other issue, as HIV could infect perhaps a billion people over the next half-century. Said differently, more lives could be saved by stopping the spread of AIDS than by all medicine's surgery, drugs, and high-tech interventions.

From this perspective, *global bioethics* clamors for attention. Even domestic questions about resources at the end of life seem related: how can Americans spend so much at the end of life when so many millions of the world die of preventable diseases?

If moral actions create the greatest good for the greatest number of humans, then moral people will now be fighting AIDS. In the next 10 years and if past trends continue, the 40 million people infected in 2006 could pass HIV on to another 40, 50, or even 60 million people.

Sub-Saharan Africa has the greatest pool of HIV-infection, containing 26 million infected people. South Africa, even with a relatively advanced economy, has 5.5 million infected.

China and India cause concern because of amplification systems there. Parts of China's blood supply is infected, which its officials often deny. Migratory laborers in India acquire HIV from prostitutes and pass it along to their wives and then to newborn children. In 2006, India surpassed South Africa as the country with the largest sheer number of citizens with AIDS, having 5.6 million to South Africa's 5.5 million. Asia altogether in 2006 had over 8 million infections.

Eastern Europe and central Asia (the Ukraine, Kazakhstan, etc.), with large numbers of intravenous drug-users, in 2005 had 1.6 million infected, up from 1 million in 2000.[19]

Facing the Problem Head-On

Given the vast extent of the problem, how do we stop the spread of HIV around the globe? Part of the answer is a moral one. Do we attack the behavior or the microbe in trying to stop the spread? Do we use nonmoralistic education or moralistic condemnation? Is money spent on education in developing countries helpful? Are cheap anti-AIDS drugs worthwhile when the numbers infected keep doubling and when many lack clean water? Would it be more efficient to *triage* countries with masses of infected people and then concentrate resources where they might save the most lives? These are the questions for the rest of this chapter,

The following section sketches four views of how to stop AIDS from spreading further. This section also features some exchanges between proponents of the different views.

Educational Prevention

Ultimately, humanity's only hope of preventing HIV is nonmoralistic education. Self-interested humans can learn. Learn what? To protect themselves against HIV by negotiating safe sex, using clean needles, avoiding infected blood, and taking drugs to prevent infection of newborns.

Prevention outranks cure, especially as AIDS has no cure. Not only is "an ounce of prevention worth a pound of cure," but prevention costs much less.

Cynics deride education to prevent infection, but education has worked. The number of new infections in the developed world declined rapidly in the 1990s and 2000s. Blood became safe, people routinely used condoms, and mothers stopped HIV from infecting their babies.

In the late 1980s, Thailand modeled how to arrest HIV. With a national campaign for 100 percent use of condoms, it advertised on television, hired outreach workers, ran testimonials by its royal family, and educated its sex workers, drug-users, and citizens in preventing HIV-infection. It allowed free access to testing and counseling, and protected the infected against discrimination. It gave out free AZT and championed production of generic anti-AIDS drugs for the poor. Over the next decade, new infections dropped 80 percent, preventing 200,000 HIV-infections.[20]

Similar efforts worked in Uganda. Led by President Yoweri Museveni, Uganda ran testimonials on radio and television by famous Ugandans diagnosed with HIV. Infection rates during the 1990s among Uganda's youth dropped dramatically. At the same time, the rate of HIV-infection there dropped by half in rural areas and by two-thirds among urban, pregnant women.

Perhaps the most surprising success in educational prevention is Brazil. Like Cuba, Brazil has a large commercial sex industry for both its citizens and tourists, so in 1990 its large cities had high rates of HIV-infection. In 1996, the Brazilian government funded universal access to the latest and best anti-AIDS drugs, resulting over the next decade in the creation of a national system of out-patient centers, Brazilian manufacture of generic anti-AIDS drugs, and sophisticated labs and record-keeping. As a result, deaths from AIDS in Brazil dropped in half and rates of infection in São Paulo and Rio de Janeiro dropped 54 and 73 percent, respectively.[21]

Brazil's huge population means this program is a great success. Although both Brazil and South Africa have middle-class economies, Brazil's efforts at educational prevention fared much better than South Africa's. Education and prevention do work, given the will and funding.

Feminism

The key to stopping AIDS is to empower women to prevent themselves from getting infected by HIV. The key to that is to empower women to vote, to earn money, and to reject domestic violence.

A noted physician-fighter against AIDS concluded his 2006 review of this disease over 25 years with these words: "The prime mover of the epidemic is not inadequate antiretroviral medications, poverty, or bad luck, but our inability to accept the gothic dimensions of a disease that is transmitted sexually. Only if we cease to dodge this fact will effective HIV-control programs be established. Until then, it is no exaggeration to say that our polite behavior is killing us."[22]

The gothic dimensions of AIDS include the fact that nasty behavior by men around the world infects millions of women and children, that soldiers use mass rape as a weapon, that women and children are sold into sexual slavery and that poor, powerless women cannot refuse sex from their more powerful, infected husbands. The only name for this behavior is *evil*.

This evil is the kind caused by human decisions. AIDS is not a punishment from God, but a way that sin manifests itself. Consider the case of 13-year old Rhaki in Rajasthan, India:

> From a poor, rural family, Rhaki had an arranged marriage at age 13 to a 23 year-old man who worked in the distant city of Mumbai for 11 months of the year. Once a year, her husband returned for a month, during which time he had sex with her. While he lived in Mumbai, he had sex with prostitutes and became HIV+. At age 19, she learned that she and her 2-year old son were HIV+.
>
> Despite the fact that she remained faithful to her husband and used no drugs, she was blamed for bringing shame into her family. She feared she would be ejected from the family and forced to become a prostitute in a distant city.[23]

In Namibia, one study found that 95 percent of a thousand women were forced in their first sexual encounter.[24] A third of women in Sierra Leone reported the same. In sub-Saharan Africa with two-thirds of the world's HIV infections in 2006, 60 percent of those infected are women.[25] Of those newly infected and aged 15 to 24, a whopping 77 percent are women.

Dark reasons exist for this pattern. African men perceive that sex with a young girl is unlikely to infect them with HIV and some believe that sex with a virgin will cure HIV. These practices ensure that many teenage females will become infected.

In South Africa, India, and around the world, an amplification system exists that involves truck drivers, mobile soldiers, and commuting workers. India's new diamond-shaped interstate allows millions of truck drivers to transport commodities from rural areas to cities and ports. Along the way, drivers patronize prostitutes, become infected, and then infect their wives at home, resulting soon in infected babies.

South Africa's migratory pattern built up over a century, with millions of men traveling to distant mines to be housed in dormitories. Such patterns dramatically increase nonmarital sex. In Abidjan, the richest city in the Ivory Coast, migrants compose 40 percent of the city's population, and Abidjan has the highest incidence of HIV in West Africa.[26]

Despite efforts of the United Nations and Christians to stop it, human slavery still exists in parts of northern Africa. In India, Eastern Europe, Mexico, and Korea, young women are tricked, kidnapped, and sold into distant brothels, where they become sex workers, living like slaves.

In Bosnia-Herzegovina, as many as 50,000 women were deliberately raped to make them pariahs. In East Timor, the Congo, Rwanda, Azerbaijan, and Uganda, rape became not only a spoil of war but a weapon in it. In Somalia and Darfur, marauders raped thousands of women and expelled them from their homes.

These are terrible human acts. To face a problem, you must name it. This is the human face of evil. To deal with it, you must confront it. This means that moral condemnation must be a weapon against AIDS. We cannot remain neutral against such appalling acts. We cannot merely pursue bland education and sanitized programs in public health.

Slavery of all kinds must end. Mass rape must end. Forced sex must end. Bad male behavior must end.

Tough love in stopping AIDS hasn't been tough enough. In Cuba, NuShawn Williams would have been executed. What if the government of Ethiopia condemned to die a man who infected his wife with HIV? It is time to take morally tough stands, else another 10 to 15 million women and children will die.

Triage

In some parts of the world, bad behavior is entrenched. Doctors cannot bring peace to warring countries: this is not a medical problem but a political one. Similarly, physicians cannot end slavery or famine: these are larger problems than medicine can solve. Moreover, some countries have corrupt governments, corruption going back a hundred years. It is naïve to think that do-gooder missionaries and physicians with love and education can change much there.

We need to triage countries such as South Africa where President Mbeki for a decade publicly resisted the fact that HIV causes AIDS, and where he not only did not lead the fight against spread of HIV but helped to spread it by his poor example.

Pouring money and time into some countries is a waste. The point of triage is to intervene to leverage at-risk life into saved lives. So, we ignore countries that don't need our help (North America, Europe, Thailand, Uganda) and also ignore countries where nothing we do will make much difference (the Sudan, Ethiopia, the Congo). Then we focus on countries in the middle, perhaps India, where politicians could lead and where people could change their behavior.

And as for the sterling examples of Thailand, Brazil, and Cuba, well no wonder! With their huge commercial sex industries, they successfully combated HIV-infections to avoid losing the hard currency flowing into their struggling economies.

Similarly, education and counseling will only go so far if people don't care for their own safety. After 25 years, most adults on the planet know that having unprotected sex, getting a transfusion of blood, or sharing needles can get you infected with HIV. If your own self-interest doesn't protect you now from HIV, more education certainly won't.

Besides, as gripes Jeffrey Fisher, director of Center for HIV Prevention at the University of Connecticut at Storrs, most AIDS education is bland and generic, and hence, of little value in teaching teenagers how to negotiate usage of condoms during sex or how to safely use hard drugs. "We lack the political will to implement these things," he says.[27]

Among large portions of the world, primal drives for sexual pleasure, fueled by poor judgment under the influence of alcohol and other drugs, lead people to practice unprotected sex. In Russia and China, despair over the conversion to capitalism has fueled widespread use of drugs.

All these forces swamp educational efforts to stop AIDS. Wisdom lies in recognizing that we can't control the private actions of most people. Wisdom lies in keeping a candle lit as the darkness grows.

Survivors will be fastidiously aware of what behaviors can kill them, and teach their children to be similarly aware. Sure, a billion people may die from AIDS, but humanity will go on. Plagues, flu, and floods have wiped out similar percentages of humanity before, but humanity has survived. Sadly, it is merely part of humanity's Darwinian evolution.

Structuralism

Activist groups such as Partners in Health emphasize that the cause of the spread of AIDS is not irresponsible personal behavior, but evil *structures* of society. Education and prevention will never work until these structures change. So toss out Educational Prevention, Feminism, and Triage: Educational Prevention is mere window-dressing, Feminism focuses wrongly on individuals, and Triage just breeds despair.

As some structuralists lament, "Obviously it is simpler to blame the victims for the rapid spread of AIDS in poor countries than to analyze the socioeconomic and political structures that underlie, frame, and often predetermine such personal 'choices'."[28]

What evil structures? For starters, poverty, colonialism, apartheid and its legacy, racism, class injustice, and imperialism. Anthropologist Philippe Bourgois argues that in poor communities, lack of good jobs emasculates men who want to be good providers, who then turn to self-destructive behaviors out of frustration, using drugs, selling them, addicting women, and using violence to control others. Feminism for Bourgois ignores the "objective, structural desperation of a population without a viable economy."[29]

Poverty is a major cause of the spread of HIV-infection. In the 1990s, thousands of dirt-poor farmers in China's Hena province sold their plasma each week. They did so because they could not earn a good living by farming but could do so by selling plasma.

Plasma is collected by taking blood from the donor's body, separating the plasma, and returning the rest of the blood to the donor. In this way, donors can give weekly rather than once a month, with whole blood.

Because the province's blood supply became infected with HIV, most of the donors became infected. Whole villages were wiped out. Moreover, because of the secrecy of the Chinese government, we have no idea how many Chinese patients received infected blood, plasma, or clotting factors. Millions of Chinese could be infected and not suspect it.

Too much of the world adopts a "it won't happen here approach." One commentator bemoans, "for the past 25 years, the lessons learned about HIV prevention and control in one country have failed to inform decisions in others. As a result, the world has witnessed a slow-motion domino effect, as the disease overwhelms country after country."[30] Always, leaders deny that AIDS endangers the country (our blood is safe, we don't have prostitutes) and then, when cases of AIDS surface, those who are infected are blamed as deviant or foreign. "This sort of buck passing has delayed the control of AIDS in every country. By the time the scale of the problem is finally appreciated, a mature epidemic is in place, and the cost of lives and money has increased exponentially."

The connection between the spread of AIDS and structuralism may be put conceptually: *an unjust structure is an amplification system for HIV.* Women are forced into prostitution to survive, male manual laborers use drugs to get by, poor hygiene and public health lead to diseases creating sores and infections, making HIV easier to transmit. People sell their bodies and their blood to survive.

Feminism Replies

The key to stopping AIDS is to create social structures that empower women. "Uppity women" means "down with AIDS."

Poor women around the world bear the brunt of AIDS. Such women know they are at-risk but often can do little to protect themselves. Bearing the paycheck, and hence, food and clothing and other goods of life, men control these women. We will only stop AIDS when we give these women more say over voting, jobs, and sex.

Vaccines, vaginal gels, and female condoms need technological break-throughs to be effective, and one day may be so. In the meantime, women must be allowed to say "No" to abusive infection by males and forced sexual slavery. Unless structures are created to do so, AIDS will grow and grow.

Maybe unfashionable, isn't old-fashioned Feminism better than triaging 20 million people and forgetting about them? At least, Feminism directed at people says that someone *cares* about them (versus the *belle indifference* of Triage).

Structuralism is partly correct in that many of the evil structures of the world lead to the abuse, rape, killing, and HIV-infection of women, but we can help women without having a complete revolution in every society. Realistic change may need to be step-by-step rather than cataclysmic.

So basic rights for mothers, daughters, and wives can be implemented in small, faith-based communities, such as where clergy wield power in African villages. Money, food, and supplies, combined with faith and good-will, can model sex-only-within-marriage. Such an approach will also combat slavery, sexual exploitation of women and children, and be compatible with Islam.

Secular public health proposals that emphasize education may be inappropriate for faith-based, poor communities, where many people are illiterate and ignorant of the most basic science facts. Because AIDS is lethal and because a person only has to get infected once to get a lethal disease, such populations cannot wait to be taught to read or to be taught basic science. They need a solution now, and Feminism is the answer.

Finally, we do not know that moral censure has not worked. Without it, who knows how many more millions might have died or have been infected? Fear of moral condemnation motivates many people, and maybe that is not a bad thing.

AIDS kills. AIDS is caused by HIV. It's bad to infect someone with HIV. It's heinous to do so deliberately or with indifference. What other definition of a bad person do we need? Why not be a little moralistic here? After all, we're talking about *ethics*, not sanitation or legality.

Educational Prevention Responds

The champions of Educational Prevention rejects the moralism of Feminism and Structuralism. First, what's wrong with Feminism in public health is that it really serves the emotions of the moralizer, not the one condemned. Moralizing did nothing to stop gay men from having sex after AIDS was discovered, but fear of death did. Moralizing only made matters worse.

The key claim is that Feminism can change behavior. Is that true? One argument that it won't is that a lot of "tough love" has already been directed against using drugs, much less intravenous drugs. Similarly, a lot of moralism has been directed toward not having sex outside marriage, but has it worked?

If we execute men who infect their wives, who will bring home a paycheck to feed the wives? And the children? Execution sounds like a good idea, but if thought through, it's not. Seeing what would happen to them, wives would protect their husbands and not turn them in to authorities.

For workers in public health, Triage is too pessimistic. Why not generalize that attitude and let everyone starve? Or go without penicillin? Why bother about the rest of the planet at all? Why not let the undeveloped world fight it out among themselves and let the rich nations keep them at a distance, away from their shores? Just stay in your hot tub, enjoying the scenery and sipping your wine.

But is this a *moral* point of view? Sipping wine leisurely while humanity dies? What does the Golden Rule enjoin us to do? Triage does not offer the world a moral solution but gives up on finding one.

The essence of medical morality is to fight pragmatically for the good of the many especially using the tools of medicine. If we give up on that assumption, we might as well give up on medicine.

Triage Replies

The champion of Triage replies, "You're right. If there are six billion people now on the planet and if a billion of them die of AIDS, mostly on the other side of the planet and unknown to me, I don't care. The planet already has too many people and it could easily lose a billion. When stories about AIDS appear on the news, I change the channel. In fact, to avoid such stories, I don't even watch the news anymore".

"I may be morally deficient, but I have enough moral honesty to admit that I have no moral feelings of compassion, shame, or outrage about the mass of human deaths from AIDS. It's going to happen: it's a fact; it's accelerated Darwinian evolution; I don't think governments or missionaries can do anything about it; that's just the way it is. Give me my hot tub and another glass of wine."

Structuralists like economist Jeffrey Sachs argue that if Western nations transferred $150 billion a year to developing nations, by 2025 poverty could be wiped off the planet. The musician Bono has jumped on this approach. But will simply transferring money end poverty? And will ending poverty stop the spread of AIDS?

Economist William Easterly, a senior research economist at the World Bank, in *White Man's Burden*, criticizes humanitarian planners who impose their own solutions on developing countries, especially the idea that building infrastructure with foreign aid will end poverty.[31] Too many programs are funded top-down, with no feedback from poor people. Paul Theroux, who loves Africa, agrees.[32]

With AIDS, Easterly argues that more life-years could be saved by not diverting money from antimalarial programs and childhood vaccinations and by fighting ordinary scourges such as tuberculosis. A million people still die each year from malaria in Africa.

Second, Easterly urges the West to focus on prevention rather than cure, especially by giving out condoms rather than giving the infected expensive AIDS medicines.

Third, people's kids starve while they get antiretrovirals. HIV takes almost a decade to make people sick. One infected woman said she didn't need the medicines, but a job to feed her family.

Finally, some countries may be hopeless. Twenty years ago, LiveAid concerts raised $100 million for Ethiopia, but little changed, and today, life in Ethiopia is among the worst on earth.

Educational Prevention Once Again

The champion of Educational Prevention also rejects the cynicism of Triage. Both Triage and Feminism sound like solutions, but they are not. In fact, they serve the interests of those who espouse them, not the interests of the world's vulnerable women and children.

Triage would have us not offer expensive treatment to those infected but concentrate on preventing new infections. In 2006, the standard of care for HIV-infection is HAART, Highly Active Anti-Retroviral Therapy, which costs $10,000 a person per year in developed countries and which 90 percent of HIV-infected people in the world do not get.

The knock-down argument against offering no HAART treatment at all in certain countries is that such a lack takes away the major reason for testing. When Brazil offered HAART free to all its citizens, testing for HIV zoomed and thousands came forth for treatment. Without treatment, how many would have gotten tested?

Triage is not an option. Let's call it what it is: global medical apartheid. The racial system of apartheid should not be replaced with a medical one.

Triage acquiesces to hopelessness, and hopelessness allows countries to spiral downwards in war, rape, famine, and infection. Triage is not a moral solution but giving up on finding one.

In 2001, breakthroughs occurred with the creation of the Global Fund to Fight AIDS, Tuberculosis, and Malaria as well as the Doha Agreement, allowing poor countries to buy or make generic anti-AIDS drugs. Powerful religious groups pushed the Bush administration to do more for victims of AIDS, and billions of U.S. aid poured forth. Seeing that, huge economies might be destroyed, the World Bank poured money into AIDS prevention. A similar threat to world security galvanized developed nations to respond. These efforts prevented millions of new infections and allowed two to three million people to live with HIV-infection, people who in turn support millions of children.

Conclusion

Stopping the spread of AIDS is not easy, and one reason is that dramatically different views exist about how to do it. One view's solution is another view's problem.

Some of the proposed approaches are too drastic. Structuralism says we must change everything to fix AIDS: eliminate poverty, sexism, racism, and corruption. A tall order and unlikely to happen.

Perhaps the only way to stop AIDS may be to experiment and adopt one view on a small scale, perhaps in a province, where the view can be fully implemented, top to bottom in that society. Whether that approach is Feminism, Educational Prevention, or Structuralism, given different religious backgrounds, provincial leaders, and scientific understanding, a particular approach might work better in one region rather than another. What worked in Brazil might not work in Biafra or Somalia.

The problem discussed in this chapter is unprecedented in bioethics or modern medicine. It is unimaginable to contemplate a billion human HIV-infections over the next five decades. The scale of death would dwarf the Black Plague, created hundreds of millions of orphans, bring down economies in developing nations, create despair over continents, and orphan tens of millions of children.

But the number of infected people did jump from a few hundred in 1981 to 10 million in 1990, and from there to 40 million in 2005, so who knows how many might be infected by the next edition of this text—50 million?

Hopefully, far fewer people than that number will be infected, in part because medicine, and bioethics, find a way to stem the rising tide of infections.

FURTHER READING AND RESOURCES

Alexander Irwin, Joyce Millen, and Dorothy Fallows, *Global AIDS: Myths and Facts*, South End Press, Cambridge, MA, 2003.

Randy Shilts, *And the Band Played On*, St. Martin's, New York, 1987.

Anton A. Van Niekerk and Loretta M. Kopelman, *Ethics and AIDS in Africa*, Left Coast Press, Walnut Creek, CA, 2006.

CHAPTER 18

Medicine and Inequality

This chapter focuses on inequality in health care in the United States, especially for the 46 million Americans who lack good medical coverage, a number fast approaching 50 million.[1] It also focuses on the history of Medicare, the federally financed and supervised system of health care for Americans over age 65. The chapter discusses arguments for and against expansion of Medicare to give all Americans universal access to health care.

Rosalyn Schwartz

Rosalyn Schwartz, age 47, white, lives in Ridgefield, New Jersey; she has one child, Andy. She lost her medical coverage when she and her husband divorced in 1987.[2] At that time, the gift-wrap company where she worked with five other employees (making around $19,000 a year) provided no medical coverage, though it hoped to do so soon.

When Rosalyn tried to buy an individual policy, because she had a *preexisting condition*—an ulcer—several insurance companies informed her that, if they offered her a policy at all, her premiums would be $4,000 a year and exclude treatment for ulcers.

In 1988, she found a small lump in her breast. Her physician said it might be cancerous and recommended removing it, but hoping that her employer would soon offer coverage, Rosalyn postponed the lumpectomy.

In 1989, Rosalyn felt pain tear through her hip. By then her breast cancer had metastasized and had eaten into her hip, making the bones there as fragile as glass. When she fell to the floor, her hip socket shattered. In the ambulance, she sobbed and could think only of the costs. "Andy, you've just turned 18," she said. "I have no insurance. Tell them [at the hospital] I have no insurance. But don't sign anything or you'll be responsible."

Breast and prostate cancers are cells gone wild, so they must be excised and radiated as soon as possible. If such cancers reach the bone, it's bad.

Hospitalized for 23 days, Rosalyn had surgery three times. The total cost was $40,000, half paid by charity. Rosalyn owed the rest, which she paid off at $10 a month to each of 12 physicians and hospitals.

Unable to work after her surgery, Rosalyn received disability under Medicare amounting to $10,500 a year. When she tried again to buy personal medical coverage, she found that it would still cost her $4,000 a year, and now it would not cover procedures for her cancer or for other preexisting conditions. Lacking such insurance, she didn't get physical therapy for her hip replacement, nor could she afford a bone scan every six months to make sure the cancer had not spread.

About a decade later, Rosalyn died.[3] Such is the life of middle-aged working Americans who get sick and have no medical coverage.[4]

MEDICAL COVERAGE IN THE UNITED STATES

Universal medical coverage is a medical system that covers basic health care for all citizens in a nation. Almost always a *single-payer system* administered by one and only one organization, usually a governmental agency, it is often funded by taxes. Most European countries provide universal medical coverage, including Austria, Belgium, Denmark, Finland, France, Germany, the Netherlands, Norway, Portugal, Spain, Sweden, and the United Kingdom. So do Australia, Canada, Cuba, Japan, New Zealand, South Africa, and Taiwan.

America differs from other developed countries in having high consumption and great wealth, as well as high expenditures per capita on health care, yet not providing coverage for a large percentage of its citizens. The Institute of Medicine estimates that lack of medical insurance leads to the unnecessary deaths each year of 18,000 Americans.[5]

Because the United States lacks a unified system of health care, it is difficult to explain how American medicine works. Basically, America has a five-part patchwork system that covers most serious problems for most people most of the time, but still allows many people to fall through the cracks. The five parts are described below.

1. Employment-Based Coverage and Private Medical Plans

Most Americans, 54 percent, get medical coverage though employment.[6] This includes many spouses and children (including adult children in their 20s) of people who work. Coverage in retirement varies according to the largesse of the citizen's previous employer.

Employers provide medical coverage as a benefit to employees. Employers with large numbers of employees negotiate lower rates than employers with few employees because larger numbers spread the costs of illness among more people. An increasing number of small businesses cannot obtain cheap coverage and no longer offer medical coverage.

Since World War II, private insurance plans have multiplied; they now number over 300, each with its own rules, qualifications, reimbursement rates, and forms to be filled out by patients and physicians.[7] An average physician hires two full-time personnel just to deal with billing and insurance.

The strengths of employment-based coverage appear mostly with large employers, who offer far better medical plans than small employers. Large employers receive discounts from hospitals and insurance companies. Insurance companies set different rates, based on how large an employer is and employers with over 1,000 workers pay the lowest rates. Another factor affecting insurance for many larger employers is demographics: workers tend to have fewer medical problems than other groups such as unemployed people, retired people, and children.

The weaknesses of employment-based coverage appear when we consider small employers. Many small businesses do not offer medical coverage at all, and this is not necessarily their fault. Because of demographics, insuring employees can be expensive: employers with fewer than 25 employees pay the highest rates of all. Thus small businesses trying to allocate capital for expansion—or struggling to make profits—often cannot afford to offer insurance.

A second disadvantage of an employment-based system is that when a worker leaves a job, medical coverage will eventually be cut off. Until recently, insurance was not portable to another company. Many young working people do not realize that their employer pays most of their medical coverage, and that if they quit or are fired, they must bear this cost themselves, including the employer's former share, until they find another job.

In 1985, Congress passed the COBRA law, allowing employees to continue their medical insurance at group rates by paying their share plus the employer's share of their former premiums. COBRA also covers spouses after divorce and adult children.[8] In 1996, a federal law called *Health Insurance Privacy and Portability Act (HIPPA)* required portability for workers between similar plans and not excluding preexisting conditions (without this, workers with any significant medical problems would be trapped in jobs forever).

A third disadvantage is cost-shifting. American hospitals are not reimbursed for providing medical care to the poor, but federal law forbids any hospital with an emergency room to turn patients away because of inability to pay. To make up for the cost of this care, hospitals shift costs: they charge more for services to insured patients. Employers resent such cost-shifting, as it forces them to act as charities by subsidizing health care for the indigent. (This is a reason such employers favored universal coverage in Oregon, Vermont, and Massachusetts.)

A fourth disadvantage is that American employers say the cost of insuring their employees is much too high. In 1990, over $675 of the cost of each new Ford vehicle went to pay for medical coverage for employees of Ford and its suppliers.[9] Retired employees of these companies had such generous coverage, with no co-pays or deductibles, that these companies could not compete with foreign car companies.[10] In 2006, Ford had to buy out many of its employees to get them to retire and to force retirees to pay small co-pays and deductibles for the first time.

This leads to a fifth disadvantage of employment-based insurance: in recent years, many employers have been trying to lower their costs in ways that can be harmful to workers. Some businesses reduce the number of full-time employees with benefits; instead, they replace one full-time worker with two part-time workers who have no benefits. They contract "independent consultants" without benefits to replace managers. Such policies create a two-class medical system with regular employees with salaries and good benefits versus part-time employees with no benefits.

A sixth disadvantage of the employment-based system is that many workers are pushed out of the labor force and into chronic unemployment because of an illness or injury. Many poor people are poor primarily because of medical conditions that make them risky to employers who are seeking to reduce medical costs.

People who are unemployed or work for a small company which offers no medical insurance may, of course, try to buy individual policies. About 7 percent of Americans do; they include people who are self-employed, seasonal workers, adult students, and people who are between jobs. However, as Rosalyn Schwartz discovered, individual policies are expensive because the policyholder is not part of a large pool of workers.

2. Medicare

When Americans reach age 65, Medicare covers 80 percent or more of their medical expenses. Medicare in 2005 covered 36 million Americans. Medicare is a single-payer system and thus contrasts sharply with the bewildering array of private medical plans in America.

In creating Medicare in the early 1960s, Congress took a giant step toward creating universal medical coverage. Lyndon Johnson wrangled it into law in 1965. Intended to help only poor, elderly people during illness, Congress almost immediately extended it to all Americans over 65.

Medicare gave the elderly a medical security they had never known before. Before its creation, many elderly Americans worried whether they could afford physicians and hospitalization. Before Medicare, retired workers were on their own for medical coverage.

Medicare also contains a special addition to cover people with disabilities under age 65. In 2005, this addition covered 4 million disabled Americans. Together, both parts of Medicare in 2005 covered 40 million Americans.[11] Administered by the federal government, Medicare is financed from mandatory payroll taxes—indicated on paycheck stubs as FICA (Federal Insurance Corporation of America). Medicare in 2005 cost $265 billion a year.[12] Medicaid costs state taxpayers about $35 billion.[13]

Both parts of Medicare stem from a moral belief that healthy, young people should pay for the medical care of sick and elderly citizens. A related idea lay behind the creation of the Great Society legislation of the 1960s, which created Head Start, food stamps, VISTA, and Aid to Families with Dependent Children.

3. Medicaid

A third arm of American health care is Medicaid, which began in 1965 as part of the Great Society legislation. It is run somewhat differently by each state but federal matching funds aid each state's efforts and enforce national guidelines. Eligibility for Medicaid in all states depends on low income, so it is meant to cover medical expenses only for poor people. Among the people covered are people on public assistance, children of poor parents, poor seniors, people with disabilities, and adults with mental illness.

In New York in 2005, a single parent with two children could not have resources more than $6,000 or income more than $1,000 a month and qualify for Medicaid.

Eligibility for Medicaid varies with each state. A citizen could qualify for Medicaid coverage with a much higher income in California than Alabama. Also, what Medicaid covers varies from state to state. Three of the most comprehensive programs in America over the last two decades have been Medi-Cal, MassHealth, and TennCare.

One misconception about Medicare is that it covers nursing homes and long-term care. It does not. Only Medicaid does so, and in order to qualify, a senior citizen must exhaust all personal wealth, including the sale of a personal home.

Starting in 1997, the federal government allotted over 40 billion dollars of federal matching funds in 1997 toward the State Children's Health Insurance Program (SCHIP). SCHIP is designed for the working poor who earn too much money to qualify for Medicaid yet are unable to insure their children through employment or private insurance companies. SCHIP usually works with Medicaid in each state. Under SCHIP, children of parents with low-paying jobs can obtain free regular check-ups, prescriptions, dental and eye care, as well as hospital and physician services.

Importantly, Medicaid now pays for drugs; before 2006, it did not. Before SCHIP, some parents faced the moral dilemma of going to work, losing eligibility for Medicaid, and hence, losing drugs and services of physicians for their children or staying unemployed but Medicaid-eligible.

For people with mental illnesses such as schizophrenia, Medicaid is the main source of their drugs. Since most such people must take their drugs for life, this costs states a lot of money. It also means that people with schizophrenia, some of whom can easily find good work, sometimes face a dilemma between getting their drugs free versus working a job with poor coverage for mental health.

An especially controversial aspect of American medical finance has been coverage for illegal immigrant workers. The Deficit Reduction Act of 2005 forbids Medicaid from covering services to noncitizens.

4. CHAMPUS/Tricare and the Veterans Administration Hospital System

Military personnel, their families, and veterans are covered under a different medical system than other Americans. While on active duty, they receive health care through CHAMPUS/Tricare and must go to physicians and nurses employed by the Armed Services.

According to its website, "CHAMPUS is a health benefits program that covers medical necessities only. It provides authorized in-patient and out-patient care from civilian sources, on a cost-sharing basis. Retired military are eligible, as well as dependents of active-duty, retired, and deceased military."[14]

Veterans may utilize a national system of hospitals and clinics run by the Veterans Health Administration (VHA). The system was founded after World War II in appreciation of the debt that America owed its veterans, with the moral intuition that no one who had so served should be denied health care.

The second-largest department of the federal government with a budget of more than $60 billion, the VHA is one of the largest employers of physicians and nurses in the country. In recent decades, it has shed its previous reputation for shoddy care and has emerged as a national leader of good, efficient medical care.[15]

The VHA covers veterans not only for surgery, drugs, and visits to physicians, but also for mental illness and long-term care in nursing homes. The Armed Services and VHA also run their own medical schools.

5. Health Care in Emergency Rooms

Part of America's system of health care is the Emergency Medical Treatment and Active Labor Act (EMTALA) of 1986, which forbids emergency rooms from turning away anyone who is medically unstable. All patients there must be treated and stabilized before they are released.

This federal requirement means that emergency rooms serve as a national safety net for all kinds of medical problems of the uninsured and for illegal immigrants.

Medical Coverage in Canada

Canada has a fund for national medical coverage, much like the American social security system. It covers the health care of every Canadian; it is universal, portable, publicly administered through a single-payer system, and covers all medically necessary services.

The single-payer system is financed partly by high "sin" taxes on cigarettes, alcohol, and gasoline. Each Canadian province sets its own policies and allocates health care by regulating the supply of medical services. For example, each province funds only a small number of hospitals with CT scanners and lithotripters (expensive machines that break up kidney stones with sound waves).

The Canadian system became national in 1962. Canadian physicians are not restrained by what tests they can order by private insurers. They can order whatever they like for patients and will always be paid by Canadian Medicare. Physicians in Canada do not work for the Canadian government; like independent American physicians, they work for themselves and bill on a fee-for-service basis. Unlike American physicians, Canadian physicians cannot collude to raise fees.

The Canadian system for two decades cost less than $2,000 American dollars per capita and covered all Canadians, whereas the American system cost over $6,280 per capita and left over 46 million Americans uncovered.[16] Canadians live to about 80 years of life, Americans to about 77.

Canadians boast about their medical system, especially when contrasted with the American system. Why? Here are some examples.

In Canada, every pregnant woman gets free care. As a result, Canada has one of the lowest infant morality rates of developed countries. In the United States, 17 percent of women in childbirth experience not only the natural fears of birth but also the anxiety of having no medical coverage to pay for their hospitalization or physicians' bills.[17]

In Canada, all citizens can purchase affordable, long-term nursing home care, although they must pay for a portion of such care (about $19 of the $67 which is the typical cost per day). In the United States, virtually no one has coverage for long-term care in a nursing home; to become eligible for Medicaid, which pays for bare-bones nursing home care, elderly Americans must "spend down" their assets to nothing.[18]

In one poll in 1990, only 3 percent of Canadians considered the American medical system superior to their own. In contrast, in the same poll, nearly 30 percent thought Elvis Presley might still be alive.

The system doesn't cover everything. While paying almost all costs of hospitalization or visits to physicians, it pays almost nothing for drugs or dentistry.

Canadians must wait for specialized care. In Nova Scotia, only one lithotripter exists, so patients there must wait three months for an appointment to use it. However, most stone-busting is preventive; most kidney stones eventually drop and pass safely on their own; Surgery is available as an emergency alternative to lithotripsy. Furthermore, the only way to diminish the waiting list would be to buy more machines at enormous expense—each one costs millions of dollars.

Waits for other kinds of specialized services are more annoying. Because Canada limits the number of physicians in specialties, patients in Canada must wait longer between initial referral and first appointment for oncologists and orthopedic surgeons than in the United States, 5.5 weeks to see an oncologist and 40 weeks to see an orthopedic surgeon.[19]

In June 2005, Canada's Supreme Court struck down a law outlawing citizens from buying, or physicians or private insurers from selling, essential medical services.[20] That opened Pandora's box, and institutions such as Vancouver's Cambie Surgery Center started to perform knee surgeries for cash, without the usual two year wait.[21] Canadian patients with money, who are tired for waiting years for knee, hip, and cataract surgery, are now flocking to private clinics and hospitals that are opening every week. Because the public system cannot accommodate these patients quickly, the government is allowing these new enterprises.

Canada has had trouble recruiting physicians in primary care (for that matter, so has America, which has a worse shortage). Critics now call for a mixed health care model, as most European countries have, where citizens could go to private clinics for some services. Canadian officials worry that such a system would drain the current system of its specialists.

Clinton's Health Care Security Bill of 1993–1994

In 1993, President Bill Clinton proposed his Health Care Security Act to expand Medicare for all Americans. This Act assumed two tenets: first, an *employer mandate*: all employers had to pay something toward medical insurance for their employees; second, formation of large *managed care plans*. In the latter, all employees of a business get all their medical care from just one Health Maintenance Organization (HMO), and each employee has a physician-gatekeeper, who is responsible for medical decisions for the employee.

Both assumptions had political opponents. Small businesses fought the employer mandate because they feared being made to pay an unjust amount (at the time, thought to be between $1,600 and $1,900 per employee). Many said that, rather than provide such mandated medical coverage, they would simply not hire workers.

Second, many Americans in 1993 also disliked managed care. They disliked physician-gatekeepers who often denied the medical services to which they had become accustomed.

Elderly Americans in particular feared being forced into managed care. They liked Medicare and wanted to keep it as it was. Because they voted in large numbers, politicians had to reckon with their power. Medicare has often been called by politicians the "third rail": touch it and you die (like the third rail of New York subways, which carries electricity).

The Act's greatest financial problem was that it tried to simultaneously expand medical services and reduce costs. Not only did it hope to expand Medicare to cover 46 million uninsured Americans, it also planned to increase the number of services covered by Medicare. Moreover, the Americans with Disabilities Act mandated other kinds of expansion. All this contradicted the idea of lowering costs, and owners of small businesses feared new taxes on them to pay for it all.

After a year of national discussion, the Act failed to get to the floor of Congress for a vote. Perhaps the greatest reason for this failure is that President Clinton failed to clearly justify why a rich nation such as America should cover the medical needs of all its citizens. Instead of concentrating on this question of justice, he got bogged down in the arcane financial details of how the plans would work.

Three States Fund Universal Coverage

In 1987, Oregon broadened its Medicaid plan to cover all Oregonians. Under its Oregon Health Plan (OHP), all employers, even small businesses, had to offer basic coverage by 1995 or pay a new payroll tax ("pay or play").

Oregon did not fund some expensive medical services such as in vitro fertilization, experimental therapies for people with AIDS, heart or liver transplants, or health care in intensive care units for premature babies (the latter was later reversed to comply with the Americans with Disabilities Act).

Although Oregon democratically developed OHP, when the parents of seven-year-old Coby Howard learned in 1988 that Medicaid would not pay for a bone-marrow transplant for his leukemia, they appealed to the news media for an exception to OHP. Surprisingly, Coby Howard died a few months later, a rare failure of the rule of rescue.

In 1993, OHP had spent $84 million, but only $34 million had been allocated for it and it faced a predicted $150 million, shortfall.[22] In 2003 to save money, OHP reduced benefits and required higher deductibles and co-payments for many members.[23] Afterwards, between 2003 and 2005, two-thirds of the affected members lost their insurance coverage, and over three-fourths of them went uninsured for more than six months. Despite a restoration of some coverage in 2004, many of those dropped continued to experience problems obtaining medical care. In short, OHP proved more expensive than Oregonians were willing to pay for.

Twenty years after Oregon did so, Massachusetts and Vermont decided they could not wait for the federal government and in 2006 cranked up their own systems of universal medical coverage, planned to start in 2007–2008.

The programs represented a compromise between the right, which had pushed medical savings accounts, and the left, which had pushed a government-managed, single-payer system like Canada's. The Massachusetts and Vermont programs were unique in requiring every citizen to have health insurance, like car insurance. Beginning in 2008, each citizen of these states who files a tax return will have to indicate if she or he has health insurance. Insurers who do business in these states will be required to turn over lists of their clients to the state health department.[24]

In Massachusetts, auditors will investigate which of the current half million uninsured people did not buy medical insurance, and fine them. The poorest residents (making under $10,000) would get access to such insurance with no premiums and no deductibles.

Where Massachusetts penalized noncompliance, Vermont encouraged compliance with its Catamount Health for uninsured residents. Under it, families can get the same coverage as Blue Cross Blue Shield for about $500 a month, with tiered co-pays for drugs and similar deductibles.[25] Families making up to 300 percent of the poverty level (about $30,000 for one parent and $60,000 per year for a family of four), can receive graduated subsidies from Vermont.[26]

Vermont's plan recognizes that people with chronic conditions (diabetes, heart disease, obesity, high blood pressure) consume 80 percent of health care dollars. It covers screening, counseling, and preventive services for people with these conditions in hopes of reducing later, more expensive interventions.

Employers with more than 10 employees who do not provide medical coverage for them must pay the state medical fund $295 per employee. Massachusetts Medicaid/CHIP expanded to cover all expenses of children in families up to 300 percent of the poverty level.[27]

Both plans will be costly. In Massachusetts, Medicaid payments for medical care will go to $90 million a year by 2009, about what private insurers pay. One scholar predicted that working families (who will pay $14,000 a year) won't be able to afford it and that the plan will go bankrupt because physicians and patients in the plan had no incentives to cut costs.[28]

Both plans put the lie to the idea that universal coverage must be a government-run, single-payer system. By cobbling together several plans, these states managed to provide coverage for their citizens.

Expanding Medicare? For and Against AmeriCare

Why not expand Medicare to cover all Americans regardless of age? Call such an expanded Medicare system, "AmeriCare." AmeriCare could absorb other systems of medical coverage, including Medicaid, insurance for federal employees, CHAMPUS, all government disability funds, and medical payments covered under automobile insurance.

Favoring AmeriCare #1: Greater Efficiency

AmeriCare could eliminate the overhead and waste of multiple private insurers. About 4 to 12 percent of health care costs represent fees and profits of private insurance plans;[29] by comparison, Medicare has maintained reasonable administrative expenses, about 2.5 percent of its total expenditures.[30]

The crucial concept behind AmeriCare is to transfer money now spent for overhead and profits in private companies to AmeriCare to cover services for those who presently lack medical coverage. American health insurers made $100 billion in 2005, and that money would pay for a lot of health care for many Americans.[31] If such funds could easily be reallocated, the increase of money spent on medical care might be small.

Medicare is a great American success story. Elderly Americans enjoy one of the most technologically advanced medical systems in the world. It is not the fault of Medicare that the elderly still spend 15 percent of their income on medical services; this is attributable simply to increases, first in the cost of normal services, and second in the vast increase in the number and variety of services covered.

From physicians' viewpoint, AmeriCare would eliminate hiring personnel simply to deal with the vast array of private insurers. Moreover, AmeriCare would reduce the delay of payments to physicians from many private insurers.[32]

Finally, Medicare is a system already in place. Hospitals presently get about half their revenues from Medicare patients. Expanding Medicare to AmeriCare for all age groups simply broadens Medicare, rather than creating an untried system.

Medicare could be gradually expanded, the way Congress added a drug benefit in 2006, or by age groups, first dropping eligibility from age 65 at present to, say, age 55. This would allow time for changes to be assessed and for needed modifications to be made.

Opposing AmeriCare #1: Not Another Federal Bureaucracy

AmeriCare would create a bloated, unresponsive federal bureaucracy. During the 1960s and 1970s, the Veterans Administration was such a bureaucracy. The federal government simply cannot do certain things well, and especially not health care.

An expanded Medicare system would become another End Stage Renal Disease program, with runaway costs. What everyone pays for, nobody pays for, and there is a tendency for everyone to seek his or her own advantage to the detriment of the overall good. This is an age-old story, played out long ago in England in the *tragedy of the commons*: the owner of each flock increased the number of sheep he grazed on town land—the commons—until the commons were so overgrazed that the grass simply disappeared and the commons system was destroyed.[33]

What is the proper role of the federal government with regard to health care? Not providing health care. Federal funding for end stage renal disease, artificial hearts, and AIDS is politicized and has been provided at the expense of other diseases. American government is being asked to do too many things for too many people.

With one-seventh of the American economy at stake in health care, and one-sixth of new jobs, do we want to take the chance of a federally administered system?

Favoring AmeriCare #2: Eliminating Experience Rating

Private insurers issue policies using either community or experience rating. In *community rating*, risk for a large employer, state or group is evaluated, and every policyholder in that "community" is charged the same premium. Community rating favors ill people because they cannot be excluded and their benefits are subsidized by premiums of the healthy. Systems of universal medical coverage practice community rating over an entire country.

Experience rating charges an individual or small-business rates based on the characteristics of the person or employees, such that previous illness or small numbers dramatically increase costs of premiums. In extreme cases, insurers maximize profits by selling policies to healthy young people, who are unlikely to make claims and by not selling policies to people who are sick, old, disabled, or at high risk of accidents—that is, people who are likely to make claims. Insurers out to maximize profits exclude many people from coverage.

A little bit of history about medical insurance in America is instructive here. During the 1930s, surgeons and physicians founded Blue Cross and Blue Shield to ensure that patients had enough money to pay surgeons and physicians after hospitalization for catastrophic conditions. By state law, the "Blues" were nonprofit organizations; as such, in many states they paid no state or federal taxes and no taxes on the premiums they collected. In return for their nonprofit status, Blue Cross Blue Shield (BCBS) companies were required to insure everyone who wanted to be insured, and to do this they adopted community rating. Because BCBS had a state-permitted, virtual monopoly on private medical coverage between the 1930s and the 1960s, things worked out for everyone. BCBS insured everyone who wanted insurance, and rates remained reasonable.

In the early 1970s, changes in federal regulations allowed commercial insurance companies of a new kind to come into existence. These new commercial insurers were allowed to use experience rating, and they started cherry picking the healthiest customers of BCBS, leaving BCBS as an insurer of last resort for the unhealthiest and neediest customers.[34] Under these circumstances, what eventually happened to Empire BCBS, the organization serving New York State, was predictable. Commercial insurance companies took its best customers and left it with only the sickest customers, such as those with AIDS. As a result, Empire BCBS raised premiums for all its customers by nearly 100 percent.

Another target of cherry picking, Kentucky BCBS, between the early 1960s and the late 1970s saw its share of policies statewide drop from 90 to 30 percent. Some states later made cherry picking illegal.

People have misconceptions about medical insurance, a term which can be misleading. Thirty years ago, medical insurance was simply insurance—a hedge against a dreaded but rather remote possibility. At that time, people took out medical insurance policies in the hope that they would never need to receive benefits, and policies covered mainly catastrophic situations like hospital care after an automobile accident or a diagnosis of cancer.

Gradually, medical policies evolved into something quite different, though they have continued to be called insurance: they became plans for prepaid group health care. Blue Cross Blue Shield, for example, simply adds up all its medical costs (subtracting a small amount for administration), divides by the number of policyholders, and sends out the bills. Also, medical insurance expanded to cover not just catastrophic care but all "major medical" expenses. This was a logical extension: if people were willing to pay small premiums to protect themselves against remote catastrophic risks, why not pay slightly larger premiums to protect against more common risks? Thus "insurance" grew and grew until it now includes almost any medical service; today, some people become indignant when their "insurance" doesn't cover absolutely everything and they have to pay for anything at all!

Many people also mistakenly believe that most Americans without medical coverage are *unemployed*, but this is a myth: in fact, most of the 46 million Americans without good medical coverage are employed.[35] Most waiters and waitresses, for instance, have no employer-sponsored medical insurance; many workers in small shops and small businesses, like Rosalyn Schwartz, receive no medical insurance. Only 1 of 10 businesses employing fewer than 10 people provides medical coverage.[36]

AmeriCare would ban experience rating and for-profit medical insurance. It assumes that insurance is a moral enterprise of sharing risk to help those with bad genes or who are victims of accidents. It rejects the idea that selling medical insurance is primarily a way to make money.

One other point: because Blue Cross Blue Shield was created by physicians and surgeons, it reimburses *procedures* well but not *preventive services*. In particular, specialists who do procedures receive far more than physicians in primary care who talk to patients: an ophthalmologist can get $2,000 for removing a cataract in an hour but a geriatric psychiatrist only gets $80 for talking to the same patient afterwards. No wonder then that fewer and fewer physicians go into low-paying basic areas of medicine such as geriatrics, pediatrics, internal medicine, and family medicine. Given that, isn't the American system broken, spending more and more on fewer and fewer people for less and less basic care?

Opposing AmeriCare #2: Health Care Is Not a Right

AmeriCare would make access to health care a *right* of all American citizens. Elderly Americans now think of Medicare as a right, and most Americans would come to think the same of AmeriCare.

Problems at the margins would be difficult: who is a citizen and entitled to national care? A baby born here? An immigrant? How long must one live here before becoming eligible? Would it be right to let some move here and, say, after seven years, have the same medical benefits as someone who had paid into the system for 30 years of her payroll taxes?

Supporters of AmeriCare claim that citizens have a right to *minimal* or *basic* health care. The problem here is conceptual: no one can agree on what is merely basic care. One person's minimal care is another's luxury. When American nurses and physicians visit developing countries, they despair that they cannot provide the minimal treatment of American medicine.

As medicine improves, what is minimal becomes normal, just as what was once extraordinary becomes ordinary. So in 1962 kidney dialysis was extraordinary; now it is ordinary. In the 1970s, kidney transplants were extraordinary; now they are ordinary. And so on. What this means is that there is no logical point to stop providing health care, before which coverage is a right, after which, it is not.

Favoring AmeriCare #3: Justice and Fairness

Universal medical coverage may be required as a matter of *justice*. Philosopher John Rawls believed that the term *justice* best applies to the design of a society's basic arrangements, and health care is one such arrangement. According to Rawls, principles of justice stem from a hypothetical social contract in which citizens come together to make choices under *a veil of ignorance* about their own age, race, religion, sex, health, wealth, abilities, and talents. In other words, they cannot bias their choices by considering arbitrary personal characteristics.

Under these conditions, Rawls believes that rational people would not gamble with the structure of their society but would choose those structures that gave people maximal equal liberty. But some liberty could be sacrificed to achieve greater equality. To Rawls, inequality is justifiable when it works to the advantage of those who are worst off, that is, when the worst-off group does better with the inequality than without it. This is Rawls's *difference principle*.

An essential part of Rawls's concept of justice is the recognition that the world is naturally unfair: some people are born into rich families, some into poor ones; some people are born healthy, others with spina bifida. For Rawls, government can either worsen such inequalities or lessen them. For Rawls, governments that sharpen inequality are unjust; governments that reduce it are just.

Rawls's veil of ignorance can be seen as a device for ensuring that the golden rule will become part of decisions about the structure of society. Underlying this approach is the ability to imagine ourselves as "worst off"—to see ourselves as sick, hurt, poor, uninsured; to imagine how bad it would be to have a serious illness or accident, and how much worse it would be to have no way to pay for the care we need.

How might Rawls's approach be specifically applied to our own system? The three decades, 1975–2005, have not been good for the poor in America. Between 1970 and 2001, the gap between the richest 5 percent of Americans and average Americans widened, as the former jumped from $33,000 to $265,000 while the latter only inched from $2,000 to 10,100.[37]

Over these three decades, more and more workers had to work longer and longer just to keep what they had. Some jobs that once paid $20 an hour now paid $7. If, as Rawls assumes, a just society is egalitarian, then American society became more unjust.

Our existing medical system, in which more than 46 million Americans lack coverage, is an unjust, structural inequality at a level where life-and-death decisions are made. We know that inherited genes cause many diseases and no one is responsible for the genes he or she inherits. Why allow the structure of medical finance to intensify the injustices of fate?

According to Rawls's difference principle, an unequal medical structure would be just only if the poor were better off under it than under an egalitarian system; and in the present, unequal American medical system, that is obviously not the case.

Opposing AmeriCare #3: Out-of-Control Costs

The more health care is seen as a right, the more of life becomes medicalized, that is, people tend to seek medical care in more and more circumstances. That happened in Australia, whose system covers payments for in vitro fertilization. Furthermore, people now live much longer—partly because of the care Medicare provides—and people who live to be old cost the most.

A major issue about health care is that increasing access and services entails increases in costs. Fiscal conservatives say that our experience with Medicare has taught us an important lesson: the system cannot expand the number of patients covered or the range of services offered and simultaneously decrease costs.

In 2006, the trustees of Medicare and Social Security announced that, without higher taxes, Medicare will go bankrupt in 2018, 12 years sooner than predicted when George W. Bush took office in 2001.[38] Despite this announcement, Congress passed a new benefit in 2006 for Medicare recipients, covering their drugs up to $2,250 and then again after they spend $$5,100.[39]

As libertarian University of Chicago law professor Richard Epstein empha- sizes, the cost of universalizing Medicare dramatically increases as the system moves from insuring each smaller segment of the 46 million of presently unin- sured Americans.[40] Covering most of the half who are children is relatively cheap. Covering most of the adult, working poor is not exorbitant. But covering the last 10, 5, or 1 percent is expensive, because such percentages represent the real out- liers and cost-busters that all private systems want to avoid. These are the patients with diabetes, schizophrenia, or congestive heart failure. If a national system entitles such patients to the best care, it will be difficult for it to say when a just limit of care has been reached.

Furthermore, reformers often want to increase services. Each increase in serv- ice provided to all Americans costs more money. The increases in services that are most commonly mentioned are long-term care in nursing homes, home health care, hospice care, transportation to medical facilities, dental services, and drugs for people with mental illnesses.

Libertarians such as Epstein believe Clinton's Health Security Act previewed exactly what would go wrong when the government mandated medical coverage. Clinton's Act first ran into trouble with Libertarians over its vague estimates of cost. Even its advocates said it might entail an extra tax on income of 10 percent.

Another problem was making it illegal, as Canada did, to purchase extra health care outside a nationally approved plan. It is one thing to guarantee everyone a basic minimum of health care, but it's quite another to force everyone into the same sys- tem and to deny opportunities to pay for extra care. The latter seemed un-American.

Surprisingly, many recipients of Medicare opposed Clinton's Act, perceiving that the cost-containment goals could only be obtained by limiting funds for Medicare. Put differently, the costs of giving care to the most expensive uninsured patients might conflict with the goal of giving the best care to the elderly.

In general, libertarians just do not believe that the American government can control costs and provide universal access, as happened in Canada, Germany, and Australia. They fear that governments will limit freedoms of physicians and busi- nesses, and mandate expensive services that require higher taxes.

Favoring AmeriCare #4: Market Solutions Won't Work

It is sometimes argued that health care could be provided and costs controlled by letting medicine operate as a true market, subject to the laws of supply and demand. Markets regulate other goods and services without bloated bureaucracies and wasteful costs. Why not medicine, too?

In a true market, people would buy health care, such as an operation on their knee, with their own money. There would be no medical insurance and thus no reimbursement from insurers. Because people would have to pay for their care themselves, prices would tumble.

For a routine eye examination, patients might be able to choose a nurse practitioner charging $10, a primary care physician charging $30, or an ophthalmologist charging $300. Given these alternatives, most would not choose the ophthalmologist, and so ophthalmologists would have to lower their fees to compete, unless they could somehow demonstrate that their services were worth more. On the other hand, if covered by their medical plan, most Americans would go to an ophthalmologist.

Such a true market would lower costs, but a market in medicine also has burdens, especially for sick and elderly patients. When people have just discovered they have cancer or multiple sclerosis, they do not always make good decisions. As one expert group concluded:

> The special nature of older persons and their health problems argues for caution in relying primarily on private solutions to providing health care for them. . . . In particular, the elderly are less equipped to deal with a marketplace of health care than younger, working persons. Partly because elderly persons are more likely to suffer from physical and mental impairments (including eyesight, hearing, and memory), they have more trouble than younger persons in comprehending the increasingly complex insurance arrangements now available. The elderly also usually lack the counsel of the purchasing agents and benefits representatives who serve younger, employed populations. Although some retired persons may be able to navigate our health care system, many others will not fare well in the rough and tumble of a health care marketplace.[41]

In a true market, medical professions would become hardboiled, doing "wallet biopsies" before helping anyone (read A. J. Cronin's autobiographical *The Citadel* to see how physicians once practiced this way). A real market in medicine would be a harsh, cruel system where patients and professionals no longer worked together to overcome illness but where each bargained with the other for maximal financial gain.

It is also true that if health care were provided as other commercial commodities are—rather than being subsidized as it now is—many people who could afford care would not make wise decisions. If we had to choose between a new car and a hip replacement, some would choose the car. Moreover, some people might be tempted, or pressured, to sacrifice health care for the sake of their families; a parent might give up a hip replacement and put the money toward a house for her family. In this regard, a true market is exactly what people face who lack insurance today.

In some more modest form, a mixed market may have something to offer. One intriguing idea is to make the present system more like a market by making medical coverage more like automobile insurance.[42] This is what Vermont and Massachusetts did. Because people pay for automobile insurance themselves, they usually shop around for the best policy for them for a reasonable cost.

Opposing AmeriCare #4. Intergenerational Injustice

Many elderly citizens mistakenly believe that Medicare recipients have already paid for their benefits through FICA taxes. One popular book about Medicare benefits states, "The most fundamental point is that Medicare is not a gift. You paid for it while you were working. Medicare owes you services in just the same way that the health insurer to whom you have paid premiums owes them to you."[43]

In fact, the Medicare benefits going to today's elderly people are paid for by the FICA taxes of today's workers.[44] For the first few years on Medicare, most beneficiaries receive benefits amounting to what they paid in, plus all interest; thereafter, young current workers pay for their benefits.

Richard Lamm, governor of Colorado from 1978 to 1987, once set off a national debate about exorbitant medical costs when he attacked the high costs of organ transplants and the amount spent on the last years of Americans' lives. He wrote:

> Once we accept the fact that there are limits to what the nation can afford (and increasingly, people are recognizing this truth), then we will begin a process of asking how to get the most health benefits for the most Americans for our money. We should have asked this question years ago. It is outrageous that this country spends five to eight times what other countries spend, and yet has no better health outcome. America is going to demand more accountability for the more than one billion dollars a day it now spends on health care. Many countries give a high level of health care to all their citizens for a fraction of what we spend, and yet keep them healthier. We are no longer rich enough to give a blank check to an inefficient health care industry.
>
> Once we start to apply even minimum management standards to the health care industry, we will see some substantial changes. If we ask how to get the most health benefits for the greatest number of Americans for our tax dollars, many of today's practices will not meet the test. If we zero-budget all that we now do in health care, we shall inevitably close unnecessary hospitals, close excess ICU units, and look much more closely at utilization factors and outcomes.
>
> We shall have to develop a concept of cost-effective medicine. Virtually every health care provider will agree that much of what we do today in medicine has "marginal utility." When a society faces fiscal reality and seeks to optimize its dollars, it not only starts on the road to financial sanity, but it also brings dramatic change to existing medical practices. Dialysis and transplantation will undoubtedly undergo major change. The "opportunity costs" in other areas of medicine are clearly greater than much of what is being done today. The bottom line is that we can save more lives and bring better health care to more Americans for many of the dollars we are spending today.
>
> Economist Lester Thurow suggests that, to impress upon health providers what they are doing when they order marginal services, we should require them to imagine an American worker sentenced to a period of slavery long enough to pay the medical bill for that procedure. Dr. Thomas Starzl recently gave a liver transplant to a 76-year old woman. It cost $240,000. Dr. Starzl should understand that with the average U.S. family making $24,000 a year, he has sentenced 10 U.S. families to work all year so that he could transplant a 76-year old woman.[45]

If Governor Lamm is correct, then expansion of Medicare must be done by increasing taxation on present Americans. If that is politically impossible, and if financing it is only done by long-term borrowing that future Americans must pay off, it would be unjust to young Americans to create AmeriCare.

Existing Medicare will no doubt be saved. What will likely happen is that the age of eligibility will be raised, say to 67, and later, perhaps 70. The Medicare payroll tax will increase, say from 2.9 to 3.5 percent, and then later, perhaps to 4 or 5 percent. If AmeriCare is created, this tax would almost immediately jump to 10 percent. All this will be the yoke of taxation on the backs of American's working young.

Opposing AmeriCare #5: Socialized Medicine Reduces Liberties

Democracies try to balance two competing values: equality and liberty. A system once in equilibrium with perfect financial equality must forbid inheritance of money, unequal trades, or unequal pay, else the system will soon create citizens of unequal wealth.

We might conceive of equality and individual liberty as the X and Y axes of Cartesian coordinates. The more we move to perfect equality, the more individual liberty vanishes. For example, for many decades America had no income tax: citizens kept all the money they made. The programs of the Great Society resulted from transfers via income tax from the working to the needy. Liberty of some to keep all their money was reduced to increase financial and medical equality for all.

For universal coverage to work, patients cannot be allowed to opt out of the system. This is like having a situation of perfect equality and then allowing unequal trades. As we will see below, this is the problem that has put the Canadian medical system in crisis.

Similarly, physicians would not be allowed to sell their services privately or avoid being in AmeriCare.

Finally, some epidemiologists believe that the poor will only live as long and as well as average Americans when they live in neighborhoods which are as safe, have equal incentives to stop smoking and using alcohol and drugs, and are shielded from environmental toxins. To do so requires not just health care, but transfer of money to them.

But such transfers mean more taxation, and all taxation is involuntary. Involuntary taxation to some is a kind of working slavery, where a certain portion of the year is required just to pay one's taxes, say, the first six months. Critics say the cost of AmeriCare is too high if everyone must work another month to pay for it.

Favoring AmeriCare #5: AmeriCare Is Not Socialized Medicine?

Some people would call AmeriCare "socialized medicine." Lest that emotionally powerful phrase be a thought-stopper, let us consider exactly what "socialized" means. "Socialized" could mean simply "publicly owned." If so, that is not necessarily a bad thing, or even an unusual thing. Americans are used to public ownership: highways and waterways, public schools, state colleges and universities, the armed forces, airwaves, the air, the skies, and national parks are all publicly owned. When America was founded, private toll-roads were common and some people tried to "own" rivers and ports, charging tolls on ships that came and went, until the U.S. Supreme Court decided that American waterways were public goods.

When Congress debated Medicare in 1965, the American Medical Association (AMA) opposed it as "socialized medicine." American physicians feared that government-administered care financed by taxes would mean government-controlled care,[46] and that all physicians would soon be employees of the federal government.

To placate these physicians, a crucial decision was then made: under Medicare, physicians would be reimbursed on a fee-for-service basis. Eventually, this arrangement would make physicians rich and would give them the best of both worlds: freedom to work independently rather than as government employees, and freedom to order infinite services for their patients—services that would be taken care of by government-enforced payments in the form of higher and higher FICA taxes.

So if universal coverage is not necessarily socialized medicine, what could it be? Four answers are most discussed: First, it could be a single-payer system, such as AmeriCare, in which the federal government would tax all Americans and reimburse physicians on a fee-for-service basis. Second, it could be an *American medical service*—a system in which all medical professionals work for the federal government. Third, it could be an *employer-mandated system* like Oregon and Massachusetts where federal law requires every employer to buy basic medical coverage for every employee and establishes a separate government-financed system for unemployed people. Fourth, it could be a *voucher system*, where all Americans receive government-funded vouchers to buy health care directly from hospitals or insurers.

Opposing AmeriCare #6: Illegal Immigrants

The elephant in the room of universal medical coverage is illegal immigrants. In the fall of 2006, America's population reached 300 million people, a growth of 100 million people since 1967. About 53 percent of the new Americans were recent immigrants, both legal and illegal, and their children.

The majority of these immigrants are illegal workers. Covering them for medical care will break the bank. Moreover, if they are covered, workers with expensive diseases and disabilities will flock to America to get coverage for their conditions. This is what is known in the insurance industry as *adverse selection*.

Whether hospitals admit illegal immigrants varies from hospital to hospital, state to state. Reimbursement figures show that the largest group of illegal immigrant patients are pregnant women.[47] Parkland Hospital in Dallas does not ask about immigration status and pregnant mothers from Mexico flock to it to give birth, whereas JPS Health Network in nearby Ft. Worth requires proof of American citizenship for treatment of pregnant women or admission to its hospitals.[48] In 2005, California spent over $1 billion on medical care for illegal immigrants. The other top states giving such care were Arizona, Texas, New York, and Illinois.

If children are born in America, such births are reimbursed by Medicaid and then the child is an American citizen, with K–12 public schooling available to him.

America cannot afford to open its borders and to give away medical coverage and jobs to everyone who wants to enter. This would be a tragedy of the commons.

As for Vermont and Massachusetts, how many illegal workers do they have? Vermont is one of the whitest states in the country with few jobs in meat-processing, janitoring, and other low-skilled jobs that attract immigrants.

Favoring AmeriCare #6: Illegal Immigrants

Some myths abound about illegal workers. Most Americans do not believe that such workers pay FICA and income taxes, but taxes are deducted from their paychecks.[49] So workers from Central and South America who work as janitors or cut up meat in factories subsidize Social Security checks and hospital care for senior Americans.

Anti-immigration advocates claim that illegal workers burden American's hospitals and drain resources from traditional Americans. Starting in 1996, reforms to welfare disqualified illegal immigrants from receiving welfare, food stamps, subsidized housing, Medicaid, and Medicare. If injured, immigrants must be treated and stabilized in emergency rooms.

In 1996, the Internal Revenue Service began issuing identification numbers to illegal workers to take their taxes. You can be a gangster or an illegal worker in this country, and other authorities may take their time dealing with you, but in the meantime, the IRS demands your taxes. Each year, half of the 7 million illegal workers use such ID numbers to file federal and state returns and pay the same taxes as traditional Americans.[50]

FURTHER READING AND RESOURCES

Ezekiel Emanuel, *The Ends of Human Life: Medical Ethics in a Liberal Polity*, Harvard University Press, Cambridge, Mass., 1992.

Frank Marsh and Mark Yarborough, *Medicine and Money: A Study of the Role of Beneficence in Health Care Cost Containment*, Greenwood, New York, 1990.

E. Haavi Morreim, ed., "Ethics and Alternative Health Systems," *Journal of Medicine and Philosophy*, vol. 17, no. 1 (special issue), February 1992.

Notes

Chapter 1

1. Associated Press, October 16, 1983.
2. Robert Steinbock and Bernard Lo, "The Case of Elizabeth Bouvia: Starvation, Suicide, or Problem Patient?" *Archives of Internal Medicine* 146 (January 1986), p. 161.
3. Quoted in George Annas, "When Suicide Prevention Becomes Brutality: The Case of Elizabeth Bouvia," *Hastings Center Report* 14, no. 2, (April 1984), p. 20.
4. Associated Press, in *Birmingham Post-Herald*, December 14, 1984, p. A2.
5. Quoted in Arthur Hoppe, *San Francisco Examiner*, December 20, 1983.
6. Steinbock and Lo, "The Case of Elizabeth Bouvia," p. 161.
7. *Bouvia v. County of Riverside*, California Superior Court, December 16, 1983.
8. Richard Scott, in "Patient's Suicide Wish Troubles Hospital MDs," *American Medical News*, January 20, 1984, p. 5.
9. Arthur Hoppe, *San Francisco Examiner*.
10. Annas, "When Suicide Prevention," p. 46.
11. George Annas, "Elizabeth Bouvia: Whose Space Is This Anyway?" *Hastings Center Report* 16, no. 2 (April 1986), p. 20.
12. Steinbock and Lo, "The Case of Elizabeth Bouvia," p. 162.
13. George Annas, "Elizabeth Bouvia," pp. 24–25.
14. Derek Humphry and Ann Wickett, *The Right to Die: Understanding Euthanasia*, Harper and Row, New York, 1986, p. 150.
15. Paul Longmore, "Elizabeth Bouvia, Assisted Suicide, and Social Prejudice," in *Issues in Law and Medicine*, no. 2 (Fall 1987), p. 158.
16. The hospital's rationale in its brief to Judge Deering is quoted in Annas, "Elizabeth Bouvia," p. 24.
17. *Bouvia v. Glenchur*, Los Angeles Superior Court, *California Reporter* 225 (1986), pp. 296–308.
18. *Bouvia v. Superior Court* (Glenchur), *California Reporter* 297, California Appellate 2 District, 1986.
19. Jeff Wilson (AP), "Precedent-Setter Lives On after Plea to Die," *Indianapolis Star*, December 19, 1993, p. H7.
20. B. D. Colen, "His Life, to Take or Not," *Newsday*, September 25, 1989, pp. 5–19.
21. Susan Schindehette and Gail Wescott, "Deciding Not to Die," *People*, January 18, 1993, p. 86.
22. Susan Schindehette and Gail Wescott, "Deciding Not to Die," p. 86.
23. Russ Fine, *UAB Report*, September 4, 1992, p. 4.
24. Russ Fine, *UAB Report*, September 4, 1992, p. 4.
25. Associated Press, "Thousands Retiring without Social Security," February 16, 1993.
26. Russ Fine, personal communication to author, May 16, 1994.
27. Cowart's case became the topic of a famous videotape, "Please Let Me Die," and a later film, *Dax's Case*. See also L. Kliever, *Dax's Case—Essays in Medical Ethics and Human Meaning*, SMU Press, Dallas, Texas, 1989.
28. Dax Cowart, personal communication to author at meeting of American Association of Medical Colleges, Chicago, Ill., October 1989.
29. Quotations are from Phaedo, in E. Hamilton and H. Cairns, eds., *Plato: The Collected Dialogues*, Princeton University Press, Princeton, N.J. 1961.

30. Quoted by James Rachels, "Euthanasia," in T. Regan, ed., *Matters of Life and Death*, 3d ed., McGraw-Hill, New York, 1993, p. 35.
31. Seneca, *De Ira*, quoted in Rachels, "Euthanasia."
32. Jean Paul Sartre, *Existentialism Is a Humanism*, Philosophical Library, New York, 1947.
33. Frederick Russell, *The Just War in the Middle Ages*, Cambridge University Press, Cambridge, England, 1975.
34. Quoted in James Gutman, "Death and Dying in Western Culture," *Encyclopedia of Bioethics* 1, Free Press, New York, 1978, p. 240.
35. Baruch Spinoza, *Ethics*, William White and Amelia Stirling, trans., Hafner, New York, 1949.
36. Quoted in Derek Humphry and Ann Wickett, *The Right to Die: Understanding Euthanasia*, Harper and Row, New York, 1986, pp. 8–9.
37. David Hume, "On Suicide" (1755), in Eugene Miller, ed., *Collected Essays of David Hume*, Liberty Classics, Indianapolis, Ind., 1986.
38. David Hume, "On Suicide."
39. Immanuel Kant, "On Suicide" (1755–1780*), Lectures on Ethics*, L. Enfield, trans., Harper and Row, New York, 1963, pp. 148–154.
40. Immanuel Kant, "On Suicide."
41. John Stuart Mill, *On Liberty* (1859), Appleton-Century-Crofts, New York, 1974.
42. Quoted in Humphry and Wickett, *The Right to Die*, p. 16.
43. Alan Meisel, *The Right to Die:* Cumulative Supplement 1, Wylie, New York, 1991, p. x.
44. T. Woody, "Was His Act of Mercy Also Murder?" *New York Times*, November 7, 1988.
45. Art Kleiner, "Life after Suicide," *High Wire*, Summer 1982, p. 30.
46. Tad Friend, "Jumpers," *New Yorker*, October 13, 2003.
47. H. Hendin, "Suicide in America," *Miami News*, August 30, 1982, p. B1.
48. Quoted in Humphry and Wickett, *The Right to Die*, p. 152.
49. Quoted in Humphry and Wickett, *The Right to Die*, p. 155.
50. Humphry and Wickett, *The Right to Die*, p. 154.
51. Kevin D. O'Rourke, "Value Conflicts Raised by Physician-Assisted Suicide," *Linacre Quarterly* 57, no. 3 (August 1990), pp. 38–49.
52. SUPPORT Principal Investigators, "A Controlled Trial to Improve Care of Seriously Ill Hospitalized Patients. The Study to Understand Prognoses and Preferences for Outcomes and Risks of Treatment (SUPPORT), *Journal of the American Medical Association* 274 (1995), pp. 1591–1598.
53. John Shuster, talk at UAB Medical School, August 14, 1995.
54. Paul Longmore, Column in *Electric Edge*, January/February 1997.
55. Paul Longmore, "Elizabeth Bouvia, Assisted Suicide, and Social Prejudice," in *Issues in Law and Medicine* 2, no. 2 (Fall 1987), p. 158.
56. Russ Fine, *UAB Report*, September 4, 1992, p. 12.
57. Russ Fine, *UAB Report*, September 4, 1992, p. 4.
58. "McAfee Tries to Cut Red Tape," *Birmingham Post-Herald*, June 18, 1990, p. C1.
59. J. Hogeland and L. Sellars, "McAfee Shouldn't Get Special Treatment," (letter) *Birmingham Post-Herald*, July 9, 1990.
60. Douglas Martin, "Disability Culture: Eager to Bite the Hands That Would Feed Them," *New York Times*, June 1, 1997, p. A1.

Chapter 2

1. Robert Morse, in *In the Matter of Karen Quinlan: The Complete Legal Briefs, Court Proceedings, and Decisions in Superior Court of New Jersey*, vols. 1 and 2, University Publications of America, Frederick Md., 1982, p. 236 (hereafter, *Proceedings 1*, *Proceedings 2*). The later court transcript contradicts itself about the exact drugs Karen consumed. Attending physician Robert Morse testified that, "She had some barbiturates, which was normal, 0.6 milligrams; toxic is 2 milligrams, and the toxic dose is about 5 milligrams percent"[sic]. Julius Korein, in *Proceedings 1*, pp. 34–35 Consulting neurologist Julius Korein, whom the Quinlans hired, testified that Karen's drug screen "was positive for quinine, negative for morphine, barbiturates and other substances. A subsequent test for Valium and Librium was positive." (No one else mentioned Librium.) Court prosecutor George Daggett testified that Karen had taken tranquilizers with alcohol shortly before becoming unconscious. George Daggett, *New York Times*, September 20, 1975, New Jersey sec. The Quinlans denied that the drug screen showed barbiturates: "The early urine and blood samples, taken on the day Karen was brought to the hospital, revealed only a 'normal therapeutic'

level of aspirin and the tranquilizer Valium in her system." Joseph and Julia Quinlan with Phyllis Battelle, *Karen Ann: The Quinlans Tell Their Story*, 1977, Doubleday Anchor, New York, p. 22.

2. Joseph and Julia Quinlan with Phyllis Battelle, *Karen Ann: The Quinlans Tell Their Story*, 1977, Doubleday Anchor, New York, p. 27.
3. Daniel Coburn, in *Proceedings 1*, p. 17.
4. Julius Korein, in *Proceedings 1*, p. 329.
5. Fred Plum, in Quinlan and Quinlan, *Karen Ann*, p. 198.
6. Robert Morse, in Quinlan and Quinlan, *Karen Ann*, pp 188–189.
7. Quinlan and Quinlan, *Karen Ann*, pp. 272–273 (the nun is not named).
8. Gino Concetti, quoted in Quinlan and Quinlan, *Karen Ann*, p. 284.
9. Quoted in Quinlan and Quinlan, *Karen Ann*.
10. Hentoff, "The Deadly Slippery Slope," *The Village Voice*, September 1, 1987.
11. Nat Hentoff, "The Deadly Slippery Slope."
12. *Cruzan v. Director, Missouri Dept. of Health*, 110 Sup. Ct. Reporter 2841, 1990.
13. George Annas, "Nancy Cruzan and the Right to Die," *New England Journal of Medicine* 323, no. 10 (September 6, 1990), p. 670.
14. Love and Let Die," *Time*, March 19, 1990, pp. 62ff.
15. Andrew M. Malcolm, "Nancy Cruzan: End to Long Goodbye," *New York Times*, December 29, 1990, p. A3. See also, "A Conversation with Mr. and Mrs. Cruzan," *Midwest Medical Ethics: The Nancy Cruzan Case* 5, nos. 1–2 (Winter/Spring 1989).
16. Charles Baron, "On Taking Substituted Judgment Seriously," *Hastings Center Report* 20, no. 5 (September–October 1992), p. 7.
17. John Robertson, "Cruzan: No Rights Violated," *Hastings Center Report* 20, no. 5 (September–October 1992), p. 7.
18. Ronald Cranford, lecture at UAB Medical School, January 19, 1991.
19. Joanne Lynn and Jacqueline Glover, "Cruzan and Caring for Others," *Hastings Center Report* 20, no. 5, September–October 1992, p. 11.
20. Annas, "Nancy Cruzan and the Right to Die," p. 672.
21. Irwin Molotsky, "Wife Wins Right-to-Die Case; Then a Governor Challenges It," *New York Times*, October 2, 1998, p. A20.
22. Timothy E. Quill, "Terri Schiavo—A Tragedy Compounded," *New England Journal of Medicine* 352 (April 21, 2005), pp. 1630–1633.
23. Jane Brody, "Preserving a Delicate Balance of Potassium," *New York Times*, June 22, 2004, p. 12. Low-carbohydrate high-protein diets do not create the right kind and amount of potassium for the body, nor do sports drinks replenish potassium lost in exercising nearly as well as fresh fruits and vegetables.
24. According to Kenneth Goodman, M.D., of the Department of Bioethics at the University of Miami. Personal Communication, November 14, 2004.
25. Arian-Camp-Flores, "The Legacy of Terri Schiavo," *Newsweek*, April 4, 2005, p. 26.
26. Arian-Camp-Flores, "The Legacy," p. 26.
27. Austrian physician Semmelweis correctly charged his colleagues with spreading childbirth fever by not washing their hands and going from birth to birth; he was subsequently regarded by his fellow physicians as crazy.
28. Malcolm Ritter, "Degree of Schiavo's Awareness a Point of Contention Among Doctors," Associated Press, *Birmingham News*, March 25, 2005.
29. Manuel Roig-Franzia, "Justices Decline Schiavo Case," *Washington Post*, March 25, 2005, p. A1.
30. Quoted from William Colby, *The Long Goodbye: The Deaths of Nancy Cruzan*, Hay House Publishing, 2002.
31. Manuel Roig-Franzia, "Florida High Court Overrules Governor in Schiavo Case," *Washington Post*, 24 September 2004, p. A3.
32. Manuel Roig-Franzia, "Court Lets Right-to-Die Ruling Stand," *Washington Post*, January 24, 2005, p. A12.
33. Manuel Roig-Franzia, "Court Lets Right-to-Die Ruling Stand."
34. Walter F. Roche and Same Werhover, "DeLay Family Decided to End Life of His Father After Injury in 1988," *Washington Post*, March 28, 2005, p. A3.
35. Charles Babington and Mike Allen, "Congress Passes." *Washington Post*, March 2, 2005, p. A1.
36. Democrat Jim Jordan, quoted by Charles Babington, "Viewing Videotape, Frist Disputes Fla. Doctors' Diagnosis of Schiavo," *Washington Post*, March 20, 2005, p. A3.
37. Tamara Lipper, "Between Life and Death," *Newsweek*, March 28, 2005, p. 30.

38. Manuel Roig-Franzia, 'Schiavo's Parents Take 'Final Shot' to Keep Her Alive," *Washington Post*, March 26, 2005, p. A4.

39. Nancy Weaver Teichert, "Experts: Lack of Food, Water, Does Not Cause Pain for Dying," *Sacramento Bee*, March 28, 2005; *Birmingham News*, March 29, 2005, p. A6.

40. "Report of Autopsy: Schiavo, Terri, Case #5050439," March 31, 2005, p. 5. See: http://www.sptimes.com/2005/06/15/schiavoreport.pdf#search=%22Terri%20Schiavo%20autopsy%22

41. Author's note: Colleagues in physical therapy report that "H.O." on such an autopsy probably means heterotopic ossification, formation of bone in muscle and soft tissue. It often occurs in persons with head injury and spinal cord injury and indicates that forceful passive range of motion may be a causative factor especially when there is severe spasticity. Microtrauma related to aggressive passive range of motion is only one of the theories of its etiology. It can lead to joint anklyosis, immobility and consolidation of a joint.

42. "Report of Autopsy," p. 7.

43. "Report of Autopsy," p. 8.

44. President's Commission for the Study of Ethical Problems in Medicine and Biomedical and Behavioral Research, *Defining Death*, Superintendent of Documents, Washington D.C., 1981, p. 14.

45. P. Mollaret and M. Goulon, "Le Coma Depasse," *Revue Neurologie*, vol. 101, no. 3, 1959.

46. Ad Hoc Committee of the Harvard Medical School to Examine the Definition of Brain Death, "A Definition of Irreversible Coma," *Journal of the American Medical Association* 205, no. 337 (1968).

47. The characteristics listed by the philosopher Mary Anne Warren in Chapter 4 (with regard to whether an aborted fetus is a person) might be used in a similar way to define the higher person standard: If all these characteristics are lacking we do not have a person.

48. Robert Morrison, "Death: Process or Event?" *Science* 173 (1971), pp. 694–698.

49. Lance Stell, "Let's Abolish 'Brain-Death," *Community Ethics* (University of Pittsburgh Center for Medical Ethics) 4, no. 1 (Winter 1997).

50. Multi-Society Task Force on PVS, "Medical Aspects of the Persistent Vegetative State," parts 1 and 2, *New England Journal of Medicine* 330, no. 22 (May 26, 1994; June 2, 1994), pp. 1572–1579.

51. I. Dubroja, S. et al., "Outcome of Post-traumatic Unawareness Persisting for More than a Month," *Journal of Neurological Neurosurgery Psychiatry*, 58, no. 4 (1995), pp. 465–66. R. Chen et al, "Prediction of Outcome in Patients with Anoxic Coma: a Clinical and Electrophysiologic Study," *Critical Care Medicine* 24, no. 4, (April 1996), pp. 672–78. Associated Press, "Policeman who Briefly Emerged from Coma-like State in '96 Dies," *Birmingham News*, April 16, 1997, p. 7A.

52. Her CT scan is on the web site of University of Miami Department of Bioethics at: http://www.miami.edu/ethics2/schiavo/CT%20scan.png

53. I. Dubroja, et al., "Outcome of Post-traumatic Unawareness Persisting for More than a Month," *Journal of Neurological Neurosurgery Psychiatry* 58, no. 4 (1995), pp. 465–66.

54. R. Chen et al, "Prediction of Outcome in Patients with Anoxic Coma: a Clinical and Electrophysiologic Study," *Critical Care Medicine* 24, no. 4 (April, 1996), pp. 672–78.

55. Benedict Carey, "Inside the Injured Brain, Many Kinds of Awareness," *New York Times*, April 5, 2005.

56. David Hammer, "Different Cases Cast Light on US Right-to-Die Cases," Associated Press, *Birmingham Post-Herald*, November 10, 2003, C5; Associated Press, "Arkansas Man Wakes After 19 Years in Coma," July 09, 2003; Benedict Carey, "Man Recovering from Brain Injury After 19 Lost Years," *New York Times*, July 4, 2006, reprinted in *Birmingham News*, July 4, 2006, P. A1.

57. AP, "Policeman who Briefly Emerged from Coma-like State in '96 Dies," *Birmingham News*, April 16, 1997, p. A7.

58. Benedict Carey, "Inside the Injured Brain."

59. American Academy of Neurology, amicus curiae brief in *Brophy* v. *New England Sinai Hospital, Inc.*, 1986; quoted in Ronald Cranford, "The Persistent Vegetative State: The Medical Reality (Getting the Facts Straight)," *Hastings Center Report* 18, no. 1 (1988), p. 31.

60. Multi-Society Task Force on Persistent Vegetative State, "Medical Aspects," pp. 1501–1502. The task force did not comment on the apparent contradiction between its claim that brain scans show no activity in PVS patients and the fact that seven

patients made a "good recovery" after over one year in PVS.

61. Carl Zimmer, "What If There's Something Going On in There?" *New York Times Magazine*, September 29, 2003.

62. Carl Zimmer, "What If There's."

63. Rita Rubin, "Doctors Work to Understand Vegetative States," *USA Today*, March 21, 2005, p. A3.

64. Quoted from Bob Herbert, "Cruel and Unusual," *New York Times*, June 25, 2005, p. A21.

65. Cathy Lynn Grossman, "Pope Declares Feeding Tubes a 'Moral Obligation,'" *USA Today*, April 2, 2004, A1.

66. John Paris, quoted by Lisa Greene, "At Pope's Word, New Schiavo Cases?" *St. Petersburg/Tampa Bay Times*, May 1, 2004. http://www.sptimes.com/2004/05/01/ Tampabay/At_pope_s_word__new_S.shtml

67. Charles Babington and Mike Allen, "Congress Passes Schiavo Measure," *Washington Post*, March 2, 2005, p. A1.

68. Manuel Roig-Franzia, "Catholic Stance on Tube-Feeding Is Evolving," *Washington Post*, March 27, 2005, A7.

69. Frank Savage, quoted in the *Birmingham Post-Herald*, March 28, 2005, p. D1.

70. Harriet McBryde Johnson, "Overlooked in the Shadows," *Washington Post*, 25 March 2005.

71. Lisa Belkin, "As Family Protest, Hospital Seeks End to Woman's Life Support," *New York Times*, January 10, 1991, pp. A1–2.

72. Steven Miles, "Interpersonal Issues in the Wanglie Case," *Kennedy Institute of Ethics Journal* 2, no. 1 (March 1992), pp. 61–72.

73. For a review of these cases, see *Law, Medicine, and Health Care*, 20 (1993), pp. 310–315.

74. R. Knox, "Americans' New Way of Dying: Don't Fight It," *Boston Globe*, June 5, 1994.

75. Gilbert Meillander, "On Removing Food and Water: Against the Stream," *Hastings Center Report* 14, no. 6 (December 1984), pp. 11–13.

76. Daniel Callahan, "On Feeding the Dying," *Hastings Center Report* 13, no. 5 (October 1983), p. 22.

77. W. May, R. Barry, O. Greise, et al., "Feeding and Hydrating the Permanently Unconscious and Other Vulnerable Persons," *Issues in Law and Medicine* 3, no. 3 (Winter 1987), pp. 203–217; C. Sprung, "Changing Attitudes and Practices in Forgoing Life-Sustaining Treatments," *Journal of the American Medical Association* 263, no. 16 (April 25, 1990), pp. 2211–2221.

78. American Medical Association, *Opinions of the Judicial Council*, Chicago, IL., 1973.

79. Linda Greenhouse, "Right to Reject Life," *New York Times*, June 27, 1990.

80. SUPPORT Principal Investigators, "A Controlled Trial to Improve Care of Seriously Ill Hospitalized Patients. The Study to Understand Prognoses and Preferences for Outcomes and Risks of Treatment (SUPPORT). *Journal of the American Medical Association* 274 (1995) pp. 1591–1598.

81. R. F. Uhlmann, R. A. Pearlman, and K. C. Cain, "Physicians and Spouses' Predictions of Elderly Patients' Treatment Preferences," *Journal of Gerontology* 43 (1988), pp. 115–21.

82. Rick Weiss, "Patients' Surrogates Often Wrong about Preferred Treatment," *Washington Post*, March 14, 2006, p. A3

Chapter 3

1. Johannes J. M. van Delden et al., "The Remmelink Study: Two Years Later," *Hastings Center Report* 23, no. 6 (November-December 1993), p. 24.

2. http://www.euthanasia.cc/dutch.html# remm

3. http://www.euthanasia.cc/dutch.html# remm

4. Tara Burghart, Associated Press, "1 in 18 Opt Out of Assisted Suicide," August 18, 2005, *Birmingham News*, p. A11.

5. Veronica English et al., "Ethics Briefings," *Journal of Medical Ethics, 32* (2006), pp. 371–372.

6. H. E. Sgreccia, Pontifical Academy for Life, "Legalizing Euthanasia for Children in the Netherlands," www.Vatican.curia/va.roman_ curia/pontifical_academies/documents

7. Toby Sterling, Associated Press, "Netherlands Officials Sketch a Policy for Children's Euthanasia," *Salt Lake Tribune*, September 30, 2005, p. A11.

8. Ann McFeattters, "Children Need More End-of-Life Treatment," *Birmingham Post-Herald*, August 1, 2002.

9. Jack Kevorkian, *Prescription: Medicide—The Goodness of Planned Death*, Prometheus, Buffalo, N. Y., 1991, p. 221. See also *Newsweek*, November 13, 1989.

10. Isabel Wilkerson, "Physician Fulfills a Goal: Aiding a Person in Suicide," *New York Times*, June 7, 1990.

11. Timothy Quill, "Death and Dignity: A Case of Individualized Decision Making," *New England Journal of Medicine* 327 (1992), pp. 1380–84.

12. Timothy Egan, "First Known Legal Suicide Reported in Oregon," *New York Times*, March 26, 1998, p. A1.

13. Susan Tolle, "Care of the Dying: Clinical and Financial Lessons from the Oregon Experience," *Annals of Internal Medicine* 128, no. 7 (April 1, 1998).

14. Susan Tolle, "Care of the Dying."

15. Margaret Battin and Ezentel Emanuel, "What are the Potential Cost-Savings of Legalizing Physician-Assisted Suicide?" *New England Journal of Medicine*, vol. 339, 1998, pp. 167–172.

16. Susan Tolle et al., *The Oregon Death with Dignity Act: A Guidebook for Health Professionals*, (PDF document), p. 7: http://www.ohsu.edu/ethics/toc.pdf #search=%22Susan%20Tolle%20Guidebook %20Oregon%22

17. Oregon's Death with Dignity Act, *Annual Report 2001*, Oregon Health Service, www.ohd.hr. state.or.us/chs/pas/ ar-smmry.htm

18. *Seventh Annual Report on Oregon's Death with Dignity Act,* Office of Disease Prevention and Epidemiology, Department of Human Services, State of Oregon, March 10, 2005, 800 N.E. Oregon Street, Portland, OR 97232.

19. Susan Tolle et al., *A Guidebook* pp. 23–25.

20. Dave Parks, "Study: Ill Oregonians Refuse Food to Die, Rejecting Suicide Law, *Birmingham News*, July 24, 2003, p. A12.

21. Ludwig Edelstein, *Ancient Medicine: Collected Essays of Ludwig Edelstein*, O. Temkin and L. Temkin, eds. Johns Hopkins University Press, Baltimore, Md., 1967.

22. G. E. R. Lloyd, *Hippocratic Writings*, trans. Chadwick and W. N. Mann, Penguin, New York, 1950, p. 13.

23. Leo Alexander, "Medical Science under Dictatorship," *New England Journal of Medicine* 42 (July 14, 1949).

24. Robert Jay Lifton, *The Nazi Doctors*, Basic Books, New York, 1986.

25. J. C. Wilke, *Assisted Suicide and Euthanasia: Past and Present, Hayes Publications*, 1998, p. 9. I am indebted to Stephen W. Poff, M.D., for this reference and for points made in this paragraph.

26. Shana Alexander, at "Birth of Bioethics" conference, University of Washington Medical School, Seattle, October 22, 1992.

27. Timothy Egan, *New York Times*, May 5, 1994, p. A1.

28. "Excerpts from Court's Decision," *New York Times*, June 27, 1997, p. A18.

29. Linda Greenhouse, "Justices Reject U.S. Bid to Block Assisted Suicide," *New York Times*, January 17, 2006, p. A1.

30. Gina Kolata, "'Passive Euthanasia' in Hospitals Is the Norm, Doctors Say," *New York Times*, June 28, 1997, p. A1.

31. Christine Cassell, quoted in Michael Specter, "Suicide Device Fuels Debate," *Washington Post*, June 8, 1990.

32. James Rachels, "Active and Passive Euthanasia," *New England Journal of Medicine* 29 (January 9, 1975), pp. 78–80.

33. Baruch Brody, "Ethical Questions Raised by the Persistent Vegetative Patient," *Hastings Center Report* 18, no. 1, p. 35.

34. Jean Davies, "Raping and Making Love Are Different Concepts: So Are Killing and Voluntary Euthanasia," *Journal of Medical Ethics* 14, (1988), pp. 148–149.

35. Quoted in Barnard White Stack, "Doctors Divided Over the Very Ill, *Pittsburgh Post Gazette*, June 11, 1990.

36. Timothy Quill and Margaret Pabst Battin, "Excellent Palliative Care as the Standard, Physician-Assisted Dying as a Last Resort," in Timothy Quill and Margaret Pabst Battin eds. *Physician-Assisted Dying: The Case for Palliative Care and Patient Choice*, Baltimore, Md.: Johns Hopkins Press, pp. 323–330.

37. Quoted in Alan Parachini, "A Dutch Doctor Carries Out a Death Wish," *Los Angeles Times*, July 5, 1987, sec. 6, p. 9.

38. Timothy Quill and Margaret Pabst Battin, "Excellent Palliative Care," p. 323.

39. Joan Teno and Joanne Lynn, "Voluntary Active Euthanasia: The Individual Case and Public Policy," *Journal of the American Geriatrics Society* 39 (1991), pp. 827–830.

40. Timothy Quill and Margaret Pabst Battin, "Excellent Palliative Care," p. 325.

41. Quoted in Barnard White Stack, "Doctors Divided Over the Very Ill, *Pittsburgh Post Gazette*, June 11, 1990.

42. Margaret Battin, "The Least Worst Death," *Hastings Center Report* 13. no. 2 (April 1983), pp. 13–16

43. Douglas Walton, *Slippery Slope Arguments*, New York: Oxford University Press, 1992.

44. Leo Alexander, "Medical Science Under Dictatorship," p. 47.

45. Leo Alexander, "Medical Science Under Dictatorship," p. 44.

46. Charlie LeDuff, "Prosecutors Say Ex-Doctor Killed Because It Thrilled Him," *New York Times*, September 7, 2000, p. A29.

47. Yale Kamisar, quoted in Earl Ubell, "Should Death Be a Patient's Choice?" *Parade Magazine*, February 9, 1992, p. 27.

48. Michael Specter, "Suicide Device Fuels Debate," *Washington Post*, June 8, 1990.

49. Quoted in Peter Steinfels, "Dutch Study Is Euthanasia Vote Issue," *New York Times*, September 20, 1991.

50. Nat Hentoff, "The Deadly Slippery Slope," *Village Voice*, September 1, 1987.

51. Nat Hentoff, "Decision on Euthanasia Will Create a Slippery Slope," *Washington Post,* October 6, 1992.

52. Timothy Egan, "Assisted Suicide Comes . . . ."

53. Nat Hentoff, "The Coat Hanger of Assisted Suicide," *Washington Post*, December 12, 1997.

54. Norman Paradis, "Making a Living Off the Dying," *New York Times*, April 25, 1992, p. 15.

55. Sherwin Nuland, *How We Die: Reflections on Life's Final Chapter*, Vintage, New York, 1995.

56. Christiaan Barnard, *One Life*, Macmillan, New York, 1965.

Chapter 4

1. Maggie Scarf, "The Fetus as Guinea Pig," *New York Times Magazine*, October 19, 1975, pp. 194–200.

2. Maggie Scarf, "The Fetus as Guinea Pig."

3. A. Philipson et al, 'Transplacental Passage of Erythomycin and Clindamycin," *New England Journal of Medicine* 288, no. 23 (June 7, 1973), pp. 1219–1221.

4. Paul Ramsey, *The Ethics of Fetal Research*, Yale University Press, New Haven, Conn., 1975.

5. William Nolen, *The Baby in the Bottle,* Coward, McCann, and Geoghegan, New York, 1978, p. 203.

6. William Nolen, *The Baby in the Bottle.*

7. "The Edelin Trial," transcript of a WBGH recreation of Edelin's trial for a television documentary by Bill Moyers. Project of Legal-Medical Studies, Inc., Box 8219, John F. Kennedy Station, Government Station, Boston, MA 12134.

8. William Buckley, *National Review*, March 14, 1975; quoted from Nolen, *Baby in the Bottle*, p. 221.

9. *Commonwealth* v. *Kenneth Edelin*, Mass. Supreme Court 359, N.E. 2d, 1976.

10. Kenneth Edelin, quoted in *Ob. Gyn. News*, January 1, 1977, p. 1.

11. Quoted from Paul Ramsey, *Ethics at the Edges of Life*, Yale University Press, New Haven, CT, 1978, p. 94.

12. William Nolen, *The Baby in the Bottle*, p. 174.

13. William Nolen, *The Baby in the Bottle*, p. 175.

14. Paul Badham, "Christian Beliefs and the Ethics of In Vitro Fertilization," *Bioethics News* 6, no. 2, (January 1987), p. 10.

15. Michael Luo, "On Abortion, It's the Bible of Ambiguity," *New York Times*, November 13, 2005, Ideas and Trends Section, p. 1, 3.

16. Paul Johnson, *A History of Christianity*, Atheneum, New York, 1983, Ch. 3.

17. John Connery, "Abortion: Roman Catholic Perspectives," *Encyclopedia of Bioethics* 1, MacMillan, New York, 1978.

18. Robert W. Mulligan, S. J., Jesuit Community at St. Louis University, personal letter to author.

19. Over the last 30 years, the Church has moved closer to immediate animation, especially with its emphasis on the value of the human embryo.

20. *Roe v. Wade*, Supreme Court Reporter 93, 410 US 151, pp. 709–762.

21. Barbara Ehrenreich and Deirdre English, *For Her Own Good: 150 Years' of Experts' Advice to Women*, Doubleday, New York, 1987, pp. 319–320.

22. Allan F. Guttmacher Institute, Abortion and Women's Health, New York and Washington, D. C., 1990, p. 27.

23. *A Private Affair*, a 1992 movie about this case, starred actress Sissy Spacek as Sherry Finkbine.

24. Peter Steinfels, "Papal Birth-Control Letter Retains Its Grip," *New York Times*, July 29, 1993, p. A1, 13.

25. Norma McCorvey, *I am Roe—My Life: Roe v Wade and Freedom of Choice*, Harper Collins, New York, 1993.

26. Fact Sheet: Abortion Surveillance, June 7, 2002, Centers for Disease Control, Atlanta, Ga. For updates, see: www.cdc.gov/mmwr/preview/mmwrhtml /ss5407a1.htm

27. Mary Anne Warren, "On the Moral and Legal Status of the Fetus," *Monist* 57, 1973, pp. 43–61.

28. Don Marquis and Warren Quinn, "Why Abortion Is Immoral," *Journal of Philosophy* 86 (1989), pp. 183–202.

29. John T. Noonan, Jr. "An Almost Absolute Value in History," in John T. Noonan, Jr. ed.,

The Morality of Abortion: Legal and Historical Perspectives, Harvard University Press, Cambridge, MA, 1970, pp. 51–59.

30. Judith Jarvis Thomson, "A Defense of Abortion," *Philosophy & Public Affairs* 1, vol. 1 (Fall 1971), pp. 47–66.

31. Francis Kamm, *Creation and Abortion*, Oxford University Press, New York, 1992.

32. John Connery, "Abortion: Roman Catholic Perspectives," pp. 9–13.

33. Ellen Willis, "Harper's Forum on Abortion," *Harper's Magazine* (July 1986), p. 38.

34. "Explosions Over Abortion," *Time,* January 14, 1985, p. 17.

35. Jeff Lyon, "Doctor's Dilemma: When Abortion Gives Birth to Life, Physicians Become Troubled Saviors," *Chicago Tribune,* August 15, 1982, Sec. 12, pp. 1, 3. (A 2.5 pound baby may be viable; jockey Willie Shoemaker, born prematurely, weighed this much and was kept warm in a shoebox in an oven.)

36. Linda Villanova, "Newest Skill for Future OB/GYN's Abortion Training," *New York Times,* June 11, 2002.

37. Susan Lee et al, "Fetal Pain: A Systematic Review of the Literature," *Journal of the American Medical Association,* 294 (2005), pp. 947–954.

38. Consultants to the Advisory Committee to the Director, National Institutes of Health, *Report of the Human Fetal Tissue Transplantation Research Panel,* 1, National Institutes of Health, Bethesda, Md., 1988.

39. For costs and various kinds of pills, Google "Planned Parenthood" and "Emergency Contraception."

40. Gina Kolata, "Without Fanfare, Morning-After Pill Gets a Closer Look," *New York Times* October 8, 2000, A1.

41. "Mother versus Child," Kenneth Jost, *American Bar Association Journal* (April 198), p. 86.

42. E. Abel and Robert Sokol, "Fetal Alcohol Syndrome Is Now the Leading Cause of Mental Retardation" (letter), *Lancet* 8517, pp. 898–899.

43. Associated Press, "Mother Gets 6 Years for Drugs in Breast Milk," *New York Times* October 28, 1992. p. A11.

44. *Planned Parenthood* v. *Casey,* excerpts quoted from *New York Times,* June 30, 1992, p. A8.

45. Harold Morowitz, "Roe v. Wade Passes a Lab Test," *New York Times,* November 25, 1992, p. A13.

46. "Restrictions on Young Women's Access to Reproductive Services," Center for Reproductive Rights, June 2006, Item F010. www.crlp.org/tools

47. Hadley Arkes, "Courts Strike Down Laws Against Partial-Birth Abortion," *Wall Street Journal,* December 17, 1998, p. A31.

Chapter 5

1. Joseph L. Goldstein, "Comments at the (Lasker) Awards Ceremony (for Robert Edwards)," 2001, Lasker Foundation website.www.laskerfoundation.org/award/library, 2001.

2. *Time,* August 7, 1978, p. 68.

3. *Newsweek,* August 7, 1978, p. 66.

4. *Newsweek,* August 7, 1978, p. 66.

5. Richard Blandau, quoted in *Time,* November 13, 1978, p. 89.

6. *Time,* November 13, 1978, p. 89.

7. Audrey Smith, quoted in Steptoe and Edwards, *A Matter of Life: The Story of a Medical Breakthrough,* Morrow, London, 1980, p. 48.

8. Figures lag because it takes nine months from conception to produce a baby, because some conceptions take place in late December, and because the CDC audits the self-reports of ART clinics to verify numbers, so figures for, say, 1999, don't come out until 2001.

9. *BioNews* 88 (November 12, 2000), pp. 1–2.

10. Sheryl Gay Stolberg, "For the Infertile, a High-Tech Treadmill of Despair," *New York Times,* December 14, 1997.

11. Centers for Disease Control, *Assisted Reproductive Technology Success Rates in the United States: 1996 National Summary and Fertility Clinic Reports.* (CDC Web site)

12. Sheryl Gay Stolberg, "Quandary on Donor Eggs: What to Tell the Children," *New York Times,* January 18, 1998.

13. Gina Kolata, "New Pregnancy Hope: A Single Sperm Injected," *New York Times,* August 11, 1993, p. B7.

14. Gina Kolata, "Successful Births Reported with Frozen Human Eggs," *New York Times,* October 17, 1997, p. A1.

15. David Colker, ""It's a Boy—Embryo is Viable after 1990 Freezing," *Los Angeles Times,* February 17, 1998.

16. Kirsty Horsey, "Twins Born 16 Years Apart," *Daily Mail* (England), May 30, 2006, p. A1.

17. Richard Jerome, "In the Band," *People,* July 1, 2002, pp. 48–50.

18. Seale Harris, *A Women's Surgeon: The Life Story of J. Marion Sims*, Macmillan, New York, 1950, p. 245.

19. Elaine Tyler, *Barren in the Promised Land: Childless Americans and the Pursuit of Happiness*, Harvard University Press, Cambridge, Mass., 1995, pp. 65–69.

20. "Text of Vatican's Statement on Human Reproduction," *New York Times*, March 11, 1987, pp. 10ff.

21. Bishop Kelly, quoted in G. Vecsey, "Religious Leaders Differ on Implant," *New York Times*, July 27, 1978, p. A16.

22. Joseph Fletcher, *Ethics of Genetic Control: Enduring Reproductive Roulette*, Doubleday Anchor, New York; reprinted by Prometheus, Buffalo, NY, 1984, p. 36.

23. Joseph Fletcher, "Ethical Aspects of Genetic Controls," *New England Journal of Medicine* 285, no. 14, (1971), pp. 776–781.

24. Paul Ramsey, *Fabricated Man*, Yale University Press, New Haven, CT, 1970.

25. Patrick Steptoe and Robert Edwards, *A Matter of Life*, p. 113.

26. Paul Ramsey, *The Ethics of Fetal Experimentation*, Yale University Press, New Haven, CT, 1975.

27. John Marlow, quoted in *U.S. News and World Report*, August 7, 1978, p. 24.

28. John Marshall, quoted in *Time*, July 31, 1978, p. 59.

29. Leon Kass, "The New Biology: What Price Relieving Man's Estate?" *Journal of the American Medical Association* 174 (November 19, 1971), pp. 779–788.

30. James Watson, "Moving towards the Clonal Man," *Atlantic*, May 1971, p. 53.

31. Max Perutz, quoted in Steptoe and Edwards, *A Matter of Life*, p. 117.

32. Jeremy Rifkin and Ted Howard, *Who Shall Play God?* Dell, New York, 1977. p. 115.

33. Daniel Callahan, *New York Times*, July 27, 1978, p. A16.

34. Hans Tiefel, "In Vitro Fertilization: A Conservative View," *Journal of the American Medical Association* 247, no. 23 (June 18, 1982), pp. 3235–3242.

35. Jeff Minerd, "ESHRE: Birth Defect Risk Preferable to Childlessness in IVF Survey," *MedPage Today*, June 23, 2005.

36. Sheryl Gay Stolberg, "Quandary on Donor Eggs: What to Tell the Children," *New York Times*, January 18, 1998.

37. Cynthia Cohen, "Parents Anonymous," Cynthia Cohen, (ed) *Egg Donation*, Baltimore, Md.: Johns Hopkins University Press, 1997.

38. Susan Schindelhette, "My Life as a Sperm Donor," *People*, June 5, 2006, pp. 135–37.

39. Stephanie Coontz, *The Way We Never Were*, Basic Books, New York, 1992, pp. 11–12.

40. Joanna Levy, "Conservatives Clash with Psychologists," Scripps-Howard News Service, *Birmingham Post-Herald*, August 23, 1999, p. C4.

41. Gina Kolata, "With Help of Science, Infertile Couples Can Even Pick Traits," *New York Times*, November 23, 1997, p. A1.

42. Frederic Golden, "Good Eggs, Bad Eggs," *TIME*, January 11, 1999, p. 58.

43. Mary Rutz, "Selling Eggs: Cost and Consent in the Bull Market," *Bulletin of the University of Illinois at Chicago Department of Medical Education* 5, no. 2, January, 1999, p. 3.

44. "Grandmother," *People*, June 28, 2006.

45. Henry Chu, "China: Too Many Men, Too Few Women," *The Birmingham News*, February 23, 2001.

46. Reproductive Health and Early Life Changes," http://www.unfpa.org/modules/intercenter/cycle/earlylife.htm

47. Richard Jerome, "Mortal Choices," *People*, October 7, 1996, 96–102.

48. "McCaughey Septuplets Turn Four," *Dateline NBC*, November 20, 2001, reproduced at: www.msnbc.com/news/660542.asp

49. American Society for Reproductive Medicine *Guidelines on Number of Embryos Transferred: A Practice Committee Report: A Committee Opinion*, Birmingham, Ala., January 1998.

50. Gladys White and Steven Leuthner, "Infertility Treatment and Neonatal Care: The Ethical Obligation to Transcend Specialty Practice in the Interest of Reducing Multiple Births," *Journal of Clinical Ethics* 12, no. 3 (Fall 2001), pp. 223–230.

51. M. Hansen et al., "The Risk of Major Birth Defects after Intracytoplasmic Sperm Injection and in Vitro Fertilization," *New England Journal of Medicine* 346 (March 7, 2002), pp. 725–730.

52. M. Hansen et al., "The Risk."

53. Jacqueline Stenson, "Do IVF Kids Face More Health Risks?" MSNBC, July 21, 2003.

54. Amy Docker Marcus, "Does IVF Cause Birth Defects?" *Wall Street Journal*, September 16, 2003, D1, D9.

55. Amy Docker Marcus, "A Registry for Test-Tube Babies," *Wall Street Journal*, September 16, 2003, D1, D9.

56. Rick Weiss, "Bioethics Panel Calls for Ban on Radical Reproductive Procedures," *Washington Post,* January 16, 2004.

57. Laura Mansnerus, "The Baby Bazaar: How Bundles of Joy Not for Sale Are Sold," *New York Times,* 26 October 1998.

58. Laura Mansnerud, "The Baby Bazaar."

59. The American Surrogacy Center, "Legal Overview of Surrogacy Laws by State," 2002. www.surrogacy.com

60. Mark Sauer, "Ooycte Donation: Reflections on Past Work and Future Directions," *Human Reproduction* 11, no. 6 (1996), p. 1150.

61. Yvon Englert, "Ethics of Oocyte Donation Is Challenged by the Nature of the Health System." Commentary on Mark Sauer, above, in *Human Reproduction.*

62. Gina Kolata, "Soaring Price of Donor Eggs Sets Off Debate," *New York Times,* February 25, 1998, p. A1; Adrienne Knox, "Brokers and Fertility Clinics in Bidding War for Women Willing to Sell Eggs from Ovaries," *Birmingham News,* March 15, 1998, p. A3.

63. Lisa Gerson, "Human Harvest," *Boston Magazine,* May 1999, p. 106.

64. New York State Task Force on Life and Law, *Report on Assisted Reproductive Technologies,* Albany, NY: 1998.

65. Helen Ragone, *Conception from the Heart,* Indiana University Press, Bloomington, IN, 1994.

Chapter 6

1. Maggie Scarf, "The Fetus as Guinea Pig," *New York Times Magazine,* October 19, 1975, pp. 194–200; Paul Ramsey's *The Ethics of Fetal Research,* Yale University Press, New Haven, CT, 1975.

2. Associated Press, "Ex-Husband Has Embryos Destroyed," June 16, 1993.

3. Ronald M. Green, *The Human Embryo Research Debates,* Oxford University Press, New York, 2001, p. 4.

4. Nicholas Wade, "Stem Cells May Be Key to Cancer," *New York Times,* February 21, 2006, p. D1.

5. Arnold Kriegstein, Director, University of California Institute of Regenerative Medicine, quoted in "What A Bush Veto Would Mean for Stem Cells," Nancy Gibbs and Alice Park, *Time,* July 24, 2006, p. 36.

6. Douglas Melton, quoted in "What a Bush Veto Would Mean for Stem Cells," Nancy Gibbs and Alice Park, *Time,* July 24, 2006, p. 36.

7. Justin Gillis and Rick Weiss, "NIH: Few Stem Cell Colonies Likely Available for Research," *Washington Post,* March 3, 2004, p. A3.

8. "State Cloning Laws," The National Conference of State Legislators, April 18, 2006. http://ncls.org/programs/health/Genetics/rt-shcl.htm

9. Tom Delay, quoted on CNN News, June 5, 2005.

10. Alta Charo, "Passing on the Right: Conservative Bioethics Is Closer than It Appears," *Journal of Law, Medicine & Ethics* 32, (2004), pp. 307–314.

11. Elizabeth Blackburn, "A Full Range of Bioethical Views Just Got Narrower," *Washington Post,* March 7, 2004.

12. Rick Weiss, "British to Clone Human Embryos for Stem Cells," *Washington Post,* February 9, 2005, p. A2.

13. Chee Yoke Heong, "Malaysia New Dream: Biovalley," *Asia Times,* 2003.

14. "China, a Cloning Paradise," *Asia Times,* February 24, 2005.

15. Rick Weiss, "Mature Human Embryos Cloned," *Washington Post,* 12 February 2004, p. A28.

16. Gina Kolata, "Koreans Report Ease in Cloning for Stem Cells," *New York Times,* May 20, 2005, p. A1.

17. David Stout, "In First Veto, Bush Blocks Stem Cell Bill," *New York Times,* July 19, 2006, p. A1.

18. Richard McCormick, "Who or What is a Preembryo?" *Kennedy Journal of Ethics* 1, no. 1 (March 1991), p. 5.

19. Richard McCormick, "Who or What is a Preembryo?" It is also true that some Catholic theologians hold out for personhood as beginning some short time after conception. For our purposes here, and since their view has been de-emphasized of late, that view will not be discussed.

20. Richard McCormick, "Who or What is a Preembryo?" p. 12.

21. Bonnie Steinbock, "Moral Status, Moral Value and Human Embryos: Implications for Stem Cell Research," ed. Bonnie Steinbock, *Oxford Handbook of Bioethics* Oxford University Press, New York, 2007.

22. Josephine Johnston, "The Women Behind Cloning," *Washington Post,* March 8, 2004, p. A19.

23. Judy Norsigian, "Risks to Women in Embryo Cloning," *Boston Globe*, February 25, 2005.

24. Daniel Brison and Brian Lieberman, "An Ethical Way to Provide More Embryos for Research," *BioNews* 235, No. 24 (24 November 2003), archived at: www.bionews.org.uk/commnetary.lasso?storyid=1899

25. "Therapeutic Cloning Assailed as Creation for Sake of Destruction," ZENIT News Service, October 10, 2003.

26. John Haas, "Testimony before the U. S. Senate" Subcommittee on Health and Public Safety, 17 June 1997; reprinted in *The Human Cloning Debate* (ed.) G. McGee, Berkeley Hills Books, Berkeley, Ca., 2000, p. 283.

27. Leon Kass, "How One Clone Leads to Another," *New York Times*, 24 January 2003, p. A25.

28. Kirk Semple, "U. N. to Consider Whether to Ban Some, or All, Forms of Cloning of Human Embryos," *New York Times*, November 3, 2003.

29. Michael E. Ross, "Law War: Attack of the Clone Debate," MSNBC website, February 5, 2003. Archived at: www.msnbc.com/news/854226.asp?cpl=1

30. Brian Leiberman, "Use of In-Vitro Fertilisation Embryos Cryopreserved for 5 Years or More," *Lancet* 15, no. 4, October 4, 2000.

31. http://www.snowflakes.org/

32. "Committee Decides 'Therapeutic Cloning' Can Go Ahead," *BioNews* 147, 3 May 2002, p. 2.

33. Michael Gazzaniga, *The Ethical Brain*, Dana Press, New York, 2005.

34. M. V. Viola, quoted in Howard Brody, *Ethical Decisions in Medicine*, Little Brown: Boston, MA, 1976, p. 147.

35. David Ozar, "The Case for Not Unthawing Frozen Embryos," *Hastings Center Report* 15, no. 4 (August 1985), pp. 7–12.

36. Gene Outka, "The Ethics of Human Stem Cell Research," *Kennedy Institute Journal of Ethics*, 12 (2002), pp. 175–213

37. Peter Singer and Deanne Wells, *The Reproductive Revolution: New Ways of Making Babies*, Oxford University Press, New York, 1984, Ch. 3.

38. Ronald M. Green, *The Human Embryo Research Debates*, Oxford University Press, 2001, New York, NY.

39. Ronald M. Green, *The Human Embryo Research Debates*, pp. 26–28.

40. Ronald M. Green, *The Human Embryo Research Debates.*

41. Rick Weiss, "Proponents Press Senate on Stem Cell Research Measure," *Washington Post*, June 30, 2006, p. A3.

Chapter 7

1. Gina Kolata, "Iconoclastic Genius of Cloning," *New York Times*, 3 June 1997, pp. B7, B12.

2. Michael Specter with Gina Kolata, "After Decades and Many Mistakes, Cloning Success," *New York Times*, March 3, 1997.

3. "The Science and Application of Cloning," National Bioethics Advisory Commission, *Cloning Human Beings: Report and Recommendations of the National Bioethics Advisory Commission*, Rockville, Md., June 1997, p. 20.

4. I. Wilmut et al, "Viable Offspring Derived from Fetal and Adult Mammalian Cells," *Nature* 385 (February 27, 1997), pp. 810–813.

5. "State Human Cloning Laws," April 18, 2006, The National Conference of State Legislatures. http://www.ncls.org/rorams/health/Genetics/rt-shel.htm.

6. Lee Silver, *Re-Making Eden: Cloning and Beyond in a Brave New World*, Avon, New York, 1997.

7. John Rawls, *A Theory of Justice*, Harvard University Press, Cambridge, Mass., 1971, p. 108.

8. Leon Kass, "Cloned Embryos," *First Things*, June, 2002.

9. Francis Fukuyama, *Our Posthuman Future*, Farrar Straus & Giroux, New York, 2002.

Chapter 9

1. Laurie, Tarkan, "Too Many Interventions, and Too Many Premies," *New York Times*, August 6, 2002.

2. National Center for Health Statistics, November 15, 2005, March of Dimes Press Release, same day.

3. N. Marlow, "Neurologic and Developmental Disability at Six Years of Age After Extremely Preterm Birth," *The New England Journal of Medicine* 352, no. 1 (January 6, 2005).

4. John Boswell, *The Kindness of Strangers: The Abandonment of Children in Western Europe from Late Antiquity to the Renaissance,*

Pantheon, New York, 1989; Robert Weir, *Selected Nontreatment of Handicapped Newborns*, Oxford University Press, New York, 1984.

5. William Lecky, *A History of European Morals from Augustus to Charlemagne*, II, Brazilor, New York, 1955, pp. 25–56 (originally published 1869).

6. N. Marlow, "Neurologic and Developmental Disability at Six Years of Age After Extremely Preterm Birth."

7. A famous movie in medical ethics follows a case that is a collage of these three cases: *Who Should Survive?* Produced by the Joseph P. Kennedy Foundation, Film Service, 999 Asylum Avenue, Hartford, CT 10605.

8. James Gustafson, "Mongolism, Parental Desires, and the Right to Life," *Perspectives on Biology and Medicine* 16 (Summer 1973), p. 529.

9. R. Duff and A. Campbell, "Moral and Ethical Dilemmas in the Special-Care Nursery," *The New England Journal of Medicine* 289, no. 17 (October 25, 1973), pp. 890–894.

10. John Lorber, "Results of Treatment of Myelomeningocele: An Analysis of 524 Unselected Cases, with Special Reference to Possible Selection for Treatment," *Developmental Medicine and Child Neurology* 13, no. 2 (1971), pp. 279–303.

11. Mary Tedeschi, "Infanticide and Its Apologists," *Commentary*, November, 1984, p. 34.

12. Shari Staaver, "Siamese Twins' Case Devastates MDs," *American Medical News*, October 9, 1981, pp. 15–16.

13. Bonnie Steinbock, "Whatever Happened to the Danville Siamese Twins? *Hastings Center Report* 17, no. 4 (August–September, 1987), pp. 3–4. See also John Robertson, "Dilemma in Danville," *Hastings Center Report* 11, no. 5 (October 1981), p. 7.

14. U. S. Commission on Civil Rights, *Medical Discrimination Against Children with Disabilities*, Washington, D.C., September 1989, p. 391.

15. U. S. Commission on Civil Rights, *Medical Discrimination*, p. 36, 323.

16. C. Everett Koop, "The Seriously Ill or Dying Child: Supporting the Patient and the Family," in D. Horan and D. Mall, eds., *Death, Dying and Euthanasia*, University Publications of America, Frederick, Md., 1977, pp. 537–539.

17. Adrian Peracchio, "Government in the Nursery: New Era for Baby Doe Cases," *Newsday*, November 13, 1983. Reprint, "The Baby Jane Doe Story: Winner of the 1984 Pulitzer Prize for Local Reporting," *Newsday*, 1983.

18. Kathleen Kerr, "An Issue of Law and Ethics," *Newsday*, October 26, 1983; B. D. Colen, "A Life of Love—and Endless Pain," *Newsday*, October 26, 1983. (Available from *Newsday* in the reprint "The Baby Jane Doe Story: Winner of the 1984 Pulitzer Prize for Local Reporting'); "Baby Jane Doe," *Wall Street Journal*, November 21, 1983.

19. Kathleen Kerr, "Legal, Medical Legacy of Case," *Newsday*, December 7, 1987.

20. Kathleen Kerr, "Legal, Medical Legacy of Case," *Newsday*, December 7, 1987.

21. Bonnie Steinbock, "Baby Jane Doe in the Courts," *Hastings Center Report* 14, no. 1 (February 1984), p. 15; *Hastings Center Report* 14, no. 4 (August 1984).

22. Kathleen Kerr, "Legal, Medical Legacy of Case"; see also Kathleen Kerr, "Reporting the Case of Baby Jane Doe."

23. "Baby Jane Doe Has Surgery to Remove Water from Brain," *New York Times*, April 7, 1984, p. 28.

24. "Baby Jane Doe Has Surgery," *New York Times*.

25. Kathleen Kerr, "Legal, Medical Legacy of Case."

26. Steven Baer, "The Half-Told Story of Baby Jane Doe," *Columbia Journalism Review*, November–December 1984, pp. 35–38; Mary Tedeschi, "Infanticide and Its Apologists," *Commentary*, November, 1984, p. 34.

27. *Hastings Center Report* 24, no. 3 (May–June 1984), p. 2.

28. Rhoda Amon, "A Long-Running Morality Play," www.lihistory.com/9/hs9oral.htm

29. James Gustafson, "Mongolism, Parental Desires."

30. C. Everett Koop, "The Slide to Auschwitz," *Whatever Happened to the Human Race?* Revell, Old Tappan, N.J., 1979.

31. *Who Should Survive?*

32. Fred Bruning, "The Politics of Life," *MacLean's*, December 12, 1983, p. 17.

33. James Rachels, "Active and Passive Euthanasia," *New England Journal of Medicine*, 292, Jan. 9, 1975, pp. 78–80.

34. Koop, "The Slide to Auschwitz."

35. R. McCormick, "To Save or Let Die: The Dilemma of Modern Medicine," *Journal of the American Medical Association* 229, no. 8, July 1974, pp. 172–176.

36. Peter Singer, *Practical Ethics*, Cambridge University Press, New York, 1979, p. 137; Tristam Engelhardt, "Ethical Issues in Aiding the Death of Young Children," in Marvin Kohl, ed., *Beneficent Euthanasia*, Prometheus, Buffalo, N.Y., 1975; Michael Tooley, "Abortion and Infanticide," *Philosophy and Public Affairs* 2, no. 1, Fall 1972, pp. 37–65.

37. Kerr, "Legal, Medical Legacy of Case."

38. Robert Weir, *Selected Nontreatment of Handicapped Newborns*, Oxford University Press, New York, 1984.

39. R. B. Zachary, "Life with Spina Bifida," *British Medical Journal* 2 (1977), p. 1461.

40. David Gibson, "Dimensions of Intelligence," in *Down Syndrome: The Psychology of Mongolism*, Cambridge University Press, New York, 1978, pp. 35–77; Janet Carr, "The Development of Intelligence," in David Lane and Brian Stafford, eds., *Current Approaches to Down Syndrome*, Praeger, New York, 1985, pp. 167–186.

41. Janet Carr, "The Development of Intelligence," in David Lane and Brian Stafford, eds, *Current Approaches to Down Syndrome*, Praeger, New York, 1985, pp. 167–186.

42. Tom Regan, *The Case for Animal Rights*, University of California Press, Berkeley, CA, 1985.

43. *Gleitman* v. *Cosgrove*, 227 A.2d 689, 692, 693 (New Jersey, 1967)

44. Mathew Rarey, "Wrongful-Birth Lawsuits Put Doctors in Ethical Dilemma," *Washington Times*, August 5, 1999, p. A20.

45. "High Court Rules 'Wrongful Birth' Suits Invalid," *Atlanta Journal-Constitution*, July 7, 1999, p. E1.

46. Suzanne Daley, "France Bans Damages for 'Wrongful Births'," *New York Times*, Jan. 2002, p. A8.

47. Loretta Kopelman, "Do the 'Baby Doe' Rules Ignore Suffering?" *Second Opinion* 18, no. 4 (April 1983), pp. 101–113.

48. John Robertson, "Extreme Prematurity and Parental Rights After Baby Doe," *Hastings Center Report* (July/August 2004), p. 33.

49. Brenda Coleman, "Moral Floodgates Opened by Father Pulling Plug on Son," Associated Press, May 1, 1989; 49. Gregg Levoy, "Birth Controllers," *Omni*, August 1987, p. 31.

50. *In the Matter of Baby K*, United States District Court, E. D. Virginia, July 7, 1993, no. Civ. A. 93-104-A; see also "The Case of Baby K," *Trends in Health Care, Law, and Ethics* 9, no. 1 (Winter 1994), pp. 1–48.

51. Gina Kolata, "Parents of Tiny Infants Find Care Choices Are Not Theirs," *New York Times*, September 30, 1991, p. A1.

52. Laurie Tarkan, "Too Many Interventions, and Too Many Preemies," *New York Times*, April 6, 2002.

53. John Robertson, "Extreme Prematurity and Parental Rights After Baby Doe," *Hastings Center Report* (July/August 2004), p. 34.

54. A. Gallo, "Spina Bifida: The State of the Art of Medical Management," *Hastings Center Report* 14, no. 1 (February 1984), pp. 10–13.

55. Bill Bartholomene, personal communication, who also read an earlier version of this chapter and who was a resident at the time and narrated the movie, *Who Should Survive?*; also, John Freeman, "On Learning Humility: A Thirty-Year Journey," *Hastings Center Report* (May-June, 204), pp. 13–16.

56. A. Gallo, "Spina Bifida: The State of the Art of Medical Management," *Hastings Center Report* 14, no. 1 (February 1984), pp. 10–13.

57. Spina Bifida Association, *Brief Amicus Curiae of the Spina Bifida Association of America*, *Weber* v. *Stony Brook Hospital*, New York State Supreme Court, Appellate Division, 2d Department, *New York Law Journal*, October 28, 1983; quoted in Steinbock, "Baby Jane Doe in the Courts," p. 19.

58. Bob Meadows, Lorna Grisby, "Precious Child, Impossible Choice, *People*, May 15, 2006, p. 123.

59. Anita Silvers, "Rights Are Still Rights: The Case for Disability Rights," *Hastings Center Report* (November/December 2004), pp. 39–40.

Chapter 10

1. Quoted from the tape by W. Robbins, "Animal Rights: A Growing Movement in the U.S.," *New York Times*, June 15, 1984, p. A16.

2. "The Use of Animals in Research," *New England Journal of Medicine* 313, no. 6, pp. 395–400.

3. *Evaluation of Experimental Procedures Conducted at the University of Pennsylvania Experimental Head-Injury Laboratory 1981–1984 in Light of the Public Health Science Animal Welfare Policy*, Office for Protection of Research Risks, National Institutes of Health, 1985, p. 37.

4. Quoted in "Animals in the Middle," in the television series *Innovation*, sponsored by

Johnson and Johnson on A and E Network, September 5, 1987.

5. W. Robbins, "Animal Rights: A Growing Movement in the U. S," *New York Times*, June 15, 1984, p. A16.

6. Robert Marshak, quoted in *New York Times*, July 29, 1984, p. A12.

7. Donald Abt, quoted in *New York Times*, August 12, 1984, p. B1.

8. *New York Times*, December 10, 1984, p. A10.

9. *New York Times*, December 10, 1984, p. A10.

10. "Of Pain and Progress," *Newsweek*, December 26, 1988, p. 53.

11. Edward Taub, "The Silver Spring Monkey Incident: The Untold Story," *Coalition for Animals and Animal Research Newsletter* 4, no. 1 (Winter–Spring 1991), pp. 1–8.

12. Tony Dajer, "Monkeying with the Brain," *Discover*, January 1992, p. 70–71. See also Warren E. Leary, "Sharp Brain Healing Found in Disputed Monkey Tests," *New York Times*, June 28, 1991, p. A9.

13. Joachim Liepert, Heike Bauder, Wolfgang H. R. Miltner, Edward Taub, and Cornelius Weiller, "Treatment-Induced Cortical Reorganization After Stroke in Humans," *Stroke: The Journal of the American Heart Association* 31 (June 2000), pp. 1210–1216.

14. Edward Taub, *Topics in Stroke Rehabilitation* 3, pp. 38–61.

15. Sandra Blakeslee, "Pushing Injured Brains and Spinal Cords to New Paths," *New York Times*, August 28, 2001, p. D6.

16. "Stroke Rehab Therapy Shows Benefits in 2-year Follow-up," *UAB Reporter*, April 12, 2006.

17. "Taub Wins American Psychological Association Scientific Award," *UAB Synopsis*, February 16, 2004.

18. Edward Taub, Gitendra Uswatte, Danna Kay King, David Morris, Jean E. Crago, and Anjan Chatterjee, "A Placebo-Controlled Trial of Constraint-Induced Movement Therapy for Upper Extremity After Stroke," *Stroke: The Journal of the American Heart Association* 37, (April 2006), pp. 1045–1049.

19. John Durant, quoted in John Hargrove, "Bush Signs Heflin Bill to Protect Researchers," *Birmingham Post-Herald*, August 28, 1992.

20. Madhusree Mukerjee, "Trends in Animal Research," *Scientific American*, February, 1997, p. 89. See also M. S. Russell and Rex L. Burch, *The Principles of Humane Experimental Technique*, London, Methuen, 1959; F. Barbara Orlans and Tom Beauchamp, eds.

The Human Use of Animals: Case Studies in Ethical Choice, New York, Oxford University Press, 1998.

21. Office of Technology Assessment, *Animal Usage in the United States*, Superintendent of Documents, Washington, D.C., 1986, p. 12; *Newsweek*, December 26, 1988, p. 51; Andrew Rowan, *Of Mice, Models, and Men: A Critical Evaluation of Animal Research*, State University of New York Press, Albany, 1984, pp. 67–70;

22. Bernard Rollins, *Animal Rights and Human Morality*, Prometheus, Buffalo, N.Y., 1981, pp. 97–99.

23. Nicholas Fontaine, M*emoires pour servir Ö l'histoire de Port-Royal*, vol. 2, originally published in Cologne in 1738; quoted in L. Rosenfield, *From Best-Machine to Man-Machine: The Theme of Animal Soul in French Letters from Descartes to La Mettrie*, Oxford University Press, New York, 1940, pp. 52–53; also quoted in Peter Singer, *Animal Liberation*, New York Review Books, 1975.

24. C. S. Lewis, *How Human Suffering Raises Almost Intolerable Intellectual Problems*, Macmillan, New York, 1940, pp. 131–133.

25. David Hume, *A Treatise of Human Nature*, 1789.

26. Peter Singer, *Animal Liberation*, New York Review Books, 1975.

27. Quoted in S. Isen, "Laying the Foundation for Animal Rights: Interview with Tom Regan," *Animals Agenda*, July–August, 1984, pp. 4–5.

28. Tom Regan, *The Case for Animal Rights*, University of California Press, Berkeley, 1983.

29. Quoted in "Animals in the Middle," in the television series *Innovation*, sponsored by Johnson and Johnson on the A & E Network, September 5, 1987.

30. Quoted in "Animals in the Middle," in the television series *Innovation*, sponsored by Johnson and Johnson on A & E Network, September 5, 1987.

31. Carl Cohen, "The Case for Animal Rights," *New England Journal of Medicine* 315, no. 14 (October 4, 1986), pp. 865–870.

32. Rebecca Dresser, "Measuring Merit in Scientific Research," *Theoretical Medicine* 10, no. 1, 1989, pp. 21–34. It is relevant to note that the discovery of the gene for colon cancer apparently resulted from "hard-core, undirected research" (Natalie Angier, "Scientists Isolate Novel Gene Linked to

Colon Cancer," *New York Times*, December 3, 1993, p. A10).

33. Andrew Pollack, "Paralyzed Man Uses Thoughts to Move a Cursor," *New York Times*, July 13, 2006, p. Al.

34. Quoted in J. Duschek, "Protestors Prompt Halt in Animal Research," *Science News*, July 27, 1985, p. 53.

35. F. Feretti, "Forsaken Vacation Animals," *New York Times*, September 5, 1984, p. C1.

36. I owe this point to Lee Silver's *Challenging God and Mother Nature at the Frontiers of Life* (Harper Collins, New York, 2006). Phosphorus itself has no smell itself, but it feeds microbes, which then release ammonia gas and hydrogen sulfide, the stinky culprits.

Chapter 11

1. S. Gomer, H. Powell, and G. Rolino, "Japan's Biological Weapons"; H. Powell, "A Hidden Chapter in History," *Bulletin of Atomic Scientists*, October 1981, pp. 43, 44.

2. Eugene Kogon, *The Theory and Practice of Hell*, Farrar, Straus, and Cudahy, New York, 1950; Berkeley reprint, 1980, p. 166.

3. Eugene Kogon, *The Theory and Practice of Hell*.

4. Vera Alexander, *The Search for Mengele*, HBO movie, October 1985; interviewed by Central Television (London) and quoted in Posner and Hare, op. cit., p. 37.

5. Miklos Nyiszli, quoted in R. Lifton, "What Made This Man Mengele?" *New York Times Magazine*, July 21, 1985, p. 22, See also Gerald Posner and Jerome Ware, *Mengele: The Complete Story*, McGraw-Hill, New York, 1986, p. 39.

6. William Curran, "The Forensic Investigation of the Death of Joseph Mengele," *New England Journal of Medicine* 315, no. 17, Ocober 23, 1985, pp. 1071–1073.

7. David Rothman, "Ethics and Human Experimentation," *New England Journal of Medicine* 317, no. 19 (November 5, 1987), p. 1198.

8. Robert Bazell, "Growth Industry," *New Republic*, March 15, 1993, p. 14.

9. Constance Pechura, "From the Institute of Medicine," *Journal of the American Medical Association* 269, no. 4 (January 27, 1993), p. 453.

10. David Rothman, "Ethics and Human Experimentation," p. 1198.

11. H. Beecher, "Ethics and Clinical Research," *New England Journal of Medicine* 274, 1966, pp. 1354–1360.

12. H. Pappworth, *Human Guinea Pigs*, Beacon, Boston, Mass., 1968.

13. Molly Selvin, "Changing Medical and Societal Attitudes toward Sexually Transmitted Diseases: A Historical Overview," in King K. Holmes et al., eds., *Sexually Transmitted Diseases*, McGraw-Hill, New York, 1984, pp. 3–19.

14. Alan Brandt, "Racism and Research: The Case of the Tuskegee Syphilis Study," *Hastings Center Report* 8, no. 6 (December 1978), pp. 21–29.

15. Paul de Kruif, *The Microbe Hunters*, Harcourt Brace, New York, 1926, p. 323.

16. J. E. Bruusgaard, "^ber das Schicksal der nicht spezifisch behandelten Luetiker" ("Fate of Syphilitics Who Are Not Given Specific Treatment"), *Archives of Dermatology of Syphilis* 157, April 1929, pp. 309–332.

17. H. H. Hazen, "Syphilis in the American Negro," *Journal of the American Medical Association* 63, August 8, 1914, p. 463.

18. James Jones, *Bad Blood*, Free Press, New York, 1981.p. 74.

19. James Jones, *Bad Blood*, p. 74.

20. James Jones, *Bad Blood*, p. 74.

21. Alan Brandt, "Racism and Research."

22. Quoted in E. Ramont, "Syphillis in the AIDS Era," *New England Journal of Medicine* 316, no. 25 (June 18, 1987), pp. 600–601.

23. R. A. Vonderlehr, T. Clark, and J. R. Heller, "Untreated Syphilis in the Male Negro," *Journal of the American Medical Association* 107, no. 11 (September 12, 1936), pp. 856–860.

24. Jean Heller, "Syphilis Victims in U.S. Study Went Untreated for 40 Years," *New York Times*, July 26, 1972, pp. 1, 8.

25. Or worse: in 1988, a malpractice suit brought against a hospital in Vermont was settled out of court for $2.7 million on behalf of a 28-year-old woman who had gone into a coma after being incompetently tapped by a resident. "Malpractice Suit Settled for $2.7 Million," Burlington Free Press, December 21, 1988.

26. Archives of the National Library of Medicine; quoted in James Jones, *Bad Blood*, p. 127.

27. W. J. Brown et al., *Syphilis and Other Venereal Diseases*, Harvard University Press, Cambridge, Mass., 1970, p. 34.

28. Jean Heller, "Syphilis Victims in U.S."

29. Jean Heller, "Syphilis Victims in U.S."

30. Allison Mitchell, "Survivors of Tuskegee Study Get Apology from Clinton," *New York Times*, May 17, 1997, p. A1.

31. Carol Yoon, "Families Emerge as Silent Victims of Tuskegee Syphilis Experiments, *New York Times*, May 9, 1998, p. A1.

32. Marcia Angell, "The Ethics of Clinical Research in the Third World," *New England Journal of Medicine* 337, no. 12 (September 18, 1997), pp. 847–49.

33. R. H. Kampmeier, "The 'Tuskegee Study' of Untreated Syphilis" (editorial), *Southern Medical Journal* 65, no. 10, (October 1972), pp. 1247–1251.

34. Thomas Benedek, "The 'Tuskegee Study' of Untreated Syphilis: Analysis of Moral Aspects versus Methodological Aspects," *Journal of Chronic Diseases* 31, 1978, pp. 35–50. I have drawn considerably on this excellent article.

35. R. H. Kampmeier, "The Tuskegee Study of Untreated Syphilis."

36. "The Deadly Deception" (with George Strait), *Nova*, January 28, 1992.

37. Thomas Benedek, "The 'Tuskegee Study' of Untreated Syphilis," p. 44.

38. Personal correspondence, April 25, 1985. Benjamin Friedman is Professor Emeritus of Medicine, UAB.

39. Thomas Benedek, "The 'Tuskegee Study' of Untreated Syphilis."

40. G. W. Hayes et al., "The Golden Anniversary of the Silver Bullet," *Journal of the American Medical Association* 270, no. 13 (October 6, 1993), p. 1610.

41. R. H. Kampmeier, "Final Report of the 'Tuskegee Study' of Syphilis," *Southern Medical Journal* 67, no. 11, 1974, pp. 1349–1353. Kampmeier advances a fourth argument which is somewhat more technical. Penicillin achieves seroreversal in latent syphilis, but Kampmeier insists that such seroreversal has never been proved to be associated with decreased morbidity or mortality. A related point is possible uncertainty over diagnosis and thus over therapeutic effects. (S. Edberg and S. Berger, *Antibiotics and Infection*, Churchill Livingstone, New York, 1983, pp.141–142; K. Holmes et al., *Sexually Transmitted Diseases*, McGraw-Hill, New York, 1984, p.1352; John Hotson, "Modern Neurosyphilis: A Partially Treated Chronic Meningitis, *Western Journal of Medicine* 135, September 1981, pp. 191–200; Sarah Polt, Professor of Pathology, UAB, personal correspondence.)

42. Thomas Benedek, "The 'Tuskegee Study' of Untreated Syphilis."

43. Thomas Benedek, "The 'Tuskegee Study' of Untreated Syphilis."

44. Sheryl Gay Stolberg, "U. S. Ends Overseas HIV Studies Involving Placebos," *New York Times*, February 19, 1998.

45. Marcia Angell, "Tuskegee Revisited," *Wall Street Journal*, October 28, 1997.

46. Ellen Goodman, "Is Tuskegee Study OK Abroad?" *The Boston Globe*.

47. Public Citizen News Release, April 22, 1997.

48. Ruth Macklin, "Ethics and International Collaborative Research, Part I," *American Society for Bioethics and Humanities Exchange* 1, no. 2, p.1

49. Ellen Goodman, "Is Tuskegee OK Abroad?"

50. D. Bagenda and P. Musoke-Mudido, "We're Trying to Help Our Sickest People, Not Exploit Them," *Washington Post*, September 28, 1997, p. C3.

51. Ruth Macklin, "Ethics and International Collaborative Research."

52. Marcia Angell, "Tuskegee Revisited," *Wall Street Journal*, October 28, 1997.

53. Ellen Goodman, "Is Tuskegee OK Abroad?"

54. Sheryl Gay Stolberg, "U. S. Ends Overseas HIV Studies."

55. Dan Stober, Knight-Ridder Newspapers, "Dr. Hamilton Was Enthusiastic Experimenter in Radiation," *Birmingham News*, February 20, 1994, p. 10A; "America's Nuclear Secrets," *Newsweek* December 27, 1993, p. 15.

56. Keith Schneider, "Scientists Are Sharing the Anguish over Nuclear Experiments on People," *New York Times*, March 2, 1994, p. A9.

57. Robert Burns, "Radiation Experiments Were Far-Reaching," Associate Press, August 18, 1995, *Birmingham Post-Herald*, p. E6.

58. Dennis Domerzalski, Scripps-Howard News Service, "Radiation 'Guinea Pigs' Tell Stories," *Birmingham Post-Herald*, February 3, 1994, p. A8.

59. Philip J. Hilts, "U.S. Is Urged to Repay Some in Radiation Tests," *New York Times*, July 17, 1995, p. A9. See also *Final Report*, Advisory Committee on Human Radiation Experiments, Washington, D.C.: US Government Printing Office.

60. Arthur Caplan, "Rethinking the Cost of War," *Due Consideration*, New York: N.Y.: 1998, pp. 123–124.

61. Manuel Roig-Franzia, "Probe Opens on Study Tied to Johns Hopkins," *Washington Post*, August 23, 2001; p. B1.
62. Tamar Levin, "U.S. Investigating Johns Hopkins Study of Lead Paint Hazard," *New York Times*, August 24, 2001.
63. Tamar Levin, "U.S. Investigating."
64. Richard Jerome, "Death by Research," *People*, February 21, 2000, 123.
65. Deborah Nelson and Rick Weiss, "Hasty Decisions in the Race to a Cure? Gene Therapy Proceeded Despite Safety, Ethics Concerns," *Washington Post*, November 21, 1999, A1.
66. Arthur Caplan is quoted extensively in Complaint for Civil Action filed by John Gelsinger for estate of Jesse Gelsinger against Trustees of University of Pennsylvania et al., www.sskrplaw.com/ links/healthcare2.html.
67. Deborah Nelson and Rick Weiss, "Hasty Decisions."
68. Rick Weiss, "Research Volunteers Unwittingly at Risk," *Washington Post*, August 1, 1998, A1. See also this article from the online journal *Target Health*, June 14, 1998. http://www.targethealth.com/
69. Institute of Medicine, *Responsible Research: A Systems Approach to Protecting Research Participants*, National Academy Press, Washington, D.C., 2002.
70. For psychiatrists who abused patients in psychiatric research on schizophrenia, see Robert Whitaker, "Lure of Riches Fuels Testing," *Boston Globe*, November 17, 1998, p. A1; for the UAB story about abuse of subjects and fraud in medical research, see Douglas M. Birch and Gary Cohn, "How a Cancer Drug Trial Ended in Betrayal," *Baltimore Sun*, June 24, 2001.
71. Steve Stecklow and Laura Johannes, "Drug Makers Relied on Clinical Researchers who Now Await Trial," *Wall Street Journal*, A1, August 15, 1997.

Chapter 12

1. Thomas Starzl, *The Puzzle People: Memoirs of a Transplant Surgeon*, Pittsburgh University Press, 1992, p. 151.
2. Obituary of Norman Shumway, *The Independent* (London, England), February 16, 2006.
3. Christiaan Barnard and Curtiss Bill Pepper, *One Life*, Macmillan, New York, 1969, p. 372.
4. Christiaan Barnard and Curtiss Bill Pepper, *One Life*, p. 406.
5. "The Ultimate Operation," *Time*, December 15, 1967, p. 65; "Heart Transplant Keeps Man Alive in South Africa," *New York Times* December 4, 1967, p. A1.
6. Christiaan Barnard and Curtiss Bill Pepper, *One Life*, p. 444.
7. Quoted in Connie Chung, "Knife to the Heart," television documentary on heart transplant surgery, January 27, 1997.
8. Christiaan Barnard, *The Second Life*, Vlaeberg Publishers, South Africa, 1993.
9. Francis Moore, M.D. quoted in interview with Connie Chung, "Knife to the Heart."
10. Andre Courmand, *New York Times*, December 6, 1967.
11. Norman Staub, quoted in Peter Hawthorne, *The Transplanted Heart*, Keartland Publishing, Johannesburg, South Africa, 1968, p. 188.
12. Denise Grady, "Summary of Discussion of Ethical Perspectives," in Margery Shaw, ed, *After Barney Clark*, University of Texas Press, Austin, Tx, p. 52.
13. *Time*, December 9, 1982, p. 43.
14. *Time*, March 14, 1983, p. 74.
15. Thomas Preston, "Who Benefits from the Artificial Heart?" *Hastings Center Report* 15, no. 1 (February 1985), p. 5; *New York Times*, December 5, 1988, p. A2.
16. *Washington Post*, May 1, 1983, p. A2.
17. William A. Check, "Lessons from Barney Clark's Artificial Heart," *Health*, April 1984, pp. 22, 26.
18. Gideon Gill, "Burcham Dies After Blood Accumulates in Chest," *Louisville Courier-Journal*, April 26, 1983.
19. Gideon Gill, "Burcham Dies."
20. Michael Vitez, "Marriage of Two Minds: 'World's Smartest Couple' Nears First Anniversary," Knight-Ridder Newspapers, July 3, 1988.
21. Steve Ditlea, "Robert Jarvik Returns," *Red Herring*, October 11, 2002.
22. "Profile: Dr. William C. DeVries, Surgeon," Linda Kozaryn, *Defend America*, American Armed Forces Press Service, August, 2002.
23. Some surgeons such as Donald Kahn of Birmingham, Al., say Shumway tacitly consented to Barnard's operation, but this claim is controversial.
24. William Pierce, "Permanent Heart Substitution: Better Solutions Ahead," editorial, *Journal of the American Medical Association* 259, no. 6, February 12, 1988, p. 891.

25. Werner Forssmann, quoted in Christiaan Barnard and Curtiss Bill Pepper, *One Life*, p. 360.

26. Thomas Starzl, *The Puzzle People*, p. 148.

27. *New York Times*, editorial, December 16, 1982, p. A26.

28. "The Dracula of Medical Technology," Editorial, *New York Times*, May 16, 1988.

29. Transplants in the U.S. by Recipient Gender," *The Organ Procurement and Transplantation Network*, June 30, 2006, http://www.optn.org/latestData/rptData.asp, (July 10, 2006).

30. David Benatar, Don A. Hudson, "A Tale of Two Novel Transplants Not Done: The Ethics of Limb Allografts," *British Medical Journal*, 324 (April 20, 2002), pp. 971–975.

31. According to Dr. Nadey Hakim, of London, interviewed by Lawrence K. Altman, "A Pioneering Transplant, and Now an Ethical Storm," *New York Times*, December 6, 2005.

32. Marco Lanzetta et al., "International Registry on Hand and Composite Tissue Transplantation," *Transplantation* 79, no 9 (May 15, 2005).

33. Ariane Bernard and Craig S. Smith, "French Face-Transplant Patient Tells of Her Ordeal," *New York Times*, February 7, 2006.

34. Susan Okie, "Brave New Face," *New England Journal of Medicine*, 354, no. 9 (March 2, 2006).

35. Lawrence K. Altman, "A Pioneering Transplant, and Now an Ethical Storm," *New York Times*, December 6, 2005.

36. Ariane Bernard and Craig S. Smith, "French Face-Transplant Patient Tells of Her Ordeal," *New York Times*, February 7, 2006.

37. Craig S. Smith, 'As a Face Transplant Heals, Flurries of Questions Arise," *New York Times*, December 14, 2005, p A1.

38. Lawrence K. Altman, "Patient Opted for Transplant as Method to Mend Face," *New York Times*, December 12, 2005, p. A6.

39. Lawrence K. Altman, "A Pioneering Transplant, and Now an Ethical Storm," *New York Times*, December 6, 2005, p. D1.

40. Marilynn Marchione, "French Face Transplant Detailed, " Associated Press, *Birmingham News*, July 4, 2006, p. C6.

41. Reuters, "China Performs Its First Human Face Transplant," April 14, 2006.

42. Neil Osterwell, "Face Transplant Recipient's Habit Could Jeopardize Recovery," *MedPage Today*, January 19, 2006. www.medpagetoday.com/surgery/PlasticSurgery/th/2516

43. Stacy Burling, "Widow Sues Artificial-Heart Maker," *Philadelphia Inquirer*, October 17, 2002; Sheryl Gay Stolberg, "On Medicine's Last Frontier: The Last Journey of James Quinn," *New York Times*, October 8, 2002.

44. Lauran Neegaard, "FDA Advisers Reject Abiomed's Artificial Heart," Associated Press, *Birmingham News*, June 24, 2005, p. A14.

45. "FDA Approves Artificial Heart Implant," *USA Today*, October 14, 2004, A1.

46. Norman Shumway, quoted in *Transplant News*, July 13, 2001, from an interview in the *San Francisco Chronicle*.

47. NIH website, www.nhlbi.nih.gov/health/public/heart/other/hrt_lung.htm#Cost

48. D. P. Lubeck and J. P. Bunker, Office of Technology Assessment, *Case Study 9, The Artificial Heart: Costs, Risks, and Benefits*, U.S. Government Printing Office, Washington, D.C., 1982.

49. *Progressive*, February 1983, pp. 12–13.

50. Rene Fox and Judith Swazey, *The Courage to Fail: A Social View of Organ Transplants and Dialysis*, 2nd ed., rev., University of Chicago Press, Chicago, IL, 1974, 1978.

51. P. M. Park, "The Transplant Odyssey," *Second Opinion* 12, November 1989, pp. 27–32; quoted in Rene Fox and Judith Swazey, *Spare Parts: Organ Replacement in American Society*, Oxford University Press, New York, 1992,, p. 202.

52. A. J. Moskowitz, "The Cost of Long-Term LVAD Implantation," *Annals of Thoracic Surgery* 71, Supplement 3 (March 2001) pp. S195–98, S203–4.

53. Sandeep Jauhar," "The Artificial Heart," *New England Journal of Medicine*, February 5, 2004, 542–44.

54. "Norman Shumway, Heart Transplantation Pioneer, Dies at Age 83," Press Release, February 10, 2006, Stanford Medical Center.

Chapter 13

1. Dale H. Cowan, ed., *Human Organ Transplantation: Social, Medical-Legal, Regulatory, and Reimbursement Issues*, Health Administration Press, Ann Arbor, Mich. 1987, p. 60.

2. James Childress, "Who Shall Live When Not All Can Live?" *Soundings* 53, no. 4 (Winter 1970).

3. Belding Scribner, unpublished manuscript, quoted in Renée Fox and Judith Swazey, *The*

Courage to Fail: A Social View of Organ Transplants and Dialysis, 2d ed. rev., University of Chicago Press, Ill., 1974, 1978, p. 227.

4. Renée Fox and Judith Swazey, *The Courage to Fail*, p. 235.

5. One of the first organized interdisciplinary conferences to discuss such issues took place in 1967, funded by a company, CIBA.

6. H. M. Schmeck, Jr., "Panel Holds Life-or-Death Vote in Allotting of Artificial Kidney," *New York Times*, May 6, 1962, pp. 1, 83.

7. Shana Alexander, "They Decide Who Lives, Who Dies: Medical Miracle Puts a Burden on a Small Committee," *Life* 53, no. 102, (November 9, 1962).

8. Renée Fox and Judith Swazey, *The Courage to Fail*, p. 209.

9. Judith Swazey at "The Birth of Bioethics" conference, University of Washington Medical School, Seattle, WA, September 24, 1992.

10. David Sanders and Jesse Dukeminier, "Medical Advance and Legal Lag: Hemodialysis and Kidney Transplantation," *UCLA Law Review* 15 (1968), pp. 357–412.

11 http://www.cms.hhs.gov/ ESRDGeneralInformation/Downloads/2004 ProgramHighlights.pdf

12. Renée Fox and Judith Swazey, *The Courage to Fail*, p. 232.

13. David Sanders and Jesse Dukeminier, "Medical Advance and Legal Lag."

14. George Annas, "The Prostitute, the Playboy, and the Poet: Rationing Schemes for Organ Transplantation," *American Journal of Public Health* 75, no. 2, 1985, pp. 187–189.

15. Renée Fox and Judith Swazey, *The Courage to Fail*, chapter 9.

16. Renée Fox and Judith Swazey, *The Courage to Fail*, p. 234.

17. Herbert Fingarette, *Heavy Drinking*, University of California Press, Berkeley, 1988.

18. Alvin Moss and Mark Seigler, "Should Alcoholics Compete Equally for Liver Transplantation?" *Journal of the American Medical Association* 265, no. 10, March 13, 1992, p. 1295.

19. C. Cohen and M. Benjamin, "Alcoholics and Liver Transplantation," *Journal of the American Medical Association* 265, no. 10, March 13, 1992, pp. 1295–1301.

20. Nicholas Rescher, "The Allocation of Exotic Medical Lifesaving Therapy," *Ethics* 79 (April 1969).

21. Tracy E. Miller, "Multiple Listing for Organ Transplantation: Autonomy Unbounded," *Kennedy Institute of Ethics Journal* 2, no. 1 (March 1992) pp. 43–57.

22. Munson, Ronald, *Raising the Dead*, Oxford University Press, New York, 2002, pp. 26–45.

23. Munson, Ronald, *Raising the Dead* p. 29.

24. Munson, Ronald, *Raising the Dead*, p. 30.

25. Munson, Ronald, *Raising the Dead*, p. 36.

26. Munson, Ronald, *Raising the Dead*, p. 45.

27. Tracy E. Miller, "Multiple Listing for Organ Transplantation."

28. M. Michaels et al., "Ethical Considerations in Listing Fetuses as Candidates for Neonatal Heart Transplantation," *Journal of the American Medical Association* 269, no. 3, January 20, 1993, pp. 401–402.

29. Rene Fox and Judith Swzey, *Spare Parts: Organ Replacement in American Society*, Oxford University Press, New York, 1992.

30. Albert R. Jonsen, "(Bentham in a Box)," *Law, Medicine and Health Care* 14 (1986), pp. 172–174.

31. "Newsroom Fact Sheets," United Network for Organ Sharing, November 21, 2005, http://www.unos.org/inthenews/ factsheets.asp, July 10, 2006.

32. Michael Stoll, "A New Waiting Game for Hearts," *Philadelphia Inquirer*, February 7, 2000.

33. Kahn, Jeffrey and Susan Parry, "Organ and Tissue Procurement," *Encyclopedia of Bioethics*, 3rd ed. MacMillan. 2004. p. 1936; see also, "A Science Odyssey: People and Discoveries: First Successful Kidney Transplant Performed," http://www.pbs.org/wgbh/aso/databank. entries/dm54ki.html

34. I distinguish here between donors and organs. More organs still come from cadavers (brain dead patients). Cadavers yield 1.7 kidneys on average, but live donors can of course give only one kidney. Each year, about 8,500 kidneys come from cadavers and about 5,500 from live donors. See www.unos.org.

35. A. Bass, "New Liver Transplants; Pressure on Parents," *Boston Globe*, December 17, 1989, 1, 75; quoted in Rene Fox and Judith Swazey, *Spare Parts*.

36. Norman Fost, "Conception for Donation," *Journal of the American Medical Association* 291, no. 17, May 5, 2004, p. 2126.

37. Huddleston, Charles B. et al., "Lung Transplantation in Children," *Annals of Surgery*. 236, no. 3: pp. 270–276, September 2002.

38. S. Quattrucci et al., "Lung Transplantation for Cystic Fibrosis: 6-Year Follow-Up," *Journal of Cystic Fibrosis* 2005 May; 4 (2): pp. 107–14.
39. V. Fourbister, "Living Donors Dramatize Risk vs. Need," *American Medical News*, September 20, 1999, vol. p. 1.
40. The death was confirmed by Dr. Jean Edmond in V. Fourbister, "Living Donors Dramatize Risk vs. Need," *American Medical News*, 20 September 1999, p. 1.
41. Debra Shelton's update is "Donor Has Physical Pain, But Peace About Decision," and "Man's Second Chance Hasn't Turned Out Like He Expected," *St. Louis Post-Disptach*, December 21, 2003.
42. Mary Ellison, et al. "Living Kidney Donors in Need of Kidney Transplants," *Transplantation*, November 15, 2002, pp. 1349–1351. These 56 patients were out of 140,00 patients. Also, UNOS elevates to top of the list for receiving a kidney anyone who previously donated one and who now needs one.
43. Carole Tarrant, "For Family, Selfless Act Goes Awry," *New York Times*, March 12, 2002.
44. Richard D. Lamm, "Health Care as Economic Cancer," *Dialysis and Transplantation* 16 (1987), p. 433.
45. Fox and Swazey, *Spare Parts*, p. 10.
46. Fox and Swazey, *Spare Parts*, p. 45.
47. Interview, *Good Morning America*, July 9, 1993.
48. Walter Robinson, *Medical Ethics* (Lahey Clinic Medical Ethics Newsletter) 11, no. 2 (Spring 2004), p. 8.
49. Walter Robinson, *Medical Ethics*, p. 6.
50. Peter Landers, "Longer Dialysis Offers New Hope But Poses a Dilemma," *Wall Street Journal*, October 2, 2003, p. A1.

Chapter 14

1. Rene Fox and Judith Swazey, *The Courage to Fail: A Social View of Organ Transplants and Dialysis*, 2d ed., rev., University of Chicago Press, Ill., 1974, 1978; Harmon Smith, "Heart Transplantation," *Encyclopedia of Bioethics*, Free Press, New York, 1978.
2. Richard Howard and J. Najarian, "Organ Transplantation—Medical Perspective," *Encyclopedia of Bioethics* 3, Free Press, New York, 1978, pp. 1160–1165.
3. *Animals Voice* 2, no. 3 (December 1984).
4. Charles Krauthammer, "The Using of Baby Fae," *Time*, December 3, 1984, p. 14.
5. Quoting Kenneth P. Stoller, M.D., "The Baby Fae: The Unlearned Lesson," *Perspectives on Medical Research* 2 (1990), www.curedisease.com/Perspectives/vol.2_1990/BabyFae.html
6. "Baby Fae Stuns the World," *Time*, November 12, 1984, p. 72.
7. "Baby Fae Stuns the World," p. 70.
8. Tom Regan, "The Other Victim," *Hastings Center Report* 15, no. 1, February 1985, pp 9–10.
9. Thomasine Kushner and Raymond Belotti, "Baby Fae: A Beastly Business," *Journal of Medical Ethics* 11 (1985), pp. 178–183.
10. Denise Breo, "Interview with 'Baby Fae's' Surgeon," *American Medical News*, November 16, 1984, p. 18.
11. "Interview with Dr. Jack Provonsha," *U.S. News and World Report*, November 12, 1984, p. 59.
12. Dan Chu and Eleanor Hoover, "Helped by a Baboon Heart, An Imperiled Infant, 'Baby Fae,' Beat the Medical Odds," *People* November 18, 1984.
13. Denise Breo, "Interview with," p. 18.
14. Dan Chu and Eleanor Hoover, "Helped by a Baboon Heart, p. 74.
15. Dan Chu and Eleanor Hoover, "Helped by a Baboon Heart, p. 74.
16. Thomas Starzl, *The Puzzle People: Memoirs of a Transplant Surgeon,* University of Pittsburgh Press, Pa., 1992, p. 123.
17. Denise Breo, "Interview with," p. 18.
18. Paul Ramsey, "The Enforcement of Morals: Nontherapeutic Research on Children," *Hastings Center Report* 6, no. 1 (August 1976), pp. 21–30.
19. 31. Richard McCormick, "Proxy Consent in the Experimentation Situation," *Perspectives in Biology and Medicine* 18, no. 1 (Autumn 1974), pp. 2–20.
20. Alexander Capron, "When Well-Meaning Science Goes Too Far," *Hastings Center Report* 15, no. 1, February 1985, pp. 8–9.
21. George Annas, "The Anything Goes School of Human Experimentation," *Hastings Center Report* 15, no. 1, February 1985, pp. 15–17.
22. "Celebrity surgery" was a term coined in a *New Republic* editorial, December 17, 1984.
23. Keith Reemtsma, *Hastings Center Report*, 15, no. 1 February 1985, p. 10.
24. Alex Capron, *Hastings Center Report*, 15, no. 1 February 1985, p. 8.
25. Charles Krauthammer, "The Using of Baby Fae," *Time,* December 3, 1984, pp. 87–88.

26. Denise Breo, "Interview with," p. 18.
27. Denise Breo, "Interview with," p. 13.
28. Thomas Starzl, *The Puzzle People,* p. 123.
29. "Baby Fae Stuns the World," p. 70.
30. Jacques Loman, *Journal of Heart Transplantation* 4, no. 1, (November 1984), pp. 10–11.
31. George Annas, "The Anything Goes School."
32. *Nature* 88, no. 312 (November 8, 1984), p. 5990.
33. Charles Krauthammer, "The Using of Baby Fae."
34. "Judicial Council Offers New Guidelines," *American Medical News* 27, December 14, 1984, p. 46.
35. Associated Press, "Hospital Sets Policy on Organ Donor Use," February 23, 1988.
36. Joan Heilman, "Tiny Gabriel's Gift of Life," *Redbook,* December 1988, p. 162. (Article given to me by Lynn Bondurant.)
37. J. Peabody et al., "Experience with Anencephalic Infants as Prospective Organ Donors," *New England Journal of Medicine.* 321, no. 6 (August 10, 1989), pp. 344–350.
38. Debra Berger, "The Infant with Anencephaly: Moral and Legal Dilemmas," *Issues in Law and Medicine* 5, no. (1989), p. 68.
39. Medical Task Force on Anencephaly, "The Infant with Anencephaly," *New England Journal of Medicine* 332, no. 10 (March 8, 1990), p. 669.
40. Robert D. Trough and John D. Fletcher, "Can Organs Be Transplanted before Brain Death? *New England Journal of Medicine* 321, no. 6 (1989), p. 388.
41. A. Kantrowitz et al., "Transplantation of the Heart in an Infant and an Adult," *American Journal of Cardiology* 22, no. 782 (1968).
42. Associated Press, "Ethicists Debate Death and Baby's Lacking Brain," March 31, 1992; in *Birmingham News,* p. A1.
43. Brian Udell, quoted in *USA Today,* March 30, 1992, p. 3A.
44. *In Re T. A. C. P., Southern (Law) Reporter,* 2d Series, Supreme Court of Florida, November 12, 1992, pp. 588–595.
45. D. Shewmon, "Anencephaly: Selected Medical Aspects," *Hastings Center Report* 18, no. 5, 1988, pp. 11–9.
46. Laurie Abraham, "The Use of Anencephalic Infants as Organ Sources," *American Medical News* 261, no. 12 (March 24–31, 1989), pp. 1773–1781.
47. Debra H. Berger, *Issues in Law and Medicine* 67, 1989, pp. 84–85; quoted by Estella Moriarty in *In Re T. A. C. P.,* p. 595.
48. D. Medearis and L. Holmes, "On the Use of Anencephalic Infants as Organ Donors," *New England Journal of Medicine* 321, no. 6 (August 10, 1989), p. 392.
49. Beth Brandon, "Anencephalic Infants as Organ Donors: A Question of Life and Death," *Case Western Law Review* 40 (1989–199), p. 781; quoted by Estella Moriarty in *In Re T. A. C. P.*
50. *In Re T. A. C. P.,* p. 590.
51. A. Capron, "Anencephalic Donors: Separate the Dead from the Dying," *Hastings Center Report* 17, no. 1, February 1987, pp. 5–8; John Arras, "Anencephalic Newborns as Organ Donors: A Critique," *Journal of the American Medical Association* 259, no. 15, (April 15, 1986), pp. 2284–2285.
52. D. Shewmon, "Anencephaly: Selected Medical Aspects."
53. Alice Dregger, *One of Us: Conjoined Twins and the Future of Normal,* Harvard University Press Cambridge, MA, 2004.
54. Alice Dregger, "Jarring Bodies: Thoughts on the Display of Unusual Anatomies," *Perspectives in Biology and Medicine* 43, no. 2, (Winter 2000), pp. 161–172.
55. Ben Carson, *Gifted Hands: The Ben Carson Story,* Zondervan Press, Grand Rapids, MI, 1990.
56. Press Release, "Conjoined Twin Fact Sheet," Johns Hopkins Children's Center, www.hopkinschildrens.org/pages/news/twins_factsheet.html
57. Alice Dregger, *One of Us:* p. 66, quoting Rowena Spencer, *Conjoined Twins: Developmental Malformations and Clinical Implications* Johns Hopkins University Press, Baltimore, MD, 2003, pp. 310–311.
58. Alice Dregger, *One of Us,* Dregger, p. 67.
59. Press Release "Hopkins Team Separates Conjoined Twins," Johns Hopkins International, September 16, 2004.
60. Alice Dregger, *One of Us,* p. 63.
61. David Wasserman, "Killing Mary to Save Jodie: Conjoined Twins and Individual Rights," *Philosophy and Public Affairs Quarterly* 21, no. 1 (Winter, 2001), pp. 9–14.
62. Alice Dregger, *One of Us,* p. 93.
63. Alice Dregger, *One of Us,* p. 65

Chapter 15

1. *New York Times,* November 6, 1987, p. B1.
2. *New York Times,* November 6, 1987, p. B1.
3. *New York Times,* November 13, 1987, p. B21.
4. *New York Times,* November 13, 1987, p. B21.

5. *New York Times,* November 13, 1987, p. A1.
6. *New York Times,* November 13, 1987, p. A1.
7. "Brown versus Koch," *60 Minutes,* interview with Ed Bradley, 1988.
8. "Court Backs Treatment of Woman Held under Koch Plan," *New York Times,* December 19, 1987, p. A1.
9. "Brown versus Koch," *60 Minutes.*
10. "Brown versus Koch," *60 Minutes.*
11. *New York Times,* January 20, 1988, p. A16.
12. Julian Jaynes, *The Origin of Consciousness and the Breakdown of the Bicameral Mind,* Houghton Mifflin, Boston, 1976.
13. Thomas Szasz, "Involuntary Mental Hospitalization: A Crime against Humanity," in *Ideology and Insanity,* Doubleday, New York, 1970.
14. D. Rosenhan, "On Being Sane in Insane Places," *Science* 179, (1973), pp. 250–258.
15. *O'Conner v. Donaldson,* 422 U.S. 563. 95 S. Ct. 2486, June 26, 1975.
16. John Petrilia, "Mental Health Therapies," *Biolaw,* University Publications of America, Frederick, Md. 1986, pp. 177–215.
17. Quoted in Charles Krauthammer, "How to Save the Homeless Mentally Ill," *New Republic,* February 8, 1988, p. 24.
18. Saul Feldman, "Out of the Hospitals, into the Streets: The Overselling of Benevolence," *Hastings Center Report* 13, no. 3 (June 1983), pp. 5–7.
19. C. Dugger, "Judge Orders Homeless Man Hospitalized," *New York Times,* December 23, 1992, p. B1.
20. www.pscyhlaws.org/PressRoom/stmt% 20subwayperez.htm
21. Treatment Advocacy Center, "State Standards for Assisted Treatment: State by State Chart," December 12, 2004. www.psychlaws.org
22. E. Rosenthal, "Who Will Turn Violent? Hospitals Have to Guess," *New York Times,* April 7, 1993, p. A1.
23. *"Tarasoff v. Regents of University of California,"* 17 Cal. 3d 425, 551 P.2d 334, 131 *California Reporter* 14 (Cal. 1976).
24. Virginia Abernethy, "Compassion, Control, and Decisions about Competence," *American Journal of Psychiatry* 141, no. 1 (1984), pp. 53–58.
25. Virginia Abernethy, "Compassion, Control, and Decisions about Competence."
26. *New York Times,* November 13, 1987, p. A1.
27. Robert Levy and Robert Gould, "Psychiatrists as Puppets of Koch's

Round-Up," *New York Times,* November 27, 1987.
28. Paul Chodoff, "The Case for Involuntary Hospitalization of the Mentally Ill," *American Journal of Psychiatry* 133, no. 5 (May 1976).
29. Ellen Goodman, "Before They Die with Their Rights On," *Washington Post,* November 21, 1987.
30. J. Livermore, C. Malmquist, and P. Meehl, "On the Justification of Civil Commitment," *University of Pennsylvania Law Review* 117, (November 1968), pp. 75–96.
31. Alice Baum and Donald Burnes, *A Nation in Denial: The Truth about Homelessness,* Westview, Boulder, Colo., 1993
32. Clifford J. Ivy, "The State is Failing the Mentally Ill in Adult Homes, 'Pataki Administration Study Says'" *New York Times,* September 15, 2002, p. 21.

Chapter 16

1. "Maria Lopez" is a composite, based on a four-part series in the *New York Times* on the emerging epidemic in diabetes, January 9–12, 2006.
2. N. R. Kleinfield, "Diabetes and Its Awful Toll Quietly Emerge as a Crisis," *New York Times,* January 9, 2006, p. A1.
3. Marc Santora, "East Meets West, Adding Pounds and Peril," *New York Times,* January 12, 2006, p. A1.
4. World Health Organization, Department of Noncommunicable Disease Surveillance. *Definition, Diagnosis and Classification of Diabetes Mellitus and its Complications.* Geneva: WHO, 1999.
5. N. R. Kleinfield, "Diabetes and Its Awful Toll."
6. N. R. Kleinfield, "Living at the Epicenter of Diabetes, Defiance and Despair," *New York Times,* January 10, 2006, p. A1.
7. N. R. Kleinfield, "Diabetes and Its Awful Toll."
8. "Diabetes Gene Detected," *Sydney Morning Herald,* January 19, 2006.
9. Web page on Francis Collins at National Human Genome Research Initiative of the National Institutes of Health, http://www.genome.gov/10001018.
10. Benjamin A. Pierce, *Genetics: A Conceptual Approach,* 2nd ed., New York: W. H. Freeman, 2006, p. 123.
11. Natalie Angier, "Team Reports Genetic Cause of Huntington's, *New York Times,* March 24, 1993, p. A1.

12. Daniel Kevles, *In the Name of Eugenics: Genetics and the Uses of Human Heredity*, Knopf, New York, 1985, pp. 3–19.
13. Daniel Kevles, *In the Name of Eugenics*, pp. 93–94.
14. Robert Lacey, *Ford: The Man and the Machine*, Little, Brown, New York, 1987.
15. Daniel Kevles, *In the Name of Eugenics*, p. 97.
16. Daniel Kevles, *In the Name of Eugenics*, p. 97.
17. Herman Muller, *Out of the Night: A Biologist's View of the Future*, Vanguard, New York, 1935; quoted in Kevles, op. cit., p. 164.
18. Ronald W. Clark, *The Life and Work of J. B. S. Haldane*, Coward-McCann, New York, 1968, p. 70; quoted in Kevles, p. 127.
19. B. S. Haldane, "Toward a Perfected Posterity," *The World Today* 45, December 1924; quoted in Kevles, p. 127.
20. Denise Grady, "Study Shows Few Women Rue Preventive Breast Operation," *New York Times*, April 17, 1999, p. A14.
21. Paul Recer, "Studies May Have Exaggerated Breast Cancer Risk," August 21, 2002, *Birmingham News*, p. 5A.
22. Denise Grady, "The Ticking of a Time Bomb in the Genes," *Discover*, June 1987, p. 34.
23. G. Meissen et al., "Predictive Testing for Huntington's Disease with Use of a Linked DNA Marker," *New England Journal of Medicine* 318, no. 9 (March 3, 1988), pp. 538ff.
24. G. Meissen et al., "Predictive Testing."
25. Danish Council of Ethics, *Ethics and Mapping of the Human Genome*, 1993.
26. Catherine Hayes, "Genetic Testing for Huntington's Disease—A Family Issue," *New England Journal of Medicine* 327, no. 20, (November 11, 1992), pp. 1449–1451.
27. Catherine Hayes, "Genetic Testing for Huntington's Disease;" Natalie Angier, "Vexing Pursuit of Breast Cancer Gene, *New York Times*, July 12, 1994.
28. C. Muir, *Cancer Incidence in Five Continents* 5, Lyon: International Agency for Research on Cancer, 1987, Table 12–2.
29. N. R. Kleinfield, "Diabetes and Its Awful Toll."
30. "Cancer Genetics," Benjamin A. Pierce, *Genetics: A Conceptual Approach*, 2nd ed., New York: W. H. Freeman, 2006, pp. 627–637.
31. D. Craufurd and R. Harris, "Ethics of Predictive Testing for Huntington's Disease: The Need for More Information," *British Medical Journal* 293 (July 26, 1986), pp. 249–251.
32. M. Waldoz, "Probing the Cell: The Diagnostic Power of Genetics Is Posing Hard Medical Choices, " *Wall Street Journal*, April 1986, p. A1.
33. Denise Grady, "The Ticking of a Time Bomb."
34. Denise Grady, "The Ticking of a Time Bomb."
35. Arthur Beaudet of Baylor College of Medicine, quoted in M. Waldoz, "Probing the Cell."
36. President's Commission for the Study of Ethical Problems in Medicine and Biomedical and Behavioral Research, *Screening and Counseling for Genetic Conditions: The Ethical, Social, and Legal Implications for Genetic Screening, Counseling, and Educational Problems*, U.S. Government Printing Office, Washington, D.C., 1983.
37. C. Norton, "Absolutely Not Confidential," *Hippocrates*, March–April 1989, pp. 53–59; see also, *Medical Records: Getting Yours*, Public Citizen, Washington, D.C., 1986.
38. John Rennie, "Grading the Gene Tests," *Scientific American*, June 1994, p. 91.
39. Ian Urbina, "In the Treatment of Diabetes, Success Often Does Not Pay," *New York Times*, January 11, 2006, p. A1.
40. Ian Urbina, "In the Treatment of Diabetes."
41. Natalie Angier, "Gene For Mental Illness Proves Elusive," *New York Times*, January 13, 1993, p. B3.
42. Miron Baron, quoted in Natalie Angier, "Gene for Mental Illness Proves Elusive," *New York Times*, January 13, 1993, p. B3.
43. "New Research Shows Second-hand Smoke Raises Diabetes Risk, *British Medical Journal*, April 17, 2006.

Chapter 17

1. Barbara Tuchman, *A Distant Mirror*, Knopf, New York, 1978, p. 119.
2. B. Hahn, G. Shaw, F. Gao, *Nature* 397 (February 4, 1999), pp. 436–441. The authors also offered proof that the three major phylogenetic groups of HIV-1 (M, N, and O) arose from three independent transmissions to man of simian immunodeficiency virus, SIVcpz, which they hypothesized had existed in chimps for hundreds of thousands of years.
3. Centers for Disease Control, "Overview of HIV/AIDS" and "Human Immunodeficiency Virus Type 2," www.cdc.gov/hiv/hivinfo.

4. Randy Shilts, *And the Band Played On*, St. Martin's, New York, 1987.
5. Greg Dixon, "Stop Homosexuals before They Infect Us All," *USA Today*, January 16, 1983.
6. "Television evangelists Jerry Falwell and Pat Robertson, two of the most prominent voices of the religious right, said liberal civil liberties groups, feminists, homosexuals and abortion rights supporters bear partial responsibility for Tuesday's terrorist attacks because their actions have turned God's anger against America." "'God Gave U.S. 'What We Deserve,' Falwell Says," John F. Harris, *Washington Post*, September 14, 2001, p. C3.
7. Charles Stanley, quoted in Scripps-Howard News Service, *Birmingham Post-Herald*, January 21, 1986.
8. Interviewed on *Cross Fire*, CNN, November 16, 1987.
9. Quoted in Randy Shilts, *And the Band Played On*, p. 311.
10. Jonathan Lieberson, "The Reality of AIDS," *New York Review of Books*, January 16, 1986.
11. Margaret Heckler, quoted in Randy Shilts, *And the Band Played On*, p. 345.
12. Joseph Bove, quoted in Randy Shilts, *And the Band Played On*, p. 345.
13. Joseph Bove, quoted from Randy Shilts, *And the Band Played On*, p. 345.
14. John Boswell, Christianity, *Social Tolerance, and Homosexuality; Gay People in Western Europe from the Beginning of the Christian Era to the Fourteenth Century*, University of Chicago Press, 1980.
15. 539 U.S. 558 (2003) http://www.law.cornell.edu/supct/html/02-102.ZS.html
16. Larry Kramer, "Who Says AIDS Is Hard to Get?" *Newsweek*, 1992.
17. Nick Wadhams, "World Falls Short on AIDS Goals, U.N. Warns," June 2, 2006, *Birmingham News*, p. A4.
18. Figures on AIDS in Africa and worldwide are notoriously vague and political. See Alan Whiteside, "AIDS in Africa: Facts, Figures and the Extent of the Problem," pp.1–15. Anton A. Van Niekerk and Loretta M. Kopelman, *Ethics and AIDS in Africa*, Walnut Creek, CA: Left Coast Press, 2006.
19. "A Global Menace," *Newsweek*, May 15, 2006, p. 52.
20. Alexander Irwin, Joyce Millen, and Dorothy Fallows, *Global AIDS: Myths and Facts*, Cambridge, MA; South End Press, 2003, p. 52.
21. Alexander Irwin, Joyce Millen, and Dorothy Fallows, *Global AIDS*, p. 55.
22. Kent Sepkowitz, "One Disease, Two Epidemics—AIDS at 25," *New England Journal of Medicine* 354, no. 23, (June 8, 2006), pp. 2413–14.
23. The case is taken from Alexander Irwin, Joyce Millen, and Dorothy Fallows, *Global AIDS*: pp. 21–22.
24. Quoted in Alexander Irwin, Joyce Millen, and Dorothy Fallows, *Global AIDS:* pp. 21–22,
25. Michael Merson, "The HIV-AIDS Pandemic at 25—The Global Response," *New England Journal of Medicine* 354, no. 23 (June 8, 2006), p. 2414.
26. J. Decosas et al, "Migration and AIDS," *Lancet* 346, no. 8978 (1995): 826–228. Quoted in Alexander Irwin et al, *Global AIDS*.
27. Jeffrey Fisher, quoted in L. A. McKeown, "Preventing AIDS in the Next Generation," *WebMD Medical News*, December 1, 1999.
28. Quoted in Alexander Irwin, Joyce Millen, and Dorothy Fallows, *Global AIDS:* pp. 21–22.
29. Philippe Bourgois, "In Search of Horatio Alger: Culture and Ideology in the Crack Economy," in *Crack in America: Demon Drugs and Social Justice*, eds, B. Rienarman and H. Levine Berkeley, Ca.: University of California Press, 1997.
30. K. Sepkowitz, "One Disease, Two Epidemics," p. 2413.
31. William Easterly, *White Man's Burden;* New York, NY: Penguin, 2006.
32. Paul Theroux, *Dark Star Safari* New York, NY: Houghton Mifflin, 2003.

Chapter 18

1. Stuart Altman and Michael Doonan, "Can Massachusetts Lead the Way in Health Care Reform?" *New England Journal of Medicine* 354, no. 20 (May 18, 2006), p. 2093.
2. Lisa Belkin, "Twice a Victim: of Both Cancer and Care System," *New York Times*, March 26, 1993, p. B12.
3. Personal communication from Lisa Belkin to author, June 17, 2006.
4. This case stemmed from a 1993 (above) story by Lisa Belkin. In 2006, an email to her revealed that one of her children said that Rosalyn had died "several years before."
5. Quoted by Paul Krugman, "Death by Insurance," *New York Times*, May 1, 2006, p. A25.

6. Robert Steinbrook, "Health Care Reform in Massachusetts—A Work in Progress," *New England Journal of Medicine* 543, no. 20 (May 18, 2006), p. 2095.

7. This has been repeatedly claimed by members of Physicians for a National Health Program; see, e.g., John V. Walsh, *Providence Journal* (Scripps-Howard), column, July 14, 1993. See also Paul Krugman, "Death by Insurance," *New York Times*, May 1, 2006, p. A25.

8. The Act allows both workers and their immediate family members who had been covered by a health care plan to maintain their coverage if a "qualifying event" causes them to lose coverage. Among the "qualifying events" listed in the statute are loss of benefits coverage due to (1) the death of the covered employee, (2) a reduction in hours (which can be the result of resignation, discharge, layoff, strike or lockout, medical leave or simply a slowdown in business operations) that causes the worker to lose eligibility for coverage, (3) divorce, which normally terminates the ex-spouse's eligibility for benefits, or (4) a dependent child reaching the age at which he or she is no longer covered. COBRA imposes different notice requirements on participants and beneficiaries, depending on the particular qualifying event that triggers COBRA rights. COBRA also allows for longer periods of extended coverage in some cases, such as disability or divorce, than others, such as termination of employment or a reduction in hours. COBRA does not apply, on the other hand, if employees lose their benefits coverage because the employer has terminated the plan altogether." Consolidated Omnibus Budget Reconciliation Act of 1985, Wikpedia. http://en.wikipedia.org/wiki/Consolidated_Omnibus_Budget_Reconciliation_Act_of_1985

9. Jack K. Shelton and Julia Mann Janosi, "Unhealthy Health Care Costs," *Journal of Medicine and Philosophy* 17, no. 1 (February 1992), p. 8.

10. Jack K. Shelton and Julia Mann Janosi, "Unhealthy Health Care Costs," p. 8.

11. Medicare Enrollment Reports," December 14, 2005, http://www.cms.hhs.gov/MedicareEnrpts/, July 11, 2006.

12. Kaiser Family Foundation, "Medicare Spending and Financing", April 2005,

http://www.kff.org/medicare/upload/7305.pdf, July 10, 2006.

13. "Health Care Costs," *USA Today*, May 12, 1993, p. A2.

14. www.tricare.mil

15. Paul Krugman, "Health Care Confidential," *New York Times*, January 26, 2006, p. A23.

16. Robert Steinbrook, "Health Care Reform in Massachusetts—A Work in Progress," *New England Journal of Medicine* 543, no. 20 (May 18, 2006), p. 2095.

17. Allan Guttmacher Institute, quoted in Associated Press, December 15, 1987.

18. Consumers Union, "The Crisis in Health Insurance," *Consumer Reports*, August 1990, p. 543.

19. Clifford Krauss, "In Blow to Canada's Health System, Quebec Law Is Voided," *New York Times*, June 10, 2005, p. A3.

20. Clifford Krauss, "In Blow to Canada's Health System, Quebec Law Is Voided," *New York Times*, June 10, 2005, p. A3.

21. Clifford Krauss, "In Blow to Canada's Health System, Quebec Law Is Voided," *New York Times*, June 10, 2005, p. A3.

22. Courtney S. Campbell, "Gridlock on the Oregon Trail," *Hastings Center Report* 23, no. 4 (July–August 1993), p. 6.

23. Carson, Matthew J.,"Results of Oregon Health Plan Study Released," *The Commonwealth Fund*, July 29, 2005. http://www.cmwf.org/newsroom/newsroom_show.htm?doc_id=288798, July 10, 2006.

24. Steve LeBlanc, "Mass. Health Care Plan Riles Some Liberals," Associated Press, April 7, 2006.

25. "Coverage," Patricia Barry, *AARP Bulletin* (July–August, 2006), pp. 8–10.

26. Stuart Altman and Michael Doonan, "Can Massachusetts Lead the Way in Health Care Reform?" *New England Journal of Medicine* 354, no. 20 (May 18, 2006), p. 2094.

27. Stuart Altman and Michael Doonan, "Can Massachusetts Lead the Way?"

28. Olga Pierce, "Analysis: Can Mass. Plan Stay Solvent?" United Press International Story, July 6, 2006.

29. Consumers Union, "Medicare for All Americans," *Consumer Reports*, September 1992, p. 592.

30. Consumers Union, "Medicare for All Americans."

31. David Leonhardt, "A Health Fix That Is Not a Fantasy," *New York Times*, April 12, 2006, p. D1.

32. Milt Freudenheim, "The Check Is Not in the Mail," *New York Times*, May 2, 2006, p. C1.

33. Garrett Hardin, "The Tragedy of the Commons," *Science*, 162, 1968, pp. 1243–1248.

34. Consumers Union, "The Crisis in Health Insurance," *Consumer Reports*, August 1990, p. 543.

35. Jack K. Shelton and Julia Mann Janosi, "Unhealthy Health Care Costs," *Journal of Medicine and Philosophy*, 17, no. 1 (February 1992), p. 8.

36. Consumers Union, "Wasted Health Care Dollars," *Consumer Reports*, July 1992, p. 436.

37. Lila Guterman, "As the Rich Get Richer, Do People Get Sicker?" *Chronicle of Higher Education*, November 28, 2003, p. A22.

38. Amy Goldstein, "Forecast Dire for Medicare Fiscal Health," *Washington Post*, May 2, 2006, reprinted in *Birmingham News*, p. A3.

39. Robert Pear, "In Medicare Debate, Massaging the Facts," *New York Times*, May 23, 2006, p. A19.

40. Richard Epstein, remarks made at UAB, Conference on the Ethics of Managed Care, April 12, 1997. See also Richard Epstein, *Mortal Peril*, Addison-Wesley Publishing Company, 1997, chs. 7–8.

41. David Blumenthal et al., "The Future of Health Care," *New England Journal of Medicine* 314, no. 11 (March 13, 1986), p. 723.

42. Michele Davis, "Make Health Insurance More Like Auto Insurance," *Birmingham News*, July 6, 1992.

43. David Orentlicher, "Rationing and the Americans with Disabilities Act," *Journal of the American Medical Association* 271, no. 4 (January 26, 1994), pp. 308–314.

44. David Orentlicher, "Rationing and the Americans with Disabilities Act."

45. Richard Lamm, "Health Care as Economic Cancer," *Dialysis and Transplantation* 16 (1987), pp. 432–433.

46. Paul Starr, *The Social Transformation of American Medicine*, Basic Books, New York, 1982.

47. Julia Preston, "Texas Hospitals' Separate Paths Reflect the Debate on Immigration," *New York Times*, July 18, 2006, p. A18.

48. Julia Preston, "Texas Hospitals' Separate Paths."

49. Shikha Dalmia, "Who's Milking Who?" *Reason*, August/September 2006, p. 44.

50. Ewardo Porter, "Here Illegally, Working Hard and Paying Taxes," *New York Times*, June 19, 2006, pp. A1–14.

Name Index

Subject Index